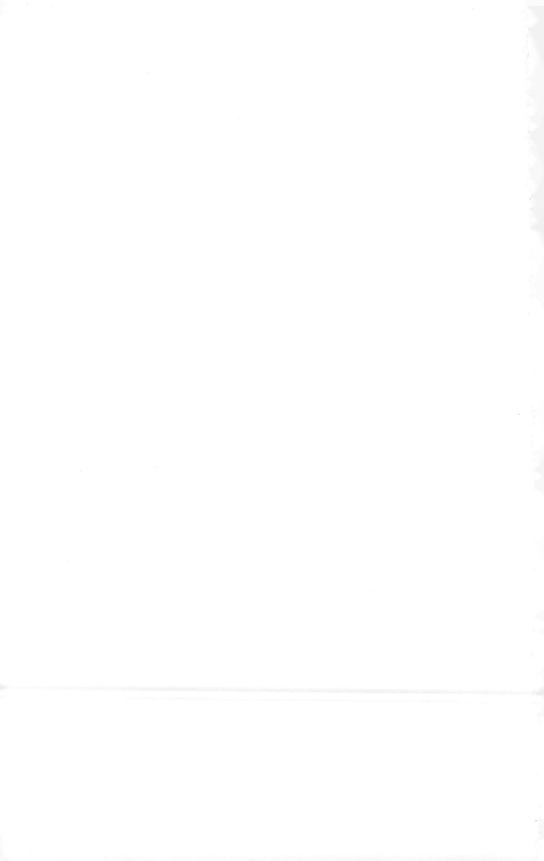

Undertaker of the Mind

MEDICINE AND SOCIETY
Andrew Scull, Editor

This series examines the development of medical knowledge and psychiatric practice from historical and sociological perspectives. The books contribute to a scholarly and critical reflection on the nature and role of medicine and psychiatry in modern societies.

Undertaker of the Mind

*John Monro and Mad-Doctoring
in Eighteenth-Century England*

Jonathan Andrews and
Andrew Scull

UNIVERSITY OF CALIFORNIA PRESS
Berkeley · Los Angeles · London

Publication of the illustrations in this book has been made possible by grants from the Scouloudi Foundation in association with the Institute of Historical Research, and from the Marc Fitch Trust.

University of California Press
Berkeley and Los Angeles, California

University of California Press, Ltd.
London, England

Library of Congress Cataloging-in-Publication Data

Andrews, Jonathan, 1961–.
   Undertaker of the mind : John Monro and mad-doctoring in eighteenth-century England / Jonathan Andrews and Andrew Scull.
       p.   cm.—(Medicine and society : 11)
   Includes bibliographical references and index.
   ISBN 0-520-23151-1 (alk. paper)
   1. Monro, John, 1715–1791.   2. Psychiatrists—England—Biography.   3. Psychiatry—History—18th century.   4. Mentally ill—England—Case studies.   5. Bethlem Royal Hospital (London, England)   I. Scull, Andrew T.   II. Title.   III. Series.
RC438.6.M66 A53   2001
616.89'0092—dc21
[B]   2001027290

Manufactured in the United States of America
10   09   08   07   06   05   04   03   02   01
10   9   8   7   6   5   4   3   2   1

The paper used in this publication meets the minimum requirements of ANSI/NISO Z39.48-1992 (R 1997) *(Permanence of Paper).* ⊗

Contents

Illustrations

Preface

This book has its origins in the discovery of a rare, if not unique, primary document, the 1766 case book kept for his private purposes by John Monro (1715–91), perhaps the most famous mad-doctor of his age.[1] Monro was visiting physician to Bethlem (or Bethlehem) Hospital, the archetypal "Bedlam," Britain's first, and for hundreds of years only, public institution for the insane. While Monro is a figure who is well known to historians of psychiatry, his case book has been virtually unknown outside of the immediate family in whose possession it remains. Some years after learning about that manuscript's existence, we decided to collaborate in producing an annotated edition for publication. Initially, we thought of our work on the case book as a relatively modest project. Once we had commenced our researches, however, it rapidly became apparent that the issues Monro's manuscript opened up called for a much more ambitious analysis than the one we had originally planned or envisaged writing.

Over our years of prior work on the history of psychiatry, we both had already accumulated a welter of information and knowledge about Monro and his career. Monro's prominence and the social standing of at least some of his clientele meant that, within months of beginning to focus on this particular project, we had enlarged these resources into a veritable treasure trove of references to him and his work. Both of us soon reached the same conclusions. We were confirmed in our earlier, more tentative suspicion: that other historians had simultaneously underestimated and misconstrued Monro's importance in the development of eighteenth-century mad-doctoring. Indeed, we became convinced that, when viewed through the various sides of the prism comprised by his career and his day-to-day practice, by his patrons and customers, and by the case book and other materials we had uncovered, the place

of madness in eighteenth-century England was revealed in a startling
new light.

As our work proceeded, we found ourselves able to draw on an as-
tonishing array of sources, both verbal and visual: the diaries, family
papers, and correspondence of England's wealthiest and best-connected
citizens; "high culture," both literary and artistic, from the poetry and
satires of writers like Swift and Pope to the paintings of Hogarth and the
sculpture of Cibber; popular culture in the form of cartoons, broad-
sheets, ballads, Grub Street Gothic novellas, and the like; the reportage
and the excesses of the daily and periodical press; the usually drier material found in hospital archives, city directories, state papers, wills,
legal documents, and trial transcripts; an array of medical treatises and
writings on madness, hypochondria, hysteria, and the spleen; and the simultaneously mute and immensely telling testimony of buildings and
their architecture. All of these materials helped us to gain a better grasp
of the viewpoints, practice, and approaches of this particular mad-doctor
and to set them in the widest possible historical context. Thus, too, we
were permitted a firm purchase on the personal and family travails and
tragedies—as well as the mundane realities of the professional career—
revealed in the case book itself. In parallel fashion, the patients' experiences and narratives and the medical interventions recorded in its pages
shed new light on the stories these other sources had to tell us.

In the latter stages of our collaboration, it became increasingly apparent that a single volume could not do justice to the complexity of the
resources we had unearthed. The case book that had originally prompted
us to work together formed a natural focus for many of our analyses
of the mad-doctor, his patients, and their families. In our view, a close
reading of its contents permitted us to develop a privileged and peculiarly revealing set of insights into the microcosm that constituted and
contained the clinical encounter with madness. Those analyses lie at the
heart of our separate discussion in the second of our two volumes, entitled *Customers and Patrons of the Mad-Trade,* where we also reprint the
text of the case book itself.[2] Yet Monro's career also played itself out on
a larger stage, and attending to his activities in the public sphere permitted us to develop a broader and more wide-ranging perspective on
Unreason and those who undertook to combat it in Augustan England.
On the whole, it is that more macrocosmic view of the place of madness
in eighteenth-century society and culture that we present here. The intimate world we encounter in the pages of Monro's case book yields up
many of its secrets only when what the mad-doctor's private notes reveal

and elide is placed in a larger context. So, too, in parallel fashion, our discussion of that larger world must link back to and ground itself in the details of day-to-day activities and practices if it is to realize all its aims.

The pages that follow are thus, on one level, an account of the career of Dr. John Monro. Chapters 1 and 2, especially, chart the progress of Monro's career from his early Oxford education and fledgling apprenticeship in the mad-business under his father's guidance to the four decades he spent at the medical forefront of England's premier lunatic hospital. Taking its lead, however, from a new generation of historical and biographical writings, this book seeks to be much more than a narrative of Monro's life and times. Ranging widely over the terrain of eighteenth-century mad-doctoring, it assesses Monro as one among a number of emerging specialist practitioners of the mad-trade, closely reading his career through the broader lens of contemporary medical practice and culture. Because we recognize that the sociocultural setting of an individual's life is at least as significant as the individual's subjectivity and particular personality traits,[3] even this portion of our two-part study of Monro and eighteenth-century madness is as much about the various contexts in which Monro practiced and his interrelations with his patients and their families and friends as it is about Monro and his own family. We are concerned not to tell this tale from above, or merely from the perspective of the mad-doctor and the profession themselves, but also to present Monro and mad-doctoring through the eyes of their clientele. Thus, while focused on Monro, this book is also about those Monro treated and was hired by: his patients and their families.

As part of our study, we have provided an extensive array of visual materials that we located in the course of our researches, much of it previously unseen even by specialists. We should emphasize that these often arresting images are included not just for decorative effect, but comprise an indispensable part of our analysis. The inclusion of a wide range of visual material appeared to us to be a vital way of ensuring the bearing and significance of a pictorial narrative accompanying and complementing the textual account we were keen to offer. Thus, in according a large and vivid space for a range of illustrative media, we have also sought to signify our conviction that a history of madness, of the mad-doctor, and of the mad patient is itself liable to be unbalanced without an active engagement with representations and incarnations in graphic and pictographic, as well as written, form. The rich resource such visual materials provide is, we believe, too often overlooked, or else treated too casually and superficially by historians.[4]

John Monro was without question one of the most famous mad-doctors of his generation. Besides his position at Bethlem Hospital, he was also a major figure in the emerging private "trade in lunacy"[5] that was so notable a feature of eighteenth-century England's burgeoning consumer society. Monro attended Bethlem at a time when the hospital's custom of exposing the insane to the eyes of sightseers reached its apogee. In the last years of his tenure as its physician, the practice was radically curtailed—though not at his initiative—after a wave of public, literary, and media protest. Recognized by contemporaries as a leading authority on insanity, Monro's close social connections with members of the aristocracy and gentry, as well as with medical professionals, politicians, and divines, ensured for him a significant place in the social, political, cultural, and intellectual world of his time.

As one measure of their prominence, John Monro and his father, James, were referred to with both approval and hostility in a disparate range of contemporary literature and correspondence. There are allusions to James, for example, in the poetry of Pope and the prose of Fielding, and to John in the prose of Smollett and the letters of Elizabeth Montagu. John Monro was not just an acquaintance of, but enjoyed friendly relations with, many aristocratic families, and was the medical confidant of some of the most prominent elements of the British political elite, including the Walpole family. Over the course of his career, embedded in the web of patronage and family ties that were the hallmark of eighteenth-century Britain, Monro provided his services as a mad-doctor to a host of the rich and famous, from Horace Walpole's nephew, Lord Orford (a detailed exploration of whose treatment comprises chapter 4 of this book), to the earl of Chatham and Sir Francis Chester. Monro's status as a specialist practitioner and physician to Bethlem saw him summoned to pronounce on the mental condition of an assortment of famous eighteenth-century mad people, including the murderous aristocrat Lord Ferrers and the attempted regicide Margaret Nicholson. While he was practically on his deathbed in 1788–89, his opinion was also solicited as to the mental condition of the allegedly "incurably mad" George III. Chapter 6 entails a comprehensive discussion of Monro's dealings with these notorious cases.

Monro's attendance (as well as his father's) on Alexander "the Corrector" Cruden, the famous compiler of a Bible concordance that remains in print to this day, brought him notoriety of a different sort: a torrent of published criticisms from the disaffected patient that constituted one of the first examples of a persistent tradition of protest literature directed against the claims of mad-doctoring (and, later, psychiatry) to be engaged upon a therapeutic enterprise. The case is examined here (in chapter 3) as part of the tangled set of relationships between religion and insanity in this period: in particular, between those who appeared to suffer from this especially problematic admixture, and the doctors, divines, and laymen who, alternately, ministered to and vilified them. The Monros' tendencies to stigmatize religious enthusiasts as crazy, and their medical treatment of Methodist madmen, was to bring down opprobrium on their heads from the movement's leaders, John Wesley and George Whitefield. (Sympathy for popular religious enthusiasm was in rather short supply among the ultra-orthodox "Bethlemetical" physicians, with their family history of high Anglican, Tory, and Jacobite sympathies.) Yet, despite such periodic controversies, and his occasional involvement in contentious cases of alleged false confinement, John Monro succeeded in staving off disrepute and carving out for himself a lucrative and successful career at the summit of the emerging "trade in lunacy."

Notwithstanding their persistent association with Jacobitism and scandal, translating themselves from Scotland to Oxford and then to London enabled the Monros to exploit their public practice and the advantages that a metropolitan residence and orbit provided in the way of sociopolitical connections. Indeed, they succeeded in generating a rewarding, if not positively roaring, trade in the treatment of nervous and mental diseases among well-heeled and well-connected families. Besides their visiting role at Bethlem, the Monros also attended and ran a host of private madhouses in the metropolitan region. These included establishments in Chelsea, Bethnal Green, and Hoxton, as well as two other madhouses, Clerkenwell House and Brooke House, Hackney, which, over the course of a century and more, were to form the lucrative core of the family's involvement in the mad-business. Chapter 5 focuses more particularly on the Monros' growing involvement in this burgeoning business.

In the late 1750s, Monro engaged in a rather exceptional and highly charged debate with the unfortunately named William Battie (1704–76), physician to the recently established rival institution of St. Luke's Hospital for Lunatics. The controversial relations between Monro and Battie were played out most overtly in Battie's *Treatise on Madness* (1758) and Monro's aggressive riposte, *Remarks on Dr Battie's Treatise* (1758)—sources that have been much quoted both by contemporary mad-doctors and by modern historians of psychiatry. The two men's complex interactions are discussed at length in chapter 2. As we shall see, Monro's case book registers his continuing tensions with Battie in the subsequent decade, the former occasionally permitting the bile of personal antipathy to seep from his quill. The careers of Monro and Battie thus make for a striking source of contrast and comparison, one that says a great deal about the particular directions the mad-trade took after 1750.

In the modern historiography of psychiatry, Battie is usually hailed as the enlightened progressive and Monro castigated as the conservative reactionary, but there is evidence that—in eighteenth-century terms, at least—the accuracy of this assessment is less clear-cut than some have claimed. Despite their crossing of swords, the professional interests of Monro and Battie also coincided at times, and they were commonly called upon to act in tandem, as when Monro testified alongside and in agreement with Battie before the 1766 Commons inquiry into private madhouses. Indeed, as the following pages show, the genuine or lasting differences between these two doctors may have been distorted and exaggerated.

A word, finally, about the book's title. William Belcher, a patient incarcerated for seventeen years in a Hackney madhouse, and freed only after the intervention of John Monro's son Thomas, referred to the institution in which he had been locked away as a "premature coffin of the mind," or "one of the graves of mind, body, and estate," confinement for him being experienced as a form of "legal death." [6] Belcher was far from the first or only contemporary to perceive (or to be represented as conceiving) confinement in a madhouse as a form of living death. Some lunatics were indeed confined for life, and literary accounts of patients such as Margaret Nicholson (discussed in chapter 6) dwelt morbidly on the departure of their hopes and spirit as they whiled away their days at Bethlem and kindred institutions. Other patients, meanwhile, were artistically represented sketching gravestones on their cell walls to signify their ineluctable entombment in the madhouse or the lunatic hospital (see figure 7 in chapter 1).

Also pertinent, we believe, is a conversation Samuel Johnson had with Fanny Burney during April of 1783 (as reported by James Boswell). Discussing the extravagant funeral of David Garrick, each asserted sharply contrasting views of the moral and emotional effects of living beside either a lunatic hospital or a graveyard. Their exchange further highlights the magnetic contiguity of madness and death: both Janus-faced subjects for sad reflection and, alternately, for avoidance in this period. It also signals, however, a transition in elite attitudes over the later decades of the eighteenth century, as—mollified by feminized sentiment—spectacles of suffering and loss were found less instructive and salutary than unpalatable, mortifying, and distressing.

> Mrs Burney wondered that some very beautiful new buildings should be erected in Moorfields, in so shocking a situation as between Bedlam and St. Luke's Hospital; and said she could not live there. JOHNSON. "Nay, Madam, you see nothing there to hurt you. You no more think of madness by having windows that look to Bedlam, than you think of death by having windows that look to a church-yard." MRS BURNEY. ". . . it is right that we should be kept in mind of death." JOHNSON. "Nay, Madam . . . it is right that we should be kept in mind of madness, which is occasioned by too much indulgence of imagination . . . a very moral use may be made of these new buildings: I would have those who have heated imaginations live there, and take warning." MRS BURNEY. "But, Sir, many of the poor people that are mad, have become so from disease, or from distressing events. It is, therefore, not their fault, but their misfortune; and, therefore, to think of them is a melancholy consideration." [7]

The arresting images and contemplations we have summarized above led us to reflect more generally upon the linkage between madness and death in this period. More specifically, we found ourselves prompted to consider the analogous kinds of service that eighteenth-century mad-houses/mad-doctors and undertakers provided for their clients. Contemporaries, both lay and medical, had long recognized a propensity for madness and death to coincide, whether a mental affliction was blamed for bringing about an individual's demise, or—as Sir Thomas Browne had emphasized as far back as the 1640s—whether physical deterioration through age and disease was observed to have culminated in a loss of one's senses.[8] Yet the intrusion of specialist caretakers into such domains was relatively rare in the Civil War era. A century or more later, however, the mad-doctor and the undertaker were both intervening with mounting regularity and determination into these sensitive and difficult arenas.

Undertakers, of course, offered (and offer) a particular and peculiar sort of assistance to others, taking on the essential, but rather unpopular, work of arranging for the handling of the corpse, the conduct of a funeral, and the interment of the body. Mad-doctors undertook the similarly burdensome and unpleasant (but increasingly necessary) task of treating, coping with, and confining difficult or impossible people. Madness, moreover, was widely portrayed as entailing a kind of social, mental, or metaphysical death, and from this perspective, mad-doctoring

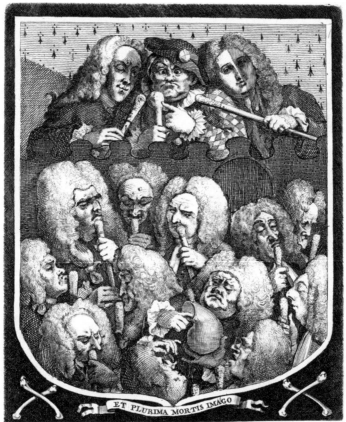

The Company *of* Undertakers

Beareth Sable, an Urinal proper, between 12 Quack-Heads of the second & 12 Cane Heads Or, Consultant. On a Chief Nebulæ, Ermine, One Compleat Doctor issuant, checkie Sustaining in his Right Hand a Baton of the Second. On his Dexter & Sinister sides two Demi-Doctors, issuant of the second, & two Cane Heads issuant of the third; The first having One Eye conchant, towards the Dexter Side of the Escocheon; the Second Faced per pale proper & Gulæ, Guardent. —
With this Motto ———— *Et Plurima Mortis Imago .*

Price Six pence

FIGURE 1. William Hogarth, *The Company of Undertakers* (1737). Hogarth's print representing the doctors of his day as a company of undertakers assumes the form of a mock coat of arms. Pictured as bewigged and cane-carrying quacks, a gallery of fellows of the Royal College of Physicians occupies the lower portion of the picture, their gentlemanly airs and (false) claims to curative prowess savagely burlesqued as they array themselves above a caption that reads *"Et Plurima Mortis Imago"* (everywhere the image of death). Nine of them nod on their gold-headed canes, while three more cluster round a flask of urine, two inspecting it, while the third dips in his finger to taste its contents. In Hogarth's own words, aping the language of heraldry: "Beneath Sable, an Urinal proper, between 12 Quack-Heads of the second & 12 Cane-Heads . . ." Above them, offering a dubious benediction to the

might be thought of as an onerous undertaking, one that was intimately associated with concerns about the corruption and death of the mind. In the dark shadowland of human fears, associations, and motivations, we might say, its practitioners were engaged in activities that closely paralleled the fashion in which undertakers made their living from the corruption and death of the body.

In the process of profiting from the provision of an essential but stigmatized service, both occupations also found themselves fending off accusations of financial corruption and of being engaged in the cruel exploitation of human misery. While contemporary undertakers were frequently condemned as "death hunters" and "cold cooks," performing a distasteful and disreputable office beneath that of even a trade, mad-doctors were castigated as traders in lunacy, "louses," and "Smiling Hyenas" whose dubious skills did little credit to their standing and claims as a profession. If mad-doctors found themselves castigated as "mad quacks" and "nostrum mongers," similar terms of opprobrium

---

assembled multitude of orthodox quacks/undertakers, is a wondrous gallery of characters whose identities would have immediately been obvious to Hogarth's audience—two "Demi-Doctors . . . dexter [and] sinister" and a "Compleat Doctor" in the center, who together were three of the most notorious and prominent self-promoting quacks in the capital: respectively (with "eye conchant"), the wandering occulist and author of "wonder cures" John Taylor, presently ministering to the king; Joshua Ward, widely known as Spot Ward, for the prominent birth mark that disfigured his face, and famous as the inventor of "Ward's Drop," a mixture of antimony and arsenic guaranteed to promote "vomits, purges and sweats," if not paralysis and death; and finally, reigning over the lot, the bone-setter Sarah Mabb, a.k.a. "Crazy Sally," the daughter of a country farrier, whose main talents lay (allegedly) in the strength of her forearms and the hardness of her heart, which inured her to the shrieks of the "beneficiaries" of her manipulations. This notorious "Harlequin Female Bone-Setter" (thus costumed here) had recently been taken up by royalty

and had attended Queen Caroline. In honor of her accomplishments, Queen Mabb herself had not long before been invited to preside over a special evening of display at Lincoln's Inn Fields—in October 1736—at which she had requested a performance of "The Worm Doctor," an unconscious reference to the close connections between medical attendance and mortality that Hogarth must surely have appreciated. Certainly, three lines of a ballad sung about her on the occasion could have directly inspired his satire on the foolishness of those who entrusted their illnesses to the tender mercies of profiteers/practitioners who would likely do no more than speed their passage to the grave:

> Zounds! Cries the dame, it hurts not me,
> Quacks without art may either blind or kill,
> But demonstrations shew that mine is skill. . . .

(Coincidentally, but delightfully so, the *New Canting Dictionary* of 1725 defines "mab" as a wench or a harlot.) Reproduced by kind permission of the British Museum/Wellcome Institute Library. Copyright © The British Museum.

were hurled at undertakers, their rivals in the embalming trade demeaning them as "quacks" and "mountebanks."[9] Yet, both these occupations were in increasing demand in an ever wealthier consumer society. Indeed, the Augustan age witnessed a marked expansion of the marketplace for both varieties of enterprise, as the growth of commerce and the parallel advance of what Norbert Elias has termed "the civilizing process" produced, in its turn, far greater rewards for those willing and able to offer a superior service to the genteel and middling sort.[10]

Both occupations, therefore, as they sought to take charge of perhaps the most irrational aspects of human experience—madness and death—underwent a considerable transformation in the Age of Reason. In common with many other lines of work, both became steadily more commercial and commercialized. In the process, though, mad-doctors and undertakers also discovered that they seemed inextricably linked to the practice and stigma of the lower forms of trade, no matter how hard they struggled to raise the status of their respective occupations by offering superior forms of specialist services and an array of facilities in return for a range of fees. To the dismay of their practitioners, both found themselves striving—and somewhat vainly—to eschew the stigma with which those perceived as securing profits from speculating in human misery were inevitably and inescapably tarred and tainted.

We are fully conscious of the danger that the title we have selected may conjure up a more negative and polemical image of the mad-doctor and mad-doctoring than we would wish to convey, and may evoke or encourage an overly literal reading of the contemporary critics of this emerging specialty. Yet, we hope that the double meaning of the term "to undertake" has also been emphatically communicated to our readers, and trust that the more positive and necessary sides of the services that the mad-doctor was performing, and that were under increasing demand in this period, are given a conspicuous and balanced assessment in the account that follows.

Acknowledgments

Our thanks to Joel Braslow, Bill Bynum, Howard Boyer, Stephen Cox, Matthew Craske, Elizabeth Foyster, Steve King, Elaine Murphy, Roy Porter, Steven Shapin, Len Smith, and Akihito Suzuki for helpful comments on various drafts of the text, and for directing us to useful materials we might otherwise have overlooked. We are grateful to staff at the Ashmolean Museum, the Bethlem Royal Archives, the Bodleian Library, the British Library, the British Museum, the Courtauld Institute, the Guildhall Library, the Hackney Archives, the House of Lords Records Office, the Public Records Office (Kew), the Wellcome Institute Library for the History of Medicine, the Interlibrary Loan Department of the University of California, San Diego Library, the Huntington Library in San Marino, and the Clark Library in Los Angeles for help with research and resources. Caroline Overy at the Wellcome was particularly helpful in obtaining illustrations for the book from the library's iconographic collections. Laura Harger and Sue Carter of the University of California Press gave the manuscript a close and enormously helpful editorial review, for which we are most grateful. Our thanks, finally, to Eilis Kennedy for her support and encouragement, and to Stanley Holwitz.

This is perhaps the place for a brief note about our collaboration. Following our initial decision to work together on this project, we have managed face-to-face contacts on a handful of occasions. For the most part, however, our mutual research and writing have depended heavily on the magic of the Internet. The ability to raise and respond to queries about particular issues, and more importantly, the capacity to exchange our work-in-progress virtually in real time have allowed us to work efficiently and seamlessly as a team, smoothing away even the potential problems raised by an eight-hour time difference. Like many historians who work in the same field, the two of us have disagreed on interpretative matters in the past. Those differences are not on display here for a simple reason: though we debated some issues vigorously as our work proceeded, ultimately we found ourselves in essential agreement on all important matters, a consensus that we would like to think flows from our mutual commitment to careful empirical work and respect for the evidence before us. We have thoroughly enjoyed working together, and though each of us originally took responsibility for individual portions of the text, every section of it reflects our joint input. Even we would have a difficult time at this point disentangling who was responsible for what piece of prose, and to attempt to do so would be to contradict the spirit of what for us has been an unusually rewarding and stimulating opportunity to work together. Not the least of the many virtues of the Internet and of electronic mail may turn out to be the way they facilitate collaborations of this sort.

It should be obvious, of course, from what we have said here that we share equally in the responsibility for any errors of omission and commission others may detect in the text that follows.

CHAPTER I

John Monro

The Making of a Mad-Doctor

What is Dr. Monro? A mad-doctor; and pray what great matter is
that? What can mad-doctors do? prescribe purging physic, letting of
blood, a vomit, cold bath, and a regular diet? How many incurables
are there? . . . physicians . . . are often poor helps; and if they mistake
the distemper, which is not seldom the case, they do a deal of mischief.

Alexander Cruden, *The Adventures
of Alexander the Corrector* (1754)[1]

"All men are mad," the raging poet cries.
Each frantic Reader, "Not quite all," replies.
Lifting his jaundic'd eye, "Not all Sir, sure,"
Cries rich Avaro, mad beyond cure.
"Not all," coy Chloe adds, by wine made bolder.
"Not all," repeats the Parrot from her shoulder.
The pensioned Peer affirms it is not so.
The mitred Politician echoes, "No."
Each for himself and friends the charge denies;
And Bedlam joins to curse poetic lies.

Quoted in Thomas Monro,
Essays on Various Subjects (1790)[2]

FORGING THE EARLY CAREER

Rare is the doctor whose very name becomes synonymous with the practice of a particular branch of the healing arts. Yet, for eighteenth-century Englishmen, the mere mention of the name "Monro" was sufficient to conjure up images of the imperious "mad-doctor" confronting and taming the fancies and furies of the madman. Consulted by the richest and most powerful families in Georgian England, John Monro (1715–91) stood at the very head of his dubious profession, the target of satirical jests and gibes, and simultaneously the repository of some of the deepest fears and most shameful secrets of "the respectable class." Even his foibles and physique were matters of common repute. When Thomas Rowlandson sought to skewer the pretensions of Charles James Fox, Whig grandee and "man of the people," he drew him strait-waistcoated and driven mad by his delusions of grandeur and the evanescence of his dreams of political power. Opposite him, peering through his quizzing glass like a connoisseur viewing some strange and suspect sculpture, Rowlandson portrayed the corpulent carcass of Dr. "M[onr]o," dispensing his diagnosis with a dismissive aside: "As I have not the least hope of his Recovery, Let him be removed amongst the Incurables."

Who was this connoisseur of insanity, this high priest of the trade in lunacy? How did he manufacture his fame and his fortune? What exactly was it that this captain of confinement did to and for those who consulted him on matters of madness? For, however familiar the man in his own time and place, in ours he is largely forgotten. Nevertheless, his life and career provide us with our own quizzing glass—a prism through which we can peer at the patrons and customers of the mad-trade, and at the mad-doctor to whom, by necessity, they paid court.

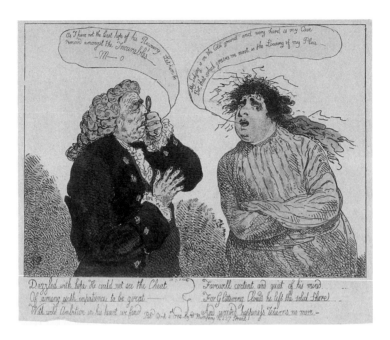

FIGURE 2. Thomas Rowlandson's political caricature of Dr. John Monro and Charles James Fox. This caricature, published on 4 April 1784 in the aftermath of the election, portrays Monro looking at Fox, a leading figure in the Whig government, driven insane at his loss of office, and the arrival of the Tory ministry of William Pitt. (Fox, in coalition with Lord North, had formed a new government in April 1783, with the Duke of Portland as prime minister.) Straitjacketed and with straw in his hair, Fox is depicted as mad beyond recovery, singing in forlorn despair:

> My Lodging is on the Cold ground and very
>   hard is my Case,
> But that which grieves me most is the Loosing
>   of my Place.

Monro stands to one side in his court dress, inspecting the patient through his quizzing glass and delivering his damning verdict:

> As I have not the least hope of his Recovery,
>   Let him be removed amongst the Incurables.

Beneath the picture, the following lines appear:

> Dazzled with hope He could not see the Cheat
> Of aiming with impatience to be great.
> With wild Ambition in his heart we find
> Farewell content and quiet of his mind
> For Glittering Clouds he left the solid Shore,
> And wonted happiness returns no more.

Reproduced by kind permission of the Wellcome Trust, London. Copyright © The British Museum.

John Monro was born on 16 November 1715 at Greenwich, the son of James Monro, M.D. (1680–1752), and his wife, Elizabeth. His family were of Scottish extraction, descended from a branch of the house of Fyrish. His grandfather was the Rev. Alexander Monro, D.D. (d. 1715?), a cadet of Foulis, and the first among that branch of the family to change

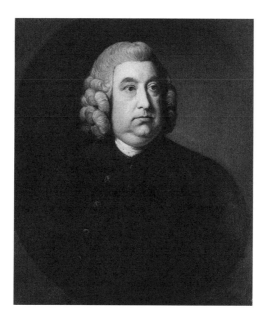

FIGURE 3. Portrait of Dr. John Monro, painted in 1769. Oil on canvas. This portrait, showing Monro in his younger days, was painted by one of the leading portrait artists of the day, Nathaniel Dance (1735–1811). It was donated to the College of Physicians by the mad-doctor's great-grandson, Dr. Henry Monro, in 1857, and is on loan to the Bethlem Royal Hospital Museum. Reproduced by kind permission of the Royal College of Physicians, London.

the traditional spelling of their surname, "Munro," to "Monro," while his grandmother was Anna Logan. Alexander was a high church minister, who was (from 1685) Principal and Professor of Divinity at Edinburgh University. John's early education was at Merchant Taylor's School. Subsequently, he followed in his father, James's, footsteps to Oxford University, graduating from St. John's College, earning his B.A. on 13 May 1737 and his M.A. on 11 July 1740. During the course of his university studies, from 1 to 22 August 1735, he conducted (in the company of four others) an extensive but lightning tour (evidently on horseback) of the towns and antiquities of England. Beginning in Oxfordshire, Monro's tour extended from Warwickshire and Staffordshire to the Midlands, Lancashire, and finally to Yorkshire. He recorded his impressions in detail in a leather-bound pocket book. This book[3] shows

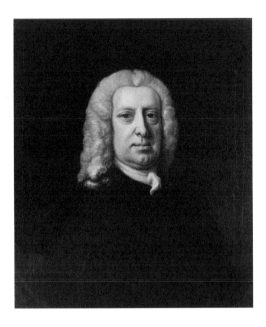

FIGURE 4. Portrait of Dr. James Monro, painted by John Michael Williams in 1747. Oil on canvas. James Monro, M.D. (1680–1752), was the father of John and the first of the family to be physician to Bethlem. James's picture was donated to the College of Physicians by his great-great-grandson, Dr. Henry Monro, in 1857, and is on loan to the Bethlem Royal Hospital Museum. Reproduced by kind permission of the Royal College of Physicians, London.

the young student voraciously consuming the culture and heritage of England, eagerly jotting down his impressions and experiences, and acquiring the cultural accoutrements of the cultivated eighteenth-century man. On display is his breadth of intellectual interest in the history, economy, industry, landscape, art, and architecture of England, and also in the houses and seats of England's aristocratic families, but the diary is notable for its lack of reference to medical matters, the only remotely relevant reference being Monro's comment that the "Matlock bath is in a very romantic situation."

The Monros' family background was not exactly the perfect foundation for a successful career in the politically charged climate of eighteenth-century London. John's grandfather, Alexander Monro, although allegedly brought up a Roman Catholic and subsequently professing Presbyterianism, had increasingly tended toward episcopacy and sided politically with the cause of James II—a damaging affiliation that severely blighted his career and prospects once the Stuarts were chased from the throne. His Jacobitism ultimately necessitated his resignation from the ministry and from the university on the Presbyterians' coming to power with the Glorious Revolution in 1688, and thereafter led to his removal to London in 1690 or 1691.[4]

The taint of Jacobitism appears to have continued to attach itself to the family even after Alexander's death. His son James was labeled "a Jacobite" by his troublesome private patient Alexander Cruden,[5] and in 1746 Walpole's friend and correspondent Sir Horace Mann (1696–1759) referred to John himself as one of a number of "Jacobites abroad" in the habit of frequenting the Pretender's Court in Italy (the young doctor evidently doing so while on a Radcliffe medical traveling fellowship). Disparaging the disloyal and opportunistic motives of Monro and his fellow travelers, whom he saw as cynically courting the possibility of future preferment, Mann informed Walpole that

> some of our travellers [*sic passim*] have so good an opinion of their success, that they are gone to Rome, to pay homage among the first. Bouverie does not act publicly as to the Pretender, but has all his people constantly to dine with him. His three companions, Holt, Phelps, and Munroe the mad doctor's son went last fryday to the Portico of the Sti Apostoli, to wait for the Pretender's coming out, to compliment him upon his Son's birthday, and went afterwards to dine at his house,—it is said with him, but I suppose with his people.[6]

Two weeks later, Mann wrote to Walpole reiterating his disapproval of the "villains" received by the Pretender at Rome, and what he regarded as Monro and company's scandalously overt political dissidence, hoping (vainly) that some action might be taken by the government: "Bouverie, Phelps, Holt and Munroe [are] in high favour because they pay their court publicly to mock-Majesty, with whom they have dined. Munroe is the mad physician's son and is himself a travelling Physician. They are all persuaded things will go as they wish; for, as I told you, they publickly frequent the Pretender and his people. Surely the Government will take notice of this behaviour."[7] Mann had heard "that Munroe's pension as a travelling physician had been taken from him" as a result of these activities, but this appears to have been wishful thinking on his part.[8]

Monro had gained election as a Radcliffe traveling fellow in April 1741, the year following his graduation with an M.A. from Oxford,[9] in a period when the University was rife with Tory and Jacobite sympathizers.[10] These fellowships, described by Webster as "the most important medical fellowships in Oxford," established at University College, were ten-year appointments worth the grand sum of £300 per annum.[11] Requiring the incumbents to pursue the study of medicine for up to five years in Britain and a further five on the continent, they were the medical equivalent of the Grand Tour. Monro was thus enabled to seek out the best of Europe's medical schools while simultaneously acquiring a range of cultural experiences and capital that would stand him in good stead in elite social circles once he set up in private practice. According to Horace Walpole (who should have known), Monro won this appointment "by my father's interest," the prime minister, Sir Robert, having "had a great regard for the old doctor" (i.e., James Monro). Sharing Mann's disdain for Jacobite sympathizers, however, the younger Walpole suggested that "if he [John Monro] has any skill in quacking madmen, his art may perhaps be of service in the Pretender's court."[12] Here, vividly encapsulated, is the predicament that was again and again to dog the careers of the Monros: namely, that mad-doctoring as a specialty conveyed a dubious professional and social status and offered an easy and regular target for gibes—all the more so when combined with questionable political allegiances and antecedents.

The trouble their political heterodoxy undoubtedly must have caused the Monros in their attempts to chart a successful course in their profession in London society may help to explain John's and his father's lack of patronage from the Hanoverian court itself. Yet its potentially damaging effects may also account for their efforts to assert their orthodoxy through other means, in particular through their apparently staunch adoption of High Church Anglicanism and their antipathetic stance toward religious sectarianism, Catholicism, and evangelicalism. John's brother, Thomas (d. 1781), was vicar of Burgate and rector of the two Worthams, Suffolk, and John had grandchildren and great-grandchildren who were also Anglican clerics. John's father, James, had evidently been appreciative of the solution that the physician Sir Edward Hulse (1682–1759) arrived at when censured for unorthodoxy, and rendered the formula in verse, which was subsequently circulated by Horace Walpole to his various correspondents:

> When Hulse for some trifling unorthodox jests
> As unchristian was censured by bigots and priests,
> He wisely resolv'd to wipe off the reproach
> And was seen by [i.e., next to] a parson six months in his coach.[13]

At Bethlem itself, however, with the ranks of the governors dominated by Tories, the Monros' politico-religious affiliations, far from
being a handicap, may even have proved helpful when James and
later John stood for election to the physicianship. Mindful of their
need to keep their fences mended, both were certainly careful in general to display no actionable signs of disaffection with the Hanoverian
régime.

It is significant that their somewhat heterodox political allegiances
do not appear to have prevented either Monro from being consulted on
medical matters by the Walpoles and other leading Whigs. There were,
after all, not so very many specialist mad-doctors about in eighteenth-
century England, and none had the advantage of such an unrivaled theater for practice as their posts at Bethlem provided the Monros. James's
medical knowledge, which was prized and defended by John later in his
career, was evidently sufficiently esteemed by Robert Walpole for him
not only to support John's appointment as a Radcliffe fellow, but also to
pass down some of the elder mad-doctor's aphorisms to his own son.
However dubiously disposed young Horace Walpole had been toward
the Monros in the 1740s, even he seems to have accorded them more
than a little respect for their professional acumen. As he put it in a letter of 1780, advising the countess of Upper Ossory that the sick Miss
Vernon "ought to go abroad" (and evidently repeating some advice
James had given his father over thirty years earlier): "Old Monro told
my father that he scarce knew anything that asses' milk and change of
air would not cure, and that it was better to go into bad air than not to
change it often." [14]

James had not only offered Sir Robert the benefit of his experience on
general matters of physical and mental health, but toward the end of his
life had also been consulted as to the mental affliction of the latter's sister, Lady Dorothy Child (d. 1786). Lady Dorothy was described in a letter from Smart Lethieullier to Charles Lyttelton in the summer of 1751
as "so ill (she brooks the loss of her coach and six, etc.) that she is really
gone out of her senses and retired with Mr Child to the Lake House,
where Dr Monroe attends her and God knows whether she will ever recover." [15] Such episodes underline not only the long-standing medical attendance of the Monros on the Walpole family and its circle, but also
the considerable ground that these mad-doctors were prepared to cover
to minister to the needs of their wealthiest and most influential clients.
Apparently, Lady Dorothy had been disturbed (or, as Conway put it in
a contemporaneous letter to Walpole, "left . . . in fits . . . and quite in-

consolable") by the sudden departure to France of her relation John (Lord) Tylney or Tilney (formerly Child; 1712–84).[16]

James Monro's friendship and occasional consultations with Sir Robert Walpole and his family, and the patronage Walpole accorded John, suggest, therefore, that politics significantly but only partially interfered with the Monros' medical practice. The memory of John's previous associations would doubtless also have faded in the years after the Jacobite rising of 1745. John's subsequent assiduous and discreet attendance on the distracted Lord Orford, Horace Walpole's nephew (a case we shall discuss at greater length in chapter 4), highly appreciated as it was by the Whig grandee, must have diminished further the importance of what could latterly, perhaps, be dismissed as the product of youthful indiscretion.

John Monro's medical education had commenced north of the border at Edinburgh, already established as the leading center of medical instruction in Augustan Britain. From here, he gravitated to Leiden, the most famous of the continental medical schools, where Herman Boerhaave (1668–1738)—among others—had lectured. After a short interruption in order to take his M.B. (Bachelor of Medicine) in Oxford on 10 December 1743, he returned to the continent, living for a period in Paris and spending much of the next eight years traveling intermittently through France, Holland, Italy, and Germany. We know that his Oxford M.D. was conferred on him in absentia by diploma on 27 June 1747, and Munk indicates that he did not return to England from France until 1751.[17] However, if the latter claim is accurate, his return from this French sojourn must have followed a second period of foreign residence, for Bethlem's records make it clear that, after becoming a governor of the hospital, he spent a large part of 1748 attending committee meetings at both Bethlem and Bridewell.[18]

The continental rite of passage John embarked on early in his career was considered virtually de rigueur in the education of elite physicians, the College of Physicians paying much mind to the cosmopolitan traditions of its founders and fellows who had pursued a continental acculturation. In his later *Harveian Oration* of 1757, Monro himself was to make much of the way in which founding fathers like Linacre and Caius had rendered themselves "learned in every branch of knowledge, [by] not lazily staying at home but going far and wide," having, in particular, "wandered throughout the beautiful lands of Italy."[19] Nor was Monro reticent in praising Radcliffe's achievements and distinguishing among them his foundation of the "travelling scholarship" for "the advancement of medicine," a bursary of which John had been an appreciative beneficiary.[20] As Orations like Monro's make clear, being a "skilled" or "learned" physician was not sufficient to provide the polish needed for success in the social circles where elite doctors sought to move. Ideally, the best physician would also be "courteous and urbane," equipped with "erudition in humane letters," and have a passing ability in or an appreciation "of poetry" and good literature, or, better still, would be, like Richard Mead, an accomplished all-rounder: "a wise philosopher, a learned student of antiquity, a patron of every kind of art and a Maecenas to all literature."[21]

On returning to reside permanently in England, John was "unanimously" elected "joint physician" to Bethlem "without salary" by his fellow governors, serving in this capacity from 21 June 1751 alongside his ailing, septuagenarian father, James.[22] The appointment was "an Honour" most contemporaries perceived as "Sufficient, as well as Gain, to counter-balance any Salary."[23] Over the course of the next year, the younger Monro set about consolidating his position, acquiring the necessary credentials for respectable medical practice from the London College of Physicians. John's Oxbridge education must have stood him in good stead. This was a time when other physicians of Scottish descent and education were encountering considerable difficulty setting up practice in London, as the College of Physicians debated whether to admit them among its members, some being of the decided opinion "that the Act of Union did not impart so extensive a Privilege."[24] Yet, although his father, James, did not rise to higher office in the College after election as candidate on 23 December 1728 and as a fellow the following year (22 December 1729), John was more successful in charting his course into the heart of the medical establishment. He was appointed as a candidate of the College on 25 June 1752, a few months before his father's death and his own appointment as sole physician at Bethlem and Bridewell. He became a fellow on the same date the following year and just four years later presented the *Harveian Oration*.[25] No doubt aided by his hospital appointment, Monro flourished over many years at the College, repeatedly serving in the capacity of censor—in 1754, 1759, 1763, 1768, 1772, and 1778, and in 1771 he was also chosen as elect.[26] That said, he never rose to the kind of prominence and influence in these circles that was achieved by his rival in mad-doctoring, William Battie, who assumed the presidency and was accorded the honor of delivering the Lumleian lectures, a series of prestigious lectures delivered annually before the Royal College of Physicians since 1583.[27]

Monro's residential addresses very much reflect his steadily increasing professional success, especially his growing private practice, and indicate the extent to which his work was concentrated around the city and its environs. Residing in his thirties at his father's house in St. Mary, Islington, in Middlesex, Monro moved subsequently to Broad Street and then to Lincoln's Inn Fields, London (ca. 1753). He settled more permanently in No. 7 Red Lion Square, in the parish of St. Andrew and St. George the Martyr, Holborn (ca. 1760), a highly fashionable and rather exclusive residential area, very popular with elite doctors and other professionals.[28] By 1769, he was paying a rental of £60 per annum for this house and 3s. in the pound for poor rates.[29] Subsequently, about 1780–81, he moved to No. 53 Bedford Square, in St. George's, Bloomsbury, an equally desirable London address, ultimately retiring (ca. 1790) to the house he kept at Hadley in Barnet, Middlesex.[30]

While at his Red Lion Square address, Monro assumed a rather controversial role in the dispensary movement, sponsoring the first children's dispensary in London in 1769. Allowing it to operate from his home,[31] Monro granted his patronage in the process to a couple of compatriot practitioners, the unpopular Scottish brothers George (1719–89) and John Armstrong (1709–79).[32] Extending support to "a self-styled surgeon (a Scot who was not qualified to practice in London) to give advice and medicine gratis within the London area"[33] might easily have brought Monro some trouble with the College and its statutes. There was, after all, significant opposition to the setting up of dispensaries among the metropolitan medical elite, and especially among some of the old guard at the London College of Physicians,[34] who saw such freely dispensed outpatient facilities as a serious threat to their income from private practice.[35] Yet Monro's sponsorship of the children's dispensary seems to have been tendered in decidedly unostentatious, charitable terms (announcements in the press, for example, did not refer to him by name), and the dispensary's backing "by [the] Voluntary Subscriptions of the Nobility and Gentry" may have helped to ensure that it operated without challenge.[36] So far as we can tell, in any event, no questions were raised about Monro's involvement in official College circles. Monro's support of the Armstrongs seems some reflection of the tendency toward social cohesion and cultural identification among Scottish doctors and literati while in London. The Armstrongs were intimately acquainted with a coterie of Scottish practitioners and writers, including the famous writer on hygiene in hospitals John Aikin (1747–1822), the surgeon and satirical novelist Tobias Smollett (1721–71), and the M.D. and author of *The Pleasures of the Imagination* (1754), Mark Akenside (1721–70).[37]

THE MAD-DOCTOR AND THE THRONE OF FOLLY: JOHN MONRO AT BETHLEM AND BRIDEWELL

John's father, James Monro, was effectively the founder of the Monro dynasty at Bethlem. In 1728, in a hotly contested election against seven other candidates, he became the first of four successive family members to gain appointment as visiting physician to the hospital.[38] While medical dynasties by which whole families pursued the same profession from one generation to the next were by no means uncommon in the eighteenth century,[39] and the proprietorship of particular private madhouses was sometimes passed down through several generations of the same family,[40] there seems to have been no equivalent to the Monros' domination of the Bethlem physicianship for 125 years at any other contemporary public institution. By the 1750s, when John took up his position as his father's co-practitioner at the hospital, the family patronymic was already firmly identified with the treatment of the mad: first, as a result of James's association with Bedlam, and second, due to the widespread disposition to employ madness and folly as metaphorical vehicles for satirizing the moral, social, political, and religious ills of the times. James was rather dubiously immortalized in Pope's *Dunciad* (1729) as the main foe of the forces of folly that Pope (and other contemporary satirists) depicted as assaulting the British nation. Here he stands, a kind of Hippocratic King Canute, vainly attempting to hold back the stormy seas of unreason:

> Close to those walls where Folly holds her throne,
> And laughs to think Monro would take her down,
> Where, o'er the gates, by his famed father's hand,
> Great Cibber's brazen brainless brothers stand.[41]

Pope also referred to James Monro in his *Book of Horace* when attacking a favorite target of the Augustan satirists, the folly of talentless writers who did not know when to stop:

> Sure I should want the care of ten Monroes,
> If I would scribble rather than repose.[42]

Pope's lines may seem to anticipate the view of the Monros that was later to form itself rather more clearly among their critics: namely, that as long-standing physicians of Bethlem they were able to enjoy a

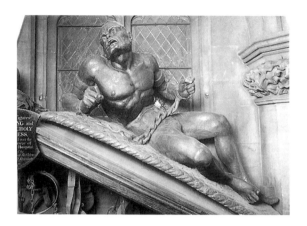

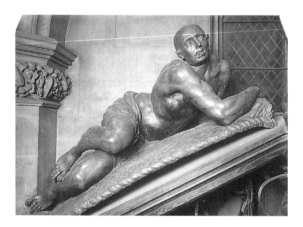

FIGURES 5A and 5B. Caius Gabriel Cibber, *Raving and Melancholy Madness.* These famous statues, which were carved out of Portland stone by Cibber ca. 1676, stood guard over the entrance gates to Bethlem at Moorfields. Powerfully evoking stereotypical images of insanity, they served both to advertise and to admonish visitors as to the madness that resided within the hospital (and also, perhaps, within themselves). The figures, which lay on replicas of straw matting and were mounted on the ends of a broken pediment, must originally have been seen at a height of about fourteen feet above ground. It was not until the early nineteenth century that the statues became popularly known as *Raving and Melancholy Madness.* With changing ideas about insanity and social decorum, the statues were relegated from 1815 to special discreet viewings behind curtains in the entrance hall to the new Bethlem building at St. George's Fields, Southwark, before they were banished to the South Kensington (Victoria and Albert) Museum in 1858 and subsequently to the Guildhall Museum. They are currently on display at the Bethlem Royal Hospital (or rather crammed into the cramped quarters of its museum), having been returned to the twentieth-century incarnation of the hospital in 1967. Reproduced by kind permission of the Bethlem Royal Hospital Archives and Museum, Beckenham, Kent.

somewhat monopolistic authority over the treatment of madness, and yet were little prepared to publish the fruits of their experience. This was one of the grounds on which William Battie was to censure John's father in his *Treatise on Madness* (1758) (see chapter 2). While the Monros' monopoly over Bethlem and the institutional treatment of madness has been exaggerated (for who could truly monopolize any branch of the inchoate profession that was medicine in this period?), there can be no doubt that it helps to explain the somewhat hidebound character of therapeutics at the hospital. Just as surely, it was also an important source of the complacency with which the hospital authorities greeted the evidence that surfaced over the years of palpable abuses and disregard of its patients.

When John Monro's career at the Bethlem and Bridewell Hospitals formally began, in 1751, he presumably was already quite familiar with both institutions. James had been careful to groom his only son to follow in his footsteps (just as John, in his turn, would nurture first one and then another of his sons as his successor). Not only had John served an apprenticeship as assistant to his father prior to his appointment, but James had also, probably, engineered his election as a governor of Bridewell and Bethlem. John was elected on 14 October 1748, having been nominated on 29 April by the prominent Tory governor and Oxonian antiquarian Dr. Richard Rawlinson (1690–1755).[43] John was also a frequent presence at subcommittee meetings during the late 1740s, attending twelve such committees, for example, during his first year as a governor. The governorship and the invitation to assist his father provided him with a brief but ideal form of sponsorship, placing him in the natural line of succession. And, sure enough, on the death of his father on 4 November 1752, John succeeded him as sole physician, receiving his appointment on 5 November 1752, after a period of about eighteen months learning the ropes. Four months later, he was granted precisely the same salary that his father had enjoyed before him.[44]

At this time, a significant faction among the Bridewell and Bethlem governors supported the enlargement of the medical establishment at the hospitals. Possibly, they were keen to see the physicianship taken out of the hands of a single incumbent, or rather a single family; or perhaps they wanted medical attendance opened up at Bethlem. Certainly they were more appreciative of the considerable demands on that office. In 1751, a successful motion for a second physician to be elected jointly with James Monro[45] was trumped by a further motion "for a Trinaty of Physicians"; and on James's death the following year, still another motion was made for "a joint Physitian."[46] In the end, however, neither of the latter two motions commanded a sufficient number of votes, a majority of the governors apparently agreeing with the assessment of the *London Evening Post* that the ministrations of a single "Coadjutor" (or else of one or both Monros) would suffice to fulfill the responsibilities of the physicianship in a "very agreeable" way.[47] Given the subsequent complaints from William Battie about how the Bethlem physicians had monopolized madness, and given his role as a governor of Bethlem since 1742, it is tempting to see the hand of a rival mad-doctor at work here. His presence is recorded only at the second poll, however, and as all such ballots were conducted in secret, one cannot be sure how he voted.[48] Majority sentiment among the governors throughout John Monro's tenure would continue to be that the hospitals could afford, and that the insane required, scarcely more than the minimum medical attention.

Bethlem was not unique in this regard, however. Even those lunatic hospitals founded after mid-century that challenged certain of its orthodoxies generally adhered to the same barely adequate provision of salaried medical staff: a single physician, apothecary, and surgeon. Reflecting some degree of acknowledgment of this insufficiency, both James and John Monro were on the Bethlem grand committee, which, in 1750–51, reconstituted the role of the apothecary, establishing an apothecary's shop at the hospital (on the model recently introduced at St. Bartholomew's Hospital) and requiring that the apothecary be a (more or less) resident officer.[49] While the precise role of the Monros in these initiatives is unclear, provisions for the apothecary's constant attendance ("once every day in the Week except Sunday")[50] were clearly designed to enlarge significantly that officer's role and the overall scope of medical attendance at Bethlem. Concurrently, the need for a second physician would have been appreciably reduced, while the erection of an apothecary's shop would also mean that medicines could be more conveniently and cheaply dispensed and more control exerted on this officer's bills. No doubt, it was felt that a hospital with a steadily mounting number of lunatics could do with a medical officer more permanently at hand.

John Monro advised again on this issue in 1769, when the grand committee he was called to assist reiterated that the apothecary "should be constantly Resident."[51] When the new apothecary resigned three years later, it was once again John Monro who was asked to direct the fitting up of the shop (as his father had been asked to do before him), and it was Monro too, along with the other medical officers, who advised the grand committee on the regulations necessary for the new incumbent.[52] The resolutions of this committee[53] furthered the trends of the previous two decades by making even more stringent the conditions requiring the apothecary to be resident and give constant attendance (possibly another delayed response to initiatives at St. Luke's, where the apothecary had been resident from the hospital's foundation). According to this system, although the primacy of Monro's authority as physician over the Bethlem medical department was firmly enshrined, it was clearly the apothecary who from now on was to be the medical officer most comprehensively in charge of the daily medical care of the patients and the medical oversight of their keepers.[54] These provisions would create controversy in 1815, when the House of Commons Select Committee graphically exposed appalling conditions and medical negligence at Bethlem, raising the question of whether the physician or the apothecary bore primary responsibility. (In the event, both were forced to resign.)[55]

Once he was made sole physician in 1752, John Monro appears to have done what was asked of him at Bethlem and Bridewell, although just how much more he did is open to doubt. The subcommittee minutes document his regular attendance, vetting virtually every Bethlem admission on official "views" of patients on Saturdays between 10 and 12 A.M. and coming to Bethlem, on average, at least three times a week, as he was required to do by the hospital's rules. His Bridewell duties were rather less onerous, most of the medical oversight there being provided by the apothecary and surgeon.[56] Besides this attention to his routine obligations, Monro was also a regular presence at court and other committee meetings, and probably had an important role in a number of the reforms in Bethlem's administration that took place in the second half of the century.

Alexander Cruden (a patient, as we shall see, of both Monros), alleged that in James's time the physician of Bethlem had virtual carte blanche at committee meetings because of the small numbers of governors who attended them: "It's said that there are only three Governors and Dr Monro, who are commonly present at the common Meetings on Saturdays at Bethlehem, and that the Doctor can bring to pass what he pleases."[57]

Almost invariably, decisions about admission had indeed been taken by the Monros and the Bethlem Committee at these Saturday views ever since the early eighteenth century. Only exceptionally was the Court of Governors involved in such deliberations, and even then it seems to have relied on the Bethlem physician to determine a doubtful case. A good example is the case of Margaret Lewis, who in 1763 was brought before the governors on an alderman's warrant, having been charged by Dr. Hugh Smith (1736?–89) of Mincing Lane "for coming to his House in a riotous Manner and Making a great Disturbance there and Collecting a large crowd of People there . . . & for being a loose Idle & Disorderly p[er]son."[58] At the court's request, John Monro examined her. While he was certainly prepared to assist a fellow professional in this instance, there is no evidence of any bias on his part, nor any reason to contradict his verdict that she was "insane . . . and a proper Object for Bethlem."[59]

It was understandably considered quite appropriate that the physician should have the major say in vetting admissions and discharges at Bethlem, and both Monros were evidently sufficiently discriminating to reject the occasional applicant as unsuitable. On the other hand, Cruden clearly underestimated both the numbers and the commitment of Bethlem's committee members.[60] Apart from admissions and other day-to-day business, most important decisions about Bethlem were taken at grand committee and court meetings where large numbers of governors were present. Smaller, subcommittee management was certainly to take over more of the running of Bethlem and other London hospitals as the eighteenth century wore on. Yet, if the Monros dominated decisions over admissions, they were nonetheless seen very much as the governors' loyal officers, and in other respects their influence was rather limited. One should be careful to keep in perspective the influence any doctor was able to bring to bear on men who seem to have regarded the management of the hospital as primarily a matter for themselves, collectively, in the exercise of their civic duty, and who were socially the equals or betters of the Bethlem physician. Nor was this situation in any sense exceptional: the subordination of medical officers to the authority of lay governors was, after all, the standard pattern at most hospitals until well into the nineteenth century.

Of course, by modern standards Monro's attendance at the hospital (just three times a week and for roughly two or three hours at a time) seems a perfunctory performance, a meager commitment of time that scarcely accords with what one would expect of the chief medical officer of such a sizable and important institution. In contemporary terms, though, far from suggesting a dereliction of duty, this pattern of attendance accorded with the customary model for hospital service. Monro, like his father and generations of Bethlem doctors before him, had been appointed to Bethlem only in a visiting, quasi-honorary capacity. Attendance at medical charities like Bethlem, as was the case with comparable positions at other London hospitals, was regarded as a part-time activity. Although posts were highly valued and often hotly contested, they most definitely were not meant to interfere with a physician's private practice and other gentlemanly pursuits. Hospital appointments were not a direct source of one's professional livelihood, but a means to a number of ends. Their primary value lay in the opportunities they provided for the widening of one's contacts among the affluent and socially prominent who served as the charity's governors; in the visibility they brought among the well-to-do more generally (the potential patients whose favor could help to establish a lucrative private practice); in the bolstering of one's own powers of patronage and social status; and in the securing of some small but stable source of regular income, while one pursued the less guaranteed, but higher, financial rewards available through private practice. Hospital posts were, in other words, a route to, rather than a signification of, professional success.[61] Monro's hospital duties were understood by all to require nothing more than an intermittent attendance, leaving him ample time to prosecute a lucrative private trade in lunacy.

Monro's contemporaries who held analogous hospital posts treated them in essentially the same fashion. For example, Thomas Brookes, M.D., the physician to St. Luke's (and also a physician to the army) during the 1760s, was said to attend the hospital on Mondays and Fridays, while the rest of his days, between the hours of 10 A.M. and 4 P.M., were spent pursuing his private practice. Yet even such limited professional commitments gave his wife, Harriet (née Nelthorpe), enough opportunity to pursue an adulterous affair with Edward Hoare Esquire of Chelsea (who was also married), the melodramatic and partly staged discovery of which led to a highly public divorce proceeding.[62]

Throughout the eighteenth century in metropolitan London, those claiming the title of "physician" clung tightly to what they asserted was their status as gentlemen engaged in the practice of a noble art. In general, they strove (to be sure, with only limited success) to eschew their connection with the lower "tradesman-like" practices of their professional brethren, the surgeons and apothecaries. Like the gentlemen they were, or rather were keen to be seen as, city physicians traveled about in carriages, carried swords and gold-headed canes, and wore wigs and robes—the external stigmata of superior status. Disposed to avoid the socially contaminating effects of anything that smacked of manual labor, they diagnosed essentially by symptoms rather than signs, rarely performed physical examinations, and avoided, as far as possible, the laying of hands on patients.[63] Such menial tasks—inspection and inter-

ference with their patients' orifices, the bleeding, purging, and scarify-
ing of their clients' bodies, along with the dispensing of the prescriptions
they wrote—the lordly physicians left to the lesser branches of the
noble art, those who worked with hand rather than head, and who performed, in somewhat servile fashion, at their direction. Theirs was to be
"a calling by which a gentleman, not born to a gentleman's allowance of
good things, might ingeniously obtain the same by the exercise of his
abilities"[64]—so that considerations that bore upon social status and
standing were at least as important as those with more direct economic
consequences.

The construction of "the art of physick" as a form of professional
gentility thus profoundly affected the very practice of medicine.[65] It
influenced the ways in which physicians diagnosed and prescribed, and
manifested itself in even the most intimate details of the interaction between doctor and patient. Changes in the theory and practice of physic,
such as the introduction of more "mechanistic" medical approaches following the Scientific Revolution and the rising competitiveness and status of surgeons and surgeon-apothecaries, were accompanied by class-
mediated accusations from physicians of the old robe who carped that
the practitioners of the new philosophy of medicine were mere "mechanics"—like the surgeons they were generally keen to maintain in
a subordinate station—quite literally people who worked with their
hands.[66]

This context, and a long tradition of physicians providing consultations for genteel patients via letters and indirect, written consultations,
may itself help to explain why Monro was sometimes prepared to diag-
nose (much to some of his patients' chagrin) without even seeing those
who sought the benefit of his advice and expertise. In other respects as
well, Monro and his fellow mad-doctors adhered to the well-established
pattern of physicianly behavior outlined here—and unsurprisingly so,
since, as we shall suggest in more detail below, throughout the period
in which Monro practiced, mad-doctoring constituted in no sharp or
simple way a distinct branch of medicine.

MONRO AND THE GREAT BEDLAM EXHIBITION

The almost four decades during which Monro presided as physician at
the Bethlem and Bridewell Hospitals, 1752–91, constituted a momentous period in Bethlem's history. It was in the eighteenth century that
Bethlem as "Bedlam" truly assumed its archetypal place as a by-word

for all things mad and chaotic. Not only did Bedlam become a medium for satirizing the follies of the nation, but it was also in the same period that Bethlem really began to generate its own history of scandal and vilification. As part and parcel of such developments, the Monros themselves would be depicted as the quintessential mad-doctors by famous poets and playwrights, as well as the not so famous Grub-Street scribblers, cartoonists, and pamphleteers.

This was a time, moreover, when Bethlem was to reach perhaps the height of its exposure to the prying eyes of the public. It had long been the custom of its governors to permit outsiders a rather indiscriminate access and license as visitors to come and gaze at the insane. Yet it was in the 1760s that the quantity of visitors appears to have reached its peak, as the hospital acquired an ever greater popularity as a source of public entertainment. (This was certainly the decade when annual poor's box takings from the donations made by those viewing the hospital were at their highest, providing one telling measure of the mounting volume of visitation.) Bedlam's wards had become emblematic of Unreason, its very name synonymous with lunacy, and its crazed inmates reduced to a spectacle to which the masses reacted with mirth, mockery, and callous teasing. As one observer recorded after mid-century, ". . . a hundred people at least [were] . . . suffered unattended to run rioting up and down the wards, making sport and diversion of the miserable inhabitants [some of whom were] provoked by the insults of this holiday mob into furies of rage; [prompting in] the spectators . . . a loud laugh of triumph at the ravings they had occasioned." [67]

Yet just as more and more hoi polloi were coming to gawk or to laugh at, to pity or to receive moral instruction and edification from a sight of the lunatics,[68] more and more of those moving in influential, educated circles were beginning to raise their voices in protest. As the expression of painful sensibilities grew more legitimate, in what historians and literary critics have evocatively termed a new "age of sensibility," men and women "of feeling" gave vent to much ingenuous (and disingenuous) sorrow, mortification, and disgust over the spectacle of lunatics being shown like animals in a human zoo.[69] The fun of seeing the insane began to pale and recede. Visiting Bethlem became one of a number of evocative symbols of barbarous insensibility and vulgar showiness, alongside public executions, public dissections, grandiloquent charity, and grandiose forms of burial.

In a fluid society, differences of taste and sensibility provide a potentially invaluable mechanism for marking status boundaries. Accordingly,

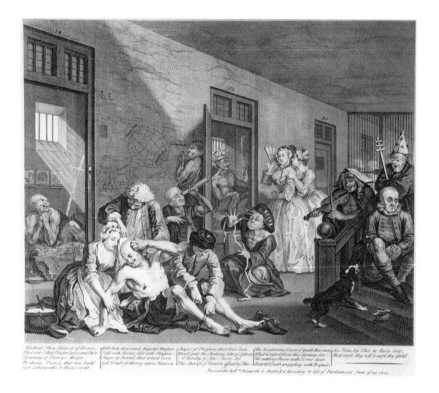

FIGURE 6. Hogarth's scene viii from *A Rake's Progress,* 1735 engraving. The artist here depicts stereotypical incurable lunatics, including the "Rake" himself, along with public visitors and hospital employees, in a chaotic melée at Bethlem Hospital. In the forefront, Tom Rakewell, maddened by his debauched rake's life, is represented in a half-naked recumbent posture, holding his head in evident distress, intentionally reminiscent of Cibber's statue "melancholy madness" (see figure 5b). His shoes having been removed, he is being manacled by a keeper, while the bewigged physician in attendance gently attempts to intervene. A plaster beneath his right breast may suggest that he has been bled. The other lunatics depicted include a mad scientist/projector (plotting longitudes on the hospital wall); a mad tailor obsessed with measurement, with tape in hand; a mad astronomer gazing at imaginary stars through his rolled-up paper telescope; a mad musician (with violin in hand and score atop his head); a crazy Papist with mitre and trinitarian staff; a lovesick moonfaced melancholic, sitting on the stairs while a dog barks at his feet (as dogs were proverbially said to do at the moon), and a mad king whose crowned head and regal aspect are contradicted by his nakedness and his act of urinating in his cell. In addition, a religious maniac (invested, like Rakewell, with allusions to Cibber—although this time "raving madness" is the evident model) is shown mistaking the light from his cell window for a revelation. Two visitors—judging by their appearance, either ladies of fashion (or a lady and her maid) or high-class courtesans—stand by the cell of the crazed king. The epitome of idle, unfeeling, and uncivilized curiosity, they gaze unsympathetically upon the lunatics, as one conceals her amusement behind her fan while the other whispers in her

over the course of the eighteenth century, significant segments of the genteel educated elite and of the emerging middle classes strove energetically to maximize the distance between polite and popular culture. The excesses of the crowd at Bethlem thus became one more occasion for drawing invidious contrasts between elite refinement, rationality, and sensitivity on the one hand, and the depraved attitudes, mindless superstition, and moral coarseness characteristic of the unwashed masses on the other. Samuel Richardson's analogous discussions of visits to Bethlem and the hanging tree at Tyburn provide a striking illustration of this process at work. According to Richardson, it was "natural" "curiosity" that drew "most people" to Tyburn; "affecting concern" was the "unavoidable" response of "a thinking person" to "the scene," which was "interesting" (or instructive) "to all who consider themselves of the same species with the unhappy sufferers." Yet "the mob" were merely motivated by "silly curiosity" and, by reacting with "noise" and "a barbarous kind of mirth, altogether inconsistent with humanity," spoiled the spectacle for the polite. Likewise, at Bethlem, Richardson

> was very much at a loss to account for the behaviour of the generality of people, who were looking at these melancholy objects. Instead of the concern I think unavoidable at such a sight, a sort of mirth appeared on their countenances; and the distemper'd fancies of the miserable patients most unaccountably produced mirth and loud laughter in the unthinking auditors; and the many hideous roarings, and wild motions of others, seemed equally entertaining to them. Nay, so shamefully inhuman were some . . . as to endeavour to provoke the patients into rage to make them sport.[70]

Initially, one observes a movement among the "better sort" away from searching out and describing the most entertaining and brutish of the inmates toward a concentration on the most moving. Soon, however, the complaints were taken a step further, and objections began to be voiced to any exhibition of the insane before the rabble. In the words of Mackenzie's "man of feeling," "I think it an inhuman practice to expose the greatest misery with which our nature is afflicted to every idle visi-

ear. These attitudes are contrasted with those of the physician and of the spurned Sarah Young, Rakewell's former sweetheart, who kneels forlornly by his side, wiping her tears with a handkerchief. Architectural details of the hospital seem accurately depicted, including the recently erected rails, which divided the "incurables'" wings from other portions of the hospital where "curables" were lodged. Reproduced by kind permission of The Wellcome Trust, London.

tant who can afford a trifling perquisite to the keeper; especially as it is a distress which the humane must see with the painful reflection, that it is not in their power to relieve it."[71]

The shifting climate of opinion among the educated classes eventually had practical consequences, and after a series of measures aimed at controlling the occasional excesses of visitors, particularly at holiday times, when the behavior of elements of the crowd bordered on the riotous, the Bethlem governors finally curtailed the practice in 1770. What Foucault called the "organized exhibition" of the "scandal" of madness[72] was radically sanitized, or rather converted into a more respectable matter: indiscriminate sightseers were outlawed and all visitors henceforth required to obtain the authority of a ticket signed by a governor, and to be attended by a hospital servant.[73]

As the hospital's physician, Monro presided over this rather dramatic, if paradoxical, rise and fall of madness as spectacle. There is scant evidence, however, that he himself exerted, or attempted to exert, much influence over the practice. Monro certainly stated, in his response to Battie's *Treatise on Madness,* that he did not think it advisable for patients to receive visitors, accepting that "there are times, when such visits are highly detrimental."[74] However, he doubted his ability to determine this matter, or that patients' relations would "put so much confidence in their physician" as to leave the decision to him, while he emphasized that visits might "sometimes be permitted without any bad consequences" and that he had "frequently known them of service." Furthermore, this rather compromised circumspection with regard to visiting is a view he seems to have applied only to his private practice. Implicitly, he appears to have advocated different rules for the inmates of Bethlem than for patients of a higher social rank.[75] If his comments represent a realistic attitude to the limits of medical authority in the more private world of paying patrons, they also amount to an elision of the issue and the main area of controversy when it came to the public sphere of hospital practice. Certainly, they seem quite pusillanimous by comparison with Battie's unequivocal repudiation of visiting at St. Luke's. It was Bethlem's governors who continued to permit the intrusions of idle visitants to occur during Monro's first two decades in office. Subsequently too, it was the governors (rather than their physician) who, increasingly concerned about the public controversy and damage to the hospital's reputation that visiting was causing, belatedly brought the practice to a close—albeit only after at least two decades of regular protest, voiced in polite magazine culture in particular.

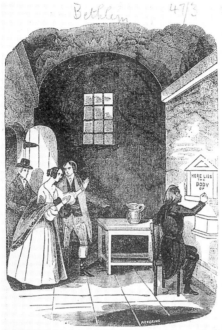

The wretched maniac was, at the time they entered the room, occupied in sketching another tomb.

FIGURE 7. Early nineteenth-century engraving by Pickering, depicting a lady visitor to Bethlem. Pickering illustrates the ineluctable nature of confinement, depicting a lady visitor, shown in by two keepers, with a gentleman patient drawing a tombstone on his cell wall inscribed "Here lies the body. . . ." In one of the authors' possession; source unknown.

To be sure, even before mass visitation was brought to an end in 1770, Monro and the other Bethlem officers had occasionally taken steps to prevent certain patients from being exposed to view: those who were naked, for example (or loosely clothed), because they were incontinent or destructive; and those who were physically debilitated or in a highly agitated state. For example, Monro's name was the second on the membership list of two grand committees that substantially expanded and reformed Bethlem's regulations as to officers and servants in 1765, and that inter alia had sought to attend to the abuses of visiting.[76] These regulations reiterated an old but "much Neglected" rule requiring the

porter and servants to limit the loitering of certain categories of unde-
sirable visitors in Bethlem, namely "Prentice Boys, Idle Girls and Jews
on a Saturday" and to "turn them out if they behave improperly." [77]

These measures, however, aimed ineffectually at reforming, rather
than actually questioning or significantly containing, the practice of public visiting, and relied on (patently unreliable) inferior officers and servants to police the character and conduct of visitants. Their promulgation hints at the degree and inveteracy of the moral blindness at Bethlem
to the deleterious consequences of exposing its inmates to the taunts and
gaze of outsiders, and to what was really in the best interests of patients.
Apparently, Monro was not at committee meetings during 1764–65
when extra muscle was hired to police the hospital's doors at Easter; he
was not at the 1766 court and grand committee meetings that banned
visitors during holidays; he was not on the 1769 committee that ordered
that the hospital's back gate be kept permanently locked (except for the
receipt of provisions, patients, and governors); he was not present in
1775, when visitors under the age of sixteen were banned; he was not
on the committees that limited visitors to four per ticket in 1779 and
barred ex-incurables as visitors; nor was he a member of the committee
that banned all Sunday visiting in 1781, "unless Attended by a Governor"; neither, finally, does he seem to have had a hand in the exclusion
of visitors (apart from relations and friends) from the infirmaries in
1786.[78] Although a 1769 grand committee convened to draw up regulations for the hospital was ordered to do so with Monro's assistance, it
is unclear how much influence he had on its resolutions, which included
restricting visitors to the hours of 10 A.M. to 3 P.M. and imposing tighter
restrictions on the access of male visitors to female patients.[79] (We know,
for instance, that he did not sign the committee's ultimate report.) He
was, however, one of those seventeen governors on a subsequent grand
committee that finally devised the ticket system, as confirmed and imposed by order of court.[80]

It seems safe to assume that Monro approved of most of the initiatives mentioned above and had some sort of role in the general moves
afoot to curtail visiting. There is no evidence, though, to suggest that
it was his opinion, or that of other medical voices, that led the governors
to conclude that the patients were suffering as a result of the practice of
visiting—something that, by the 1780s, the united hospitals' chaplain
and Bethlem's first historian, Thomas Bowen, was unequivocal about.[81]
Indeed, the decided lack of medical input into the reform of visiting at
Bethlem is suggested by the fact that it does not seem to have been until

1792, just over a month after John Monro's death, that "the Priviledge [*sic*]" was formally granted the physician "of signing Visitors to view Bethlem Hospital or personally to introduce whoever he may think proper." [82]

Hospital rules had long forbidden servants to show patients in states of semi-nudity to visitors, and such rulings were reiterated and elaborated in the 1760s. Patients judged "not fit to be Exposed" were ordered to be "kept properly Confined," with "the Wickets of their Doors kept Shut, as well as their Doors," while a baseline attention to healthy, seasonally adjusted ventilation was provided by the stipulation that their "Upper Doors" be opened during "the summer time." [83] Women patients who were "Lewdly Given" were to "be Confined to their Cells and no persons Suffered to come to them but in Company with one of the gallery Maids." [84] However, repeated orders and records of abuses that are entered in the governors' own minutes indicate that such regulations were regularly flouted. More often than not, furthermore, Monro's role seems far from central to what reforms were attempted.

Again, even during the period of allegedly indiscriminate visiting, certain classes of visitors were, on occasion, banned from seeing patients: if the prospective visitors were considered to be disturbing or unhelpful to patients, or if they were known to be troublemakers. However, while the governors strove to weed out thieves, apprentices, idlers, the young, the loose and the disorderly, and even Sabbath-day Jews and ex-incurables from the ranks of their visitors "of quality," exclusions of this sort represent a somewhat jaundiced jurisdiction of the excesses of the mob. These specific bars were, anyway, far from effective, while restrictions were rarely imposed on the visits or conduct of patients' relations. Most instances recorded in the committee minutes of patients' friends being excluded from visiting occurred after 1770.

Yet perhaps, after all, this may be a misplaced criticism. Impolitic as it may seem to raise the question, one must ask to what extent Bethlem's patients benefited from the adoption of the new exclusionary policy. For the mob seeking their entertainment and show were only one portion of Bedlam's visitors. Just how harmful to patients' interests, on the other hand, were those friends who were barred from the hospital after 1770 because they visited too often, "at all times and Seasons," or those who brought in unlicensed provisions? One wonders, similarly, how much other patients, whose friends were restricted to monthly visits, appreciated such limits, which were imposed only partially out of concern for their interests. Visitors, it seems, were often perceived by patients as a welcome relief from the monotony that inevitably accompanied their confinement. More significantly, no doubt, later abuses at Bethlem during the physicianship of John's son Thomas (1759–1833) (in particular the long and notorious confinements of William Norris and James Tilly Matthews),[85] suggest a certain value to the practice of maintaining a permeable boundary between the hospital and the outside community, not least in exposing daily institutional routines to regular external scrutiny.

HOW TO TREAT A BEDLAMITE

It may well be that, rather than his complicity in putting the inmates on display, what most indicts Monro's record at Bethlem is something else: the singularly unadventurous approach toward the treatment of patients that he and other medical officers continued to practice there for decades. Therapeutics at Bethlem was characterized by relatively uniform purges, vomits, and bleeding, administered seasonally to patients, with the occasional addition of tonics (such as alcohol), cold bathing (or other cooling applications), and warm or hot baths, all of these "heroic" interventions being supplemented by (a mostly "lowering" form of) diet and regimen. This model, whereby repletion in the system was countered by depletion, and vice versa, was founded on an essentially humoral approach to mental diseases. Overlaid since the late seventeenth century by a new, mechanistic brand of Newtonian science, older principles and even types of treatment had in reality changed remarkably little.

To be sure, John Monro was skeptical of some conventional treatments: he objected to blistering, for example. This was a form of "counter-irritation" involving the application of a chemical preparation to draw out a blister on the head, neck, shoulder, foot, or some other exposed part of the body, normally recommended to draw the peccant fluids and humors to the body's surface. Blistering often required the shaving of the patient's head, the head most commonly seen as providing the best site for the operation—not least because of the added putative benefit of cooling the brain and keeping the patient free from lice. In his *Remarks on Dr. Battie's Treatise* (1758), Monro vigorously disagreed with Battie's cautious and qualified advocacy of this treatment, maintaining that "I never saw the least good effect of 'blisters' in madness . . . except in fever," and he also repudiated the supposed advantages obtained from "rough cathartics."[86] It is possible that Monro was prepared to use other counter-irritants, and to prescribe blisters in a more limited way, though there is little documentary evidence that blistering was widely practiced at Bethlem in the second half of the eighteenth century, or by John in his private practice. However, if Monro scrupled to embrace such a practice, Hogarthian and other contemporary depictions of shaven-headed maniacs at Bethlem remind us that counter-irritants had been regularly employed at Bethlem under John's father and his predecessors. Wesley also spoke of James Monro when attending Peter Shaw, employing "a strong blister on each of his arms, with another over all his head." [87]

Whatever John Monro's doubts about blisters, moreover, one searches in vain for evidence that he was sufficiently interested in therapeutic advances to experiment with new or different forms of treatment. In his *Remarks*, Monro vigorously defended the virtues of most forms of depletion (see chapter 2). That, throughout the eighteenth century, patients were only admitted to Bethlem provided they were deemed "strong enough to undergo a course of Physic," [88] and were occasionally discharged if they became otherwise, seems sufficient indication of the "heroic," if not enervating, character of "physicking" at the hospital. Rulings during Monro's time instructing servants to assist each other with bleeding, purging, vomiting, and bathing patients (1765), and requiring that the apothecary always "attend the Administration of the Vomits and Purges on the Days appointed for them and see they are properly Administered" (1772), suggest how routine such treatments had become.[89]

However, these and other regulations also imply that doses were varied to some extent in accordance with individual patients' constitutions, a circumstance that urges us to be careful not to exaggerate the indiscriminate nature of eighteenth-century therapeutics for the insane. Monro had stressed in his *Remarks*, for example, that, however "excellent" was the "general effect" of cold bathing on the insane, due to its propensity "to hurry the spirits, it is not to be prescribed indiscriminately to every one." [90] Monro agreed in general with Cheyne and Battie that medicaments and therapies should not be applied "indiscriminately" or "too strong" and that evacuation should be "determined by the constitution of the patient," and he claimed that Battie was not the only one who did not believe "bleeding the constant and adequate cure of madness." [91] As time went on, moreover, there is some evidence that Monro may have become less convinced of the benefits of other forms of evacuation. Although he had distinguished setons and issues as serviceable in his *Remarks*, by the 1780s experience may have "induced a change of opinion"—at least that was the view of Bryan Crowther, the Bethlem surgeon during 1789–1815 (who, like Monro, had served an apprenticeship at the hospital under his father). Writing in 1811, Crowther recalled "that when patients were admitted into Bethlem with setons and issues, the late Dr. Monro directed me to heal them; alleging that he did not find any advantage from their being kept open." [92]

Yet to suggest that there were anything approaching profound doubts about evacuation among Crowther's predecessors at Bethlem would be—to choose an appropriate metaphor—clutching at straws. Eighteenth-century theories of mental pathology saw insanity—the vitiation of the higher faculties, the distortion of the fancy and the imagination, the fragmentation of mental associations—as fundamentally rooted in the body. The precise nature of the underlying somatic disorder was variously conceived: it might be traced to blockages or excesses in bodily secretions; or be attributable to debilitation of the animal spirits; or it might, depending upon its particular manifestations, correspond to excessive laxity or tautness of the nerves or fibers. Regardless, belief in the appropriateness of bleeding and various means of purging and evacuating the system was widespread in this period, and a number of contemporaries, both medical and lay, were even less sympathetic than Monro himself to metaphysical interpretations of the distemper. Lady Mary Wortley Montagu (1689–1762), for example, complained bitterly in a letter written in 1755 about Samuel Richardson's propensity to make madness an "ornament to the characters of his heroines." Casting aside the novelist's romantic notions, she insisted that

> to be carried to Bedlam . . . is really all that is to be done in that case. Madness is as much a corporeal distemper as the gout or asthma, never occasioned by affliction, or to be cured by the enjoyment of their extravagant wishes. Passion may indeed bring on a fit, but the disease is lodged in the blood, and it is not more ridiculous to attempt to relieve the gout by an embroidered slipper that to restore reason by gratification of wild desires. [93]

Although by 1820, in the wake of the 1815–16 Commons Enquiry into Madhouses, "periodical depletion" was being condemned by authorities on insanity like George Man Burrows (1771–1846) as a form of medical "charlatanry," [94] for the duration of the eighteenth century, depletion and repletion were very much the dominant therapeutic paradigm, not only for madness and at Bethlem, but also for the treatment of all kinds of diseases besides insanity outside the hospital. Nevertheless, while evacuations, tonics, diet, and regimen remained the major techniques available to contemporary physicians for madness, they seem to have

been employed with a particularly monotonous and uninspired regularity at Bethlem.

We know that the amounts of bills for medicines supplied to Bethlem
from London's Apothecary's Hall came to little more than £103–£137
per annum during the 1760s and 1770s, with an additional £16–£20
for disbursements in the apothecary's shop.[95] Yet we can only guess at
what drugs were being used, and at what Monro himself was prescribing for patients. Bethlem's records under Monro reveal very little about
the treatments patients were receiving, although this very fact, of course,
tells its own story. Mostly patients appear to have been simply allowed
to recover as best they might, and given the Monros' declared faith in
management as much as medicine,[96] this may not be surprising. The
same approach had clearly prevailed under John's father, James, and under James's predecessors. There is little sign that John Monro attempted
to vary this system or to try anything particularly new with his hospital
patients during the forty or so years of his physicianship.

One of the few departures from previous practice appears to have
been the conversion (in 1766) of the "dark cell," together with an adjoining room, into a sitting room "for the Conveniency of the Patients."[97]
(Haslam's *Observations* [1798] imply, though, that if this therapy was
indeed ever fully dispensed with, it subsequently and quite rapidly came
back into vogue at Bethlem.)[98] Another apparent innovation was the introduction of "Two Sets of Skittles for the Patients" in 1779 by a committee on which John Monro sat.[99] As for patients' diet, apart from the
addition of a weekly portion of veal and a few vegetables, it scarcely
changed during Monro's time, although the physician did occasionally
serve on committees that periodically inspected the house provisions,
sometimes declaring them "indifferent" and/or "deficient in Quality"
and taking issue with the hospitals' suppliers.[100] The leaves of absence
that, since the seventeenth century, had been quite regularly granted patients with a view to returning them to their families, and aiding or test-
ing their recoveries through a temporary stay at home or in the country,
seem to have been formalized and extended as a policy under Monro's
physicianship. Discharge registers record sojourns of several months being enjoyed by over twenty patients a year by the 1780s,[101] and committee minutes suggest that Monro and serving governors kept tabs on
some of these patients and made efforts to prioritize the readmission of
those that relapsed.[102]

The 1765 regulations for Bethlem's officers and servants, which
Monro had a definite hand in drawing up, also included new stipula-

tions augmenting the authority of the physician in some areas. These and other regulations suggest that Monro was partially responsible for the gradual (if slow) medicalization of Bethlem, making some effort to ensure that medicine exerted itself more thoroughly over the hospital's management.[103] The new rules also testify, however, to the rather harsher and more coercive side of medical supervision of patients. In that sense, rather than anticipating the moral therapeutics that became prominent at some institutions during the latter part of the century, they imply a quasi-Foucauldian stress on enhanced surveillance and forced occupational activity. The matron, for instance, was ordered to "Acquaint the Physician when ever any of the Patients (without particular Sickness) take to their Beds," while those that were "low Spirited or inclinable to be Mopish" were to be "Obliged to get up . . . Turned out of their cells, the Doors Locked, that they may not creep back again to their beds"— a provision that allowed the maidservants to go about their duties less troubled, cleaning cells and galleries.[104] Similarly, patients were to be employed "at their Needle . . . when not otherwise Busied rather than" being permitted to "Walk Idle up and down the House Shewing it to Strangers and begging Money."[105] So it was the abuses of visiting and the deficiencies and tensions of staffing, more than patients' mental or moral torpor, that were to be eased by ensuring that they be employed, as is further indicated by the requirement that patients be equally distributed among the maids so that each had "a proper number of such hands as are fit for Work to Assist her."[106]

There is evidence, too, of substantial and occasionally punitive, if selective, use of mechanical restraint and seclusion at Bethlem, both before and after mid-century. On the whole, though, the Monros seem to have taken a rather circumscribed role in such managerial decisions. Some effort was made to ensure greater oversight of restraint, for example, by requiring servants (in 1779) to notify the steward whenever it was "Necessary to confine any patients by Chains or otherwise,"[107] but the extent to which John Monro or any other medical officer attempted to, or succeeded in, controlling the resort to these forms of coercion seems limited. The Bethlem chaplain, Thomas Bowen, maintained in 1783 that the "degree of care and confinement" accorded patients was assigned by the steward "under the direction of the physician," and that it was only when patients misbehaved that they were ordered confined "immediately," but this may represent the ideal rather than the reality of restraint and seclusion. Mostly, these decisions seem to have been left to inferior officers and servants, under the supervision of the steward. The steward's accounts (which, for example, record purchases such as "4 Doz[e]n of Men & Womens Leg Locks" at £6 6s., in 1765,[108] and a further dozen leg locks and an extra dozen handcuffs less than two years later), suggest the pervasive extent of mechanical restraint at Bethlem.[109] It was the apothecary (1772–95) John Gozna (d. 1795), rather than Monro, who appears to have introduced strait waistcoats into the hospital very soon after his appointment, in preference to chains, although the latter were never fully dispensed with.[110] Nonetheless, this was an age before the fashionable nineteenth-century doctrine of non-restraint had been heard of, and it would be anachronistic to criticize Monro or any others at Bethlem too harshly for the apparent lack of interest they took in methods that were relatively universally employed in the treatment of the insane, at least before John Monro's death in the 1790s—techniques that these practitioners must have regarded as pragmatic and essential tools for the control and disciplining of unruly patients.

To a limited extent, one can observe a heightened attention to the interests, needs, safety, physical comfort, and general health of patients in the revised regulations of 1765 and in other later rulings. For example, language such as "taking particular care of patients" or attending to the "welfare" of patients began to be rather more conspicuous in court and committee minutes. A growing appreciation of the needs of physically sick patients, discernible in the addition of infirmaries during James Monro's time, was furthered under John with the erection of a second infirmary for women in 1753[111] and with instructions in 1765 for the matron to "take particular care of the Sick, and see that they are moved into the Infirmary if Judged Necessary by the Physician and there taken care of."[112] Initially, the infirmaries were very much the responsibility of the physician, but increasingly this was seen as a general responsibility of the medical staff as a whole, patients being normally on some sort of sick diet and being attended by servants while there, "so long and in such manner" as the medical officers thought "Necessary."[113]

Increased concern about the number of patients at Bethlem dying from smallpox inspired an arrangement with the London Smallpox Hospital in 1778–79 for the transfer of afflicted patients, a rather belated initiative (given that the latter hospital had been in existence since 1747 and large numbers of Bethlem's patients had contracted, and died from, the disease during this period), but, nevertheless, an initiative in which Monro's son Thomas and the Bethlem surgeon during 1769–88, Richard Crowther (d. 1788), were both involved.[114] Monro junior was also on a contemporaneous committee that required new patients to be examined and the surgeon notified of wounds and sores, another sign of (the slow pace of) medicalization at Bethlem, patients' friends having formerly been apt to "Neglect to give Notice" of this.[115] Likewise, provisions were made for the first time in 1771 for servants to strip and examine patients for lice and other vermin on their discharge from the hospital.[116]

Not only the lousy, the sick, and the dying, but corpses too were gradually accorded more attention. Instructions for more rapid notification to relatives regarding patients' deaths were made, and it was under Monro too that a "Bone/Dead House," or mortuary, was added to Bethlem. By 1765 the hospital had also acquired a "surgery."[117] Hands-on dissection, though, tended here as elsewhere to be less the province of physicians than of surgeons.[118] It is thus not surprising that, unlike subsequent medical officers such as Bryan Crowther (1765–1815), the Bethlem surgeon during 1789–1815, and John Haslam (1764–1844), the Bethlem apothecary during 1792–1815, both of whom published accounts of their inquiries into mental pathology based upon their observations in the Bethlem dissecting house,[119] Monro failed to take advantage of such facilities for any post-mortem investigations. Monro also seems to have played no explicit role in Andrew Marshall's (1742–1813) dissections of maniacs from Bethlem (and from other hospitals and lunatic establishments, including John Miles's Hoxton madhouse) during ca. 1789–94, the results of which were posthumously published in 1815.[120]

In new rules issued at Bethlem during the 1770s and 1780s, one can also observe some recognition of the need to pay more mind to patients' safety and security. There were novel requirements—for instance, for the enclosing of fireplaces, the installation of mechanical guards and servant supervision in the stove rooms, and rails on the gallery staircases[121]—precautions that were partly motivated by the desire to save money on surgery to injured patients, but that nonetheless served a protective purpose. On a related front, there were sporadic attempts to improve the healthiness and hygiene of the hospital environment and of patients' bodies, moves that reflected the real danger to health that dirt and nastiness were seen to represent in this period. Diseases (especially hospital or gaol fever) were often seen as being borne on the effluvia and bad airs of confined spaces, even if attention to this matter was little more than sporadic at Bethlem. Theodore M. Brown has pointed to the enhanced regard paid by a range of late-eighteenth-century practitioners to public hygiene and prevention in combating fevers and infectious diseases, with physicians like (Sir) John Pringle (1707–82) and Donald Monro (1727–1802) emphasizing the necessity of keeping quarters "clean and airy" and bodies "sweet and clean," particularly in the "crowded situations of jails, ships and hospitals."[122] In his *Remarks,* John Monro referred to "cleanliness" as such an obvious and "necessary article" of management in every distemper as scarce to require a mention, "since nothing but the most gross and unpardonable negligence, can leave any one to suffer by want of it."[123] At Bethlem too, the steward was instructed in 1765, for example, to conduct a thrice-weekly tour of inspection to "see that the Galleries and the cells are kept as clean and neat as the Condition of Patients will Admit," and likewise the matron was to ensure "that Patients in general are taken care of and kept as Clean as their Complaints will allow."[124] Rules (1785) requiring that patients be washed (and shaved, if male) three times per week, and specifying the amount of "clean" towels and soap servants were to be provided with, made more explicit an oft-repeated commitment at Bethlem to keeping the lunatics clean.[125] At times, though, Monro and others at Bethlem seem to have accorded more attention to the cosmetic aspects and superficial appeal of the hospital environment than they did to more pressing sanitary (and other) needs being identified by contemporary reformers such as John Aikin, M.D. (1747–1822), and John Howard (1726?–90). One sees this, for example, when the authorities required in 1765 that "windows be kept light and in good order" and free of "any rags Straw or other nastiness that may be thrust there and which shall look unseemly to the Streets"; or when, in 1778, the hospital's "very dirty" galleries and cells were belatedly ordered whitewashed.[126]

Nonetheless, on occasion, Monro could evidently be quite protective of the interests even of his poorer patients. In 1763, for example, along with the other medical officers and a committee of governors, he opposed the application of Coleman Street Ward to erect a watch-house contiguous to Bethlem[127]—and the objections raised were explicitly framed in terms of patients' health and welfare. "The patients," these medical officers contended, "will . . . be greatly Affected and prejudiced by the Noise which must Necessarily Attend at Watchhouse," and Monro and his colleagues also underlined how "Absolutely Necessary" it was "in all Cases of Lunacy and Acute Diseases that the Patients should be kept Extreamly Quiet."[128] (In his 1766 case book, as in his *Remarks on Dr. Battie's Treatise,* Monro was also to emphasize the importance of his patients "keeping quiet" and conversing "with few.")[129] The 1763 committee additionally worried about the danger of fire to the hospital, "the windows thereof not being Glazed and the Patients lying upon Straw." [130] Yet, if a modicum of effort was thus made to secure patients' safety, peace, and quiet, the numbers of visitors milling around the hospital must have severely compromised this goal, and significant numbers of patients were still exposed to the cold wind and bedded down rather like animals—however economically and pragmatically requisite this appeared.

Significantly, numerous mid- and late-eighteenth-century accounts of Bethlem in the popular touristic and magazine literature continued to obscure appreciation of patients' needs and to justify their prolonged seclusion and restraint by reference to prevailing theories about the insensibility of raving lunatics and their animalistic immunity to the ravages of the weather. Such accounts offer us a relatively precise picture of what in many quarters constituted acceptable level of provision for the poor insane at this time. In advertising the hospital in 1761–63, for example, the antiquarian Joseph Pote's (1704–87) anonymously published *Tour* through the metropolis made a particular virtue of the fact that patients had separate rooms or cells, "where they are locked up every night, and if raving, continually." [131] Similarly, distinguished for special mention were the rather basic arrangements the hospital was making for the supply of clean straw and clothing. While, for example, there was a bed place for most patients at Bethlem, "where the patients are so senseless as not to be fit to make use of one, they are every day provided with clean straw." Additionally, while friends were obliged to provide clothes, and the hospital's "wardrobe" was to supply any neglect on this front, it was only in their lucid intervals that these sorts of patients were deemed likely to be sensible of this benefit, "for though when raving or furious they suffer but little from the weather; yet in their intervals, they frequently contract other distempers, care of which is also taken, as well as of their lunacy." [132]

Nonetheless, Bethlem's governors were making a number of very pertinent new rulings at this time to attend to these very issues, requiring (in 1765) that officers and servants "be very careful" to ensure that straw be "Changed when Damp and Dirty," [133] that daily inspections be made by the matron to ensure that patients were "regularly Sheeted and Shifted as they ought to be," and that weekly inspections be made by the steward of patients' clothing and other needs (in 1757, an order repeated in 1765).[134] Subsequent enlargement of the provisioning of sheets and of the "wardrobe" for patients at the hospital also seems to have enhanced basic creature comforts.[135] This former initiative had been the inspiration of the Bethlem steward (1778–85), Henry White, but Monro had been on the Bethlem committees that annually rewarded him with gratuities "for his diligence and faithful Attention" in such work.[136] Likewise, attempts were made to ensure more effective provisioning of stoves and fires and the carrying down of vulnerable patients to stove rooms.[137] While such rulings as those detailed above may seem to modern eyes somewhat minimal as provisioning for patients, they were less so by contemporary standards of care for the poor insane. Although they may in any case have been inadequately observed, they probably still marginally improved patients' comfort and the availability and supply of clothing to them, and would have provided them with better covering against the elements. Attempts were also made to combat problems with "mortification" (or gangrene) of the extremities for patients under restraint and suffering from circulatory problems in such cold conditions. In 1778, for example, a committee on which one of John's sons seems to have sat took the initiative of instructing servants to examine, rub, and cover with flannel "the Feet of every Patient in Chains or Straw during the Winter Season" and to notify the surgeon if necessary.[138] However, the findings of the 1815–16 Enquiry into Madhouses, which uncovered a number of instances of "mortified" limbs, imply that such measures met with limited success.

Bethlem's records reveal little very explicit information as to Monro's relationship with the inferior staff. His involvement in the compilation of regulations for ancillary staff suggests that he was concerned with and realistic about their liability to abuse their trust, and keen to find ways to insure against this. The augmentation (in 1765) of the matron's authority over gallery maids, whom she was to sack (with the committee's consent) whenever she found them "negligent in their Duty, wanting in Care or otherwise Misbehaving towards the Patients,"[139] marked an effort at according more attention to staff discipline—although, in practice, dismissals remained too infrequent and staff abuses too unchecked. Monro was likewise on a 1778 committee which ordered that the hospital's internal regulations be kept in a book and perused twice yearly by its officers and servants, and it was he who, alongside the treasurer and auditor general, was made responsible for posting up inscribed regulations around the hospital in 1783.[140] Just as Monro frequently prescribed leaves of absence in the country for physically weak or sick patients, so he occasionally recommended the lodging of servants in the country when they became physically ill.[141] Although he sometimes sat on committees that reprimanded or fired hospital staff,[142] he seems to have exerted limited influence over their supervision, hiring, and firing, which was mostly left to the steward and matron and the Bethlem committee as a whole, or—in more exceptional cases—determined by the treasurer or the assembled court.[143] Likewise, although Bethlem's governors repeatedly stressed the importance, if not "Utmost Consequence that the Patients should be daily visited and attended"[144] by ancillary officers and servants, its physician does not seem to have lobbied for increasing the numbers of servants at the hospital. Indeed, neither he nor anyone else at Bethlem seems to have done a great deal to counter the deteriorating staff:patient ratio, the characteristic solution to sickness among staff being merely to get other healthy colleagues (or patients) to substitute for the shortage of hands.

During his tenure in office, Monro may well have contributed to the encouragement of greater selectivity over admissions to Bethlem, enhancing the emphasis on the treatment of the curable insane and on medical authority in general. Such policies did not actually reduce patient numbers, however, and they often had a harder edge for patients. Those patients, for instance, whose relatives were so presumptuous as to remove them against the advice of Monro and the committee were not infrequently barred from readmission, as (increasingly) were patients who had been ill for a number of years.[145] Weak and physically debilitated patients, those with infectious or other incurable diseases, and those unable to assist themselves were increasingly rejected or discharged as unfit. Medical officers and the Bethlem committee were probably concerned, among other things, to limit the demands on their servants, to avoid the expense of futile treatment, and to restrict their mortality (and keep up their cure) rates.[146] Prospective patients who were seen as idiots, mopes, consumptives, or otherwise unsuitable had been refused admission or discharged from Bethlem since at least the seventeenth century, but this exclusionary policy seems to have become even more emphatic after 1750. In 1765, for example, incurables were ordered discharged from the hospital "when they become Mopes or Consumptives," it being felt—anticipating nineteenth-century tensions in lunacy provision—that such patients could be just "as Commodiously kept in their respective Parish workhouses."[147] Bethlem also pursued the policy adopted by its rival, St. Luke's, ruling that patients who had "been Mad more than one year" were to be discharged as incurable and excluded from admission as curables, though the medical men at Bethlem (viewing lunacy as a seasonal disorder) seem to have confined this exclusion to patients presenting themselves during the unfavorable or "unhealthy" half of the year (i.e., Michaelmas to Lady Day).[148]

Despite the stress on treating curables at Bethlem, however, it must be emphasized that the continuing presence of significant numbers of incurable patients who had been maintained on separate wards at the hospital since the 1720s substantially mitigated this commitment. Those in charge at Bethlem after mid-century even prided themselves on the fact that, unlike St. Luke's, they were prepared to admit patients discharged as uncured or incurable from other hospitals. Through the 1770s, 1780s, and 1790s, efforts were made to give preference in the admission and retention of patients (especially "incurable" patients) to dangerous and "mischievous" cases—those who had a history of violence to themselves or others, or who were likely to commit "some Outrage" if discharged. Other chronic cases, though, were frequently declared "unfit."[149]

Yet despite this heightened selectivity, John Monro's physicianship was marked by a creeping growth in the numbers of both curable and incurable patients at Bethlem. By 1766, the premises contained over 270 patients, and Monro served on committees that enlarged the hospital even further. During the 1780s, Bethlem extended its incurables provision by over sixty cells.[150] The hospital's capacity had reached three hundred by 1787, and over 350 by the time of Monro's death, while admissions had risen from over 180 per annum in the 1750s to well over two hundred by the 1760s, 1770s, and 1780s.[151] Mounting numbers of inmates, an incurables waiting list of over two hundred patients by 1784,[152] and the inflation of running costs put extra pressure on Bethlem's managers. Officers became more stringent in identifying and expelling patients possessed of sufficient means to be supported elsewhere. Yet, occasional clear-outs, such as that which occurred in 1783, when the apothecary, Gozna, was ordered to prepare a list for Monro identifying which incurables were "improper Objects of this Charity," normally only skimmed the surface.[153] Once more, in 1789, Gozna and Monro (as well as his son and assistant, Thomas) were part of a special committee established to inquire into "the Health of the Incurable Patients" and the circumstances of their friends and relations. Yet, rather than contemplating any reduction in the numbers of patients, they preferred to raise the fees (especially for parish patients), concurring that "it would be highly improper to discharge or remove any."[154]

One should not exaggerate the ability of a physician like Monro to determine the environment of an eighteenth-century hospital. His role,

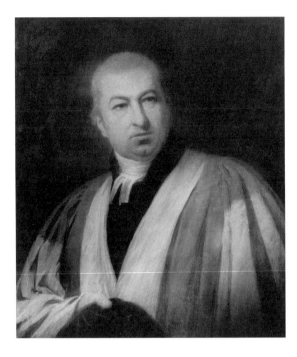

FIGURE 8. Thomas Monro (1758–1833), by Henry Monro the elder (1791–1814), ca. 1810. Portrait in pastel, paper mounted on canvas. Thomas Monro was John's youngest son (the fifth of his six children) and the third of the family to serve as physician to Bethlem. His picture was donated to the College of Physicians by his grandson, Henry Monro, in 1857, and is currently on loan to the Bethlem Royal Hospital Museum. Reproduced by kind permission of the Royal College of Physicians, London.

as we have stressed, was a visiting and in many ways rather peripheral one, the institution being run primarily by the mostly lay governors who sat on its committees and courts. Monro was neither supine nor particularly active by the standards of his era, although his own conservative instincts probably encouraged a complacency and an inertia at the hospital that would continue to characterize its régime under his son and successor.

A catalogue of abuses was unearthed by the 1815–16 House of Commons Enquiry into Madhouses: gross negligence in the care and management of patients, and heedlessness of the conditions in which they were housed; decided medical apathy toward therapeutic innovation;

excessive restraint employed by design and default, and as a means of coping with understaffing; and inadequate medical supervision of dishonest, and often brutal, ancillary staff—and it goes without saying that these practices had very deep roots that date back to John Monro's time and to that of his own father, James. After all, this inquiry took place less than twenty-five years after John Monro's death and practices and conditions at Bethlem cannot have changed substantially in the intervening period. The poor performance of Monro's son Thomas under examination by Commons' representatives; the evidently large-scale deficiencies in which he was so severely implicated; and the scandals that obliged him to tender his resignation in the aftermath of that inquiry must all, to some extent, be seen as a case of the sins of the fathers falling upon the head of the son.

On the other hand, the asylum reformers of 1815 had clearly been out to make an example of Bethlem and its officers. Thomas Monro (along with his medical colleagues and his forebears) were hung out to dry in a somewhat scapegoating or sacrificial way for charges that had as much to do with failings at the center of Bethlem's administration and with its general command and supervisory structure and governance as they did with its doctors. Furthermore, eighteenth-century society had entertained a very different view of the Monros. Without question, it was John's position at Bethlem, with the prestige and visibility it brought in its train, that anchored his reputation as the leading mad-doctor of his age and that provided the foundation on which his lucrative career in the mad-business was built.

CHAPTER 2

The "Real Use" of Discussing Madness

The Great Lunacy Debate

Madness is a distemper of such a nature, that very little of real use can be said concerning it; the immediate causes will for ever disappoint our search, and the cure of that disorder depends on *management* as much as *medicine*.

John Monro, *Remarks on Dr Battie's Treatise on Madness* (1758)[1]

When *Aesculapian* Sage assumes his seat,
When *BATTUS* thus forestalls the promis'd treat . . .
"Think, think my friends, what mischiefs threat our State,
Now ruin perches on our *College-gate* . . .
But by yon Pile, where on the chissel'd stone
The well-wrought Madman seems to live and groan,
Where on clean Straw, sequester'd in their Cells,
The Patriot, Sage, and Bard immortal dwells,
I swear, my soul detests the hated league,
And Hell, if Heav'n should fail, shall second my intrigue." . . .

Moses Mendez et al., *The Battiad* (1750)[2]

RIVALS IN MADNESS: JOHN MONRO, WILLIAM BATTIE, AND ST. LUKE'S HOSPITAL FOR LUNATICS

John Monro's accession to the physicianship at Bethlem coincided almost exactly with a development that cost the hospital its virtual monopoly over the public institutional treatment of insanity in the metropolis: the establishment of the rival institution of St. Luke's, which began to canvas for funds in 1750[3] and opened its doors to patients in 1751. Juxtaposed directly and blatantly almost adjacent to Bethlem on Moorfields, St. Luke's in many of its key features aimed to be a direct riposte to long-standing practices at Bethlem. Architecturally, for example, it adopted a stark plainness, in contrast to the opulence of the Bethlem building. Noorthouck's *New History of London* spoke of it as "a neat but very plain edifice; nothing here is expended in ornament and we only see a building of considerable length, plastered over and whitened, with ranges of small windows on which no decorations have been bestowed."[4] When rebuilt at Old Street during 1782–89, St. Luke's continued to emphasize this Spartan design ethos, advertising itself as a "new edifice" whose "plainness and simplicity are commended in buildings intended for charitable purposes."[5]

Bethlem, meanwhile, was being criticized for its grand architectural excesses, its Corinthian pilasters and luxurious ornamentation being increasingly perceived by a new generation of spectators as "more favourable to the good intentions of the founders of this charity, than their good taste, the style of architecture being very improper for an hospital for madmen. Simplicity and regularity only should have been aimed at. . . ."[6] St. Luke's distanced itself further from previous associations of charity with grandeur and spectacle by encouraging discreet subscription-based funding and anonymous donations, rejecting as vainglorious

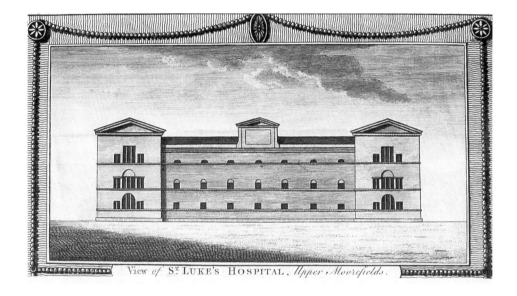

View of ST LUKE'S HOSPITAL, *Upper Moorfields.*

FIGURE 9. Engraving of St. Luke's Hospital for Lunatics in Upper Moorfields. This, the hospital's first building, was built ca. 1750–52 according to the design of George Dance the Elder (1695–1768). This engraving was made for the 1775 *New and Universal History* by Walter Harrison (pseudonym). Reproduced by kind permission of The Wellcome Trust.

the public celebration and display of the names of its benefactors mounted on large tablets on hospital walls—the custom favored at Bethlem, St. Bartholomew's Hospital, and St. Thomas's.[7] More tellingly still, from the very outset its governors totally banned indiscriminate visiting as deleterious to the welfare of patients.

While St. Luke's articulated itself in reaction to practices at Bethlem and at other charitable London institutions, Bethlem's governors responded by sniping at their rival. Bethlem's loyal organ in the press, the *London Evening Post,* defended the virtues of civic grandeur and spectacle enshrined at Bethlem, referring to the motives of St. Luke's founders as mean-spirited.[8] Rather than prompting its governors and officers to any fundamental reforms or even review of their medical régime, the challenges issued by the promoters of St. Luke's merely provoked another addition of cells at Bethlem.[9] The reasonable enough observation contained in the initial appeals for funds for St. Luke's that, while "a no-

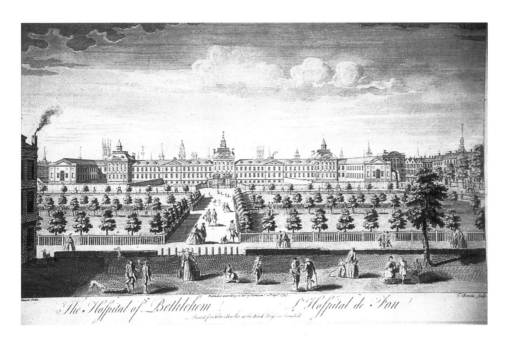

FIGURE 10. Engraving of Bethlehem Hospital at Moorfields ("l'Hospital de Fou"; post-1735). Bethlehem Hospital at Moorfields was built to Robert Hooke's design in ca. 1675–76. This engraving shows the building with its recently added incurables wards for male and female patients, situated at each end of the original façade. Also depicted in the engraving are strolling gentry, a milkmaid, dogs, and so forth, in front of the building. Reproduced by kind permission of The Wellcome Trust.

ble Charity," Bethlem was "not capable of receiving the Number of poor Objects that apply for Relief," and that there were unavoidable delays in their admission, was dismissed by the *London Evening Post* as the unjust complaint of "several ill-wishers to the Royal Hospitals." [10] Instead of accepting the invitation of the promoters of the new establishment to see their enterprise as a supplement to the provision offered at Bethlem, the latter's governors (through their mouthpiece in the press) did little but cast aspersions on what they conceived to be an upstart rival, initially attempting to negate its challenge by referring to it demeaningly as "new Bethlem."

At the outset, at least, Monro seems substantially to have shared the stubborn hostility of the Bethlem governors to this rival establishment.

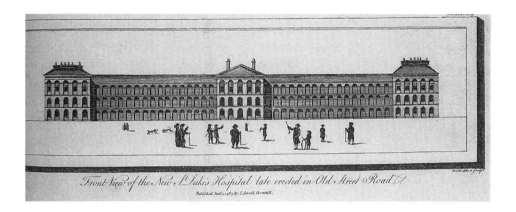

St. Luke's opened, as we have indicated, in the year before John lost his father[11] and took up sole responsibility as Bethlem's physician, momentous happenings that evidently affected him considerably. The affront to Bethlem and the practices of the Monros must have appeared all the more overt because the first physician appointed to St. Luke's was one of Bethlem's own governors, William Battie.[12] For almost a decade, beginning in 1742, Battie had been quite a prominent figure at Bethlem's committee meetings, and he was someone with whom John was presumably already well acquainted. Inevitably, as each vied for prominence among the still comparatively small array of metropolitan maddoctors, the two men became rivals, their differences on professional matters being matched by, and to some degree reflecting, contrasts in their background, character, and demeanor.

Monro, of course, came from a stable, well-heeled, and well-connected medical family of Scottish descent, with an established base in London and Greenwich. Battie, by contrast, was the son of the vicar of a small parish, Modbury, in Devonshire, and endured somewhat straitened circumstances in his early youth after his father died when Battie

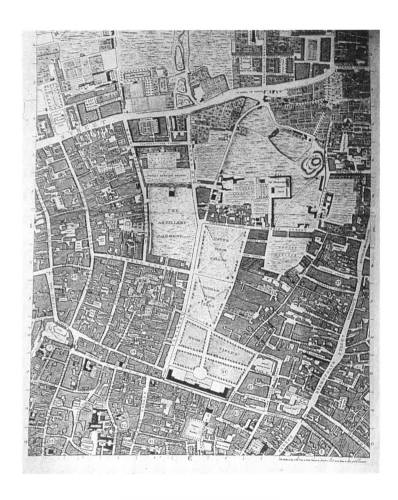

FIGURE 12. Detail from John Rocque's 1746 map of London, showing Moorfields and Bethlem Hospital, abutting London Wall, and thus just outside the city boundary. The spectacular view of Bethlem's palatial frontage afforded to visitors and passersby alike as they strolled across Moorfields is apparent from this map. It was a perspective significantly altered by the starkly contrasting St. Luke's at mid-century. This image is taken from Andrew Davies, *The Map of London, from 1746 to the Present Day* (London: Batsford and Guildhall Publications, 1987), p. 60.

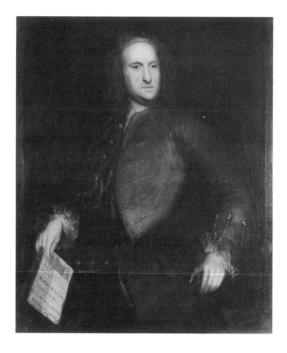

FIGURE 13. Portrait of Dr. William Battie (ca. 1752). Oil on canvas. Battie proudly clutches a copy of *Reasons for the Establishing and Further Encouragement of St Luke's Hospital for Lu-* *naticks.* Painted by Thomas Hudson (1701–79), well-known portraitist and collector. Reproduced by kind permission of the Witt Library, Courtauld Institute of Art, London.

was only ten years old.[13] Monro's medical career was almost preordained, and his progress assured through his education in London and Oxford and on the continent, while Battie, though far from poor and unprovided for,[14] had more of a struggle to settle on a profession and to secure the education and resources needed for success. Educated at Eton and Cambridge, the latter was at first inclined toward a legal career, entering Taylor's Inn Courts before shifting into medicine, and depending upon a Craven scholarship awarded when he was twenty-one to ease his passage through university. The fatherless Battie openly expressed his relief at securing these funds, writing to a friend (ca. 1725) that at last "I shall now begin to live agreeably, & have, I hope, got through the worst part of my life."[15] Battie began as a Cambridge licensee and practitioner, delivering lectures on anatomy at the university (a subject Monro displayed little interest in), and had a spell in practice in provincial Uxbridge before finally gaining his Cambridge M.D. and moving to London. Monro, as we have seen, progressed directly from his extensive continental Grand Tour into a carefully prepared position at the very forefront of his inherited specialty.

Conservatively genteel in appearance, Monro had long understood the importance of social ostentation and keeping up appearances for those who aspired to success as society physicians. Battie, by contrast, was either unwilling or unable fully to match the gentlemanly ideal, for, although he was possessed of a "vigour of . . . health," contemporaries jibed that he was but "mean of size."[16] His style of attire and behavior made things worse: he was described as "singular of dress" and as sometimes having the appearance of a "labourer." While at Eton and Cambridge, Battie acquired a reputation as a practical joker that would persist throughout his career, prompting some of his opponents to take potshots at his slightly common social origins and his alleged penchant for vulgar humor.[17] One of his patrons, Dr. Henry Godolphin (1648–1733), the elderly Eton provost,[18] early on attempted to teach him the art of self-presentation, sending him his swanky carriage to ride in—not because he was sick, but to grant him "credit in the neighbourhood"— but Battie remained at pains to avoid extravagant, flamboyant, or "vain" display of all kinds. His famously "rigid . . . frugality" and "parsimony," for example, led him in stark contrast to travel around the streets of London "in the Nestor of carriages . . . half open, to avoid the rain."[19] Although he had a reputation for frankness and cordiality alongside his "playfulness and good humour," whatever social credit this brought him was undermined by his "stern," if not "peremptory," tone and his "peculiar archness of manner." Assuredly, in the eighteenth century a forbidding demeanor was often seen as requisite for a maddoctor in clinical settings. However, unlike his rival, Battie found it difficult to vary his presentation of self when abroad and in company. As someone "never graceful" in "manners" and perpetually "serious and harsh [of] countenance," his reputation suffered accordingly, and periodically there were signs of tension between Battie and his gentrified clients, as well as between Battie and other elite physicians, including Monro.[20]

Not all was difference, of course. Both Monro and Battie were Tories and Anglicans. Both were evidently keen to show off their Greek and Latin learning in their writings and their practice, and both were loyal to the College of Physicians. Such was the nature of the marketplace for their services that they inevitably found their paths crossing and at times were virtually obliged to cooperate in significant areas of their professional lives. The two men were both highly successful and reaped handsome financial rewards from the mad-business. Monro acquired residences in fashionable districts in Holborn and Bloomsbury, as well as a fine country house in Barnet; Battie (after a spell of practice during 1732–37 in Uxbridge) divided his time between an elegant villa in Twickenham, a house on the Thames that Hardinge thought "very handsome" (although it was criticized by some as poorly built and lacking a staircase), and a large town house in Great Russell Street in Bloomsbury, where he died in 1776.[21] Even in death, there was a certain symmetry of style and self-presentation: both were buried without ceremony (Battie beside his wife and Monro beside his daughter Charlotte), in cemetery plots marked by plain, unspectacular gravestones.[22]

A VERY PUBLIC QUARREL

From the moment Battie set himself up in the metropolis at the medical forefront of a new public lunatic hospital, it would seem that future conflict with Monro was virtually guaranteed. However, existing tensions between the two doctors and their institutions were further exacerbated when, just seven years after defecting to St. Luke's, Battie published his *Treatise on Madness*.[23] Quite deliberately, and with evident desire to stir up controversy, if not to give offense, Battie seized the occasion to voice scarcely veiled criticisms of Bethlem and the Monros. "Madness," he announced, in the opening lines of his book, "though a terrible and at present a very frequent calamity, is perhaps as little understood as any that ever afflicted mankind."[24] This state of affairs was no accident:

> Our defect of knowledge in this matter is, I am afraid, in great measure owing to a defect of proper communication: and the difficulties attending the care of Lunaticks have been at least perpetuated by their being entrusted to Empiricks, or at best a few select Physicians, most of whom thought it advisable to keep the cases as well as the patients to themselves.[25]

Lest Monro fail to grasp the main object of this criticism, Battie elsewhere noted waspishly that the treatment of insanity had been "already too long confined (almost) to a single person [i.e., to James Monro, John's father]."[26]

Whereas the Monros had maintained their monopoly by neglecting to open Bethlem's doors for the instruction of less experienced members of the profession, Battie announced his intention of "introducing more Gentlemen of the Faculty to the Study and Practice of one of the most important branches of Physick" by adopting the opposite plan at St. Luke's: "admitting young Physicians well recommended to visit with me in the Hospital, and [to] freely observe the treatment of the patients there confined."[27] He provocatively asserted that "altho' Madness is frequently taken for one species of disorder, nevertheless, when thoroughly examined, it discovers as much variety with respect to its causes and circumstances as any distemper whatever." The consequences for therapeutics were plain:

> Madness, therefore, like most other morbid cases, rejects all general methods [such as those employed at Bethlem], v[ery] g[eneral] bleeding, blisters, caustics, rough cathartics, the gumms and foetid antihysterics, opium, mineral waters, cold bathing, and vomits.[28]

Battie was equally insistent that "madness . . . requires the patient's being removed from all objects that act forcibly on the nerves, and excite too lively a perception of things"[29]—a necessity that, he felt, plainly revealed the folly of Bethlem's policy on visitation. For this reason alone, "the visits therefore of affecting friends as well as enemies, and the impertinent curiosity of those, who think it a pastime to converse with Madmen and to play upon their passions, ought strictly to be forbidden."[30]

For Battie, these views did not reflect entirely new-found convictions. They are, on the contrary, of a piece with some of the ideas and sympathies that appear in his *Harveian Oration* of 1746.[31] Here, too, he advanced his firm commitment to open avenues of enquiry and debate in medicine and insisted upon the need to "speak out" against "secrecy" and selfish motivations.[32] Additionally, this earlier work criticized the medical profession for its backwardness, especially when it came to the application of remedies. While singling out earlier Bethlem physicians like Hale and Tyson for praise, his *Oration* made no mention of James Monro.[33] Instead, it assailed those practitioners who, out of financial motives or vanity, seeking to build up their wealth and reputations, kept their medicines to themselves, and others who "hawk around specious remedies for incurable diseases."[34] Identifying himself as one of the "moderns" in medicine, Battie claimed that medicine had made "almost no progress from Hippocrates himself until the last century."[35] He therefore espoused a brand of "Rational Medicine," hostile to both system and empiricism.[36] Only at the last did Battie emphasize something that would not have been so antithetical to approaches at Bethlem under Monro: quoting the example of Radcliffe's "policy of inaction," his *Oration* stressed the importance of "doing nothing" but letting nature take its course when the "solemn parade of medicaments" was likely to be unavailing, expectant waiting being the best way of restoring the patient under these circumstances.[37] Monro was to make exactly the same point in his own *Oration* (1757) (as, indeed, were many other Harveian Orators).[38]

Battie's intellectual stance may not have altered much in the twelve years between his *Oration* and his *Treatise on Madness* (1758), but the latter work, of course, threw down the gauntlet to Monro in a far more direct, comprehensive, and public fashion. The situation self-evidently required that someone from Bethlem make a spirited defense of his own institution and the tradition of medical practice it represented. Prompted by some of his friends and acquaintances among Bethlem's governors, who were doubtless keen to see this upstart rival hospital resisted and its physician and governors put in their place, John rose to the provocation. Beyond this general stimulus to action, however, the implied criticism of his father certainly gave Monro ample personal reasons "to say something in answer to the undeserved censures, which Dr. Battie has thrown upon my predecessors."[39]

In the *Harveian Oration* John himself had delivered at the College of Physicians only the year before (1757), he had contravened precedent and decorum by including a gushing paean to the memory of his father. This orational tribute—which appears to have been the first and the last to James Monro—emphasizes the depth of John's attachment and devotion to the paternal bond. It also suggests how much Battie's slurs on James's character and reputation would have stung his loyal son.

> O generous and noble soul! O delight and grief of your friends. We may worthily pronounce you a lover of this place, a fierce defender of your Alma Mater, a man most worthy of love because of the urbanity, gentleness and simplicity of your character. Happy in your natural endowments and weighty in your judgment, you ruled over the province you had made your own with a wonderful and fortunate art. You were second to none in the other parts of medicine but in this one, you were easily the leader. The illustrious Mead[40] chose you as a companion and loved you as a friend, which is not the least of your claims to praise and respect. When you were carried off he grieved you and did you the honour of following you to the grave with unfeigned tears.[41]

In his *Remarks,* John began his defense of his family, his practices, and his institution with a startling disclaimer: "my own inclination would never have led me to appear in print."[42] His own reticence, like that of those "Physicians of *Bethlem Hospital*" who had gone before him—"men no less remarkable for their honour and integrity, than distinguished by their skill and experience"—was, the reader should understand, motivated by no "selfish disposition" or desire "to keep the publick in ignorance for their own private advantage." Indeed,

> though they did not publish their thoughts on a distemper which was more immediately the object of their care, that was not owing to any secret design of keeping their manner of practice a secret, but that they thought it disingenuous, to perplex mankind, with points that must for ever remain dark, intricate, and uncertain.[43]

What in substantial measure gave warrant for their trustworthiness, and gave the lie to the aspersions Battie sought to cast upon their characters, was that theirs was the practice of gentlemen, marred by no tradesmanlike or quackish conduct:

> They made use of no mean arts, either to procure patients, or to keep them. And though the nature of their business required secrecy [because of the nature of this distemper and the interest of the patient], yet their method of practice was open and publick; they freely gave their opinion, whenever applied for, either at a consultation or in writing. Nor did they ever pretend to any particular nostrum, or make use of *antimonial vomits, strong purges, and hellebore, as SPECIFICALLY antimaniacal.*[44]

These are revealing and significant rhetorical moves. Monro's disdain for and avoidance of the publicity provided by the printed word was entirely characteristic, not just of mad-doctors of his generation and before, but of elite mid-eighteenth-century medical men more generally. What was an expected, if not an essential, element in the making of medical careers a few decades later was as yet atypical and even, perhaps, slightly suspect. Within a generation or two, publication would more generally acquire its modern guise as a primary route to professional prominence, but at mid-century, it was far from routine—apt to be interpreted as a somewhat dubious act of self-promotion and as an inappropriate opening up of properly professional issues before an audience of laymen. (It was for these reasons, among others, that many still chose, when they *did* venture into print, to prefer Latin to the vernacular—a practice Battie himself routinely adopted in his other publications.)[45]

Monro's sensitivity to charges of mercenary motives and quackery is likewise anything but idiosyncratic. Indeed, similar sentiments can once again easily be traced among all segments of the medical elite. In the business of selling something intangible—skill and expertise, rather than material goods—all professionals needed to secure a substantial measure of public approval and trust if they were to obtain not just economic rewards but the privileged place they sought in the social hierarchy. Crassly materialistic and overtly self-serving behavior thus threatened to inflict severe damage on a physician's social aspirations, not least by calling into question his claims to exercise his skills and talents in a disinterested fashion. Such concerns were felt with peculiar force, however, among those seeking to carve out a place for themselves in the treatment of madness. Mad-doctoring was perhaps the least trustworthy of any contemporary emerging specialty, for, more often than any other, it called for measures taken against the will, or without the cooperation, of the patient, and involved a more explicit threat to the patient's personal liberty, legal rights, social status, and identity. Trust[46] was an enormously difficult commodity for mad-doctors to acquire, shrouded as the specialty was by the secrecy demanded by the families of its patients, no less than it was shadowed by scandalous stories about what transpired behind the high walls and barred windows of the madhouse. The very vehemence with which Monro protested his bona fides in the face of his rival's gibes is the surest testimony to the shakiness of his specialty's social standing.[47]

Substantively, as we shall see in more detail below, Monro's rejoinder to Battie has been characterized by most historians as reactionary and narrow-minded. Whereas the St. Luke's physician suggested that many madmen were potentially curable and that the roots of their condition might be traced in the very structure of the nervous system, Monro insisted on a far darker and more pessimistic position: "Madness is a distemper of such a nature, that very little of real use can be said concerning it; the immediate causes will for ever disappoint our search, and the cure of that disorder depends on *management* as much as *medicine*."[48]

Like his father before him, John was convinced that these techniques of management were themselves the product of firsthand experience—and that the experience in question was not something that could be systematized and communicated through textbooks or other abstract means of instruction:

> [My father] knew very well [as do I], that the *management* requisite for it [i.e., madness] was never to be learned, but from observation; . . . and though

no man was ever more communicative, upon points of real use, he never
thought of reading lectures, on a subject that can be understood no otherwise
than by personal observation. . . .[49]

There was thus, he asserted, a principled reason for the silence both had
hitherto maintained on the therapeutics of insanity. Yet, however effective this defense was on one front, it raised potentially damaging questions on another: for, if effectively managing the mad rested upon the
transmission of craft-like skills, why had the Monros not given the slight-
est support to allowing medical students to walk Bethlem's galleries—a
license Battie granted and boasted of so emphatically at St. Luke's?

If this contradiction had to be awkwardly elided, elsewhere Monro
resumed his attack. Battie's discussion of the nervous origins of mental
disturbance came in for particularly tough criticism. Monro commented
scathingly that, in reality, these lengthy passages amounted to nothing
more than an exercise in verbal gymnastics, an empty assertion that "we
can discover nothing more than that the medullary substance is the *seat,*
and the nerves are the instruments of *sensation,* that I can see no benefit
is likely to arise from it." [50] The fate of Battie's entire verbose edifice, he
suggested, could be safely left "to be settled by those who are inclined
to *fight in earnest with shadows.*" [51]

Taken as a whole, Monro's brief and witheringly sarcastic rebuttal
was intended as a repudiation of the very essence of Battie's project.
Point by point, he attacked its coherence and relevance. Where his rival
had claimed to provide a detailed examination of madness that was presented as being of benefit to his fellow practitioners, to aspiring students
of madness, and to the general public, Monro countered that such discussions would only confuse a public insufficiently educated to grasp
their meaning. He heaped scorn on Battie's definition of madness as "deluded imagination," arguing, with the support of a variety of authorities
and examples, that

> it is certain that the imagination may be deluded where there is not the least
> suspicion of madness, as by drunkenness, or by hypochondriacal and hyster-
> ical affections; there may be real madness where the *imagination* is not af-
> fected; so that a *deluded imagination* is not in my opinion the true criterion
> of madness. The *judgment* is as much or more concerned than the imagina-
> tion, and I should rather define madness to be a *vitiated judgment.*[52]

(In other words, madmen "see right but judge wrong.")[53] Pointing to
the slippery way in which Battie confounded imagination, perception,
and sensation, Monro averred that "I cannot help expressing my sur-

prize, that a gentleman so ready to censure the inaccurate manner in which the generality of mankind express their thoughts, should be so careless in a matter that requires the greatest precision."[54]

In the pages that followed, whole passages of Battie's *Treatise* were held up to ridicule before being dismissed as providing "little amusement, and in my opinion as little real knowledge."[55] Still others were shown to accomplish nothing more than to dress up the most basic common sense in obscure medical jargon, prompting a sly suggestion that "it is amazing what an advantage a man of learning has over the ignorant."[56] At times the satirical commentary became positively Swiftian. Professing bewilderment about the meaning of a particularly abstruse passage, for example, Monro conceded,

> It is not impossible but my ignorance in this point may arise from the little regard I have hitherto paid to metaphysical enquiries, in which I have generally observed much labour used to cover the want of real knowledge. In order therefore to be better informed, I have selected such passages as seem to stand most in need of being explained; these I have drawn out, and have some thoughts of proposing them as prize questions, (in imitation of the *French*) to the academicians of *Bethlem,* where it is among the *senior recluses* only that I can expect to find any one, who is able to resolve them all.[57]

Two elements of Battie's *Treatise* were the focus of particularly close analysis and criticism: his attempt to unravel the causes of madness, and his discussion of its treatment, using either medicine or "management." By turns mocking and dismissive, Monro savagely burlesqued his rival's text. Discussing the etiology of insanity, for instance, Battie distinguished what he termed "original" and "consequential" madness.[58] Monro pounced: "The first of these is entirely the doctor's invention it never having been mentioned by any writer, or observed by any physician. What is the cause of *original* madness? it is unknown. What are the symptoms? there are none. The method of cure? it admits of no cure. . . ."[59] As for the twelve causes Battie listed for "consequential madness," they were so much speculative nonsense: a mixture of "vulgar error" and "conjecture" presented in prose that verged on the incoherent.[60]

Nor did Monro find the sections on treatment much more satisfactory. Battie saw only his "consequential madness" as potentially curable, and had arranged his discussion of its medical treatment in accordance with his notions about its supposed etiology. The section offering these prescriptions Monro greeted with a typically back-handed compliment. It was, he remarked, "not inferior to the rest of the performance," and contained a "very singular" set of instructions that "would be of great use to us, and save an infinite deal of trouble were it possible to put it into practice."[61] Many, however, were simply ridiculous assertions of the obvious, and others just absurd. Battie suggested, for example, that some forms of madness were caused by sunstroke. What was his proposed solution? "Though so strangely expressed, [it] is nothing more than this; we cannot prevent the sun from shining, but we may sometimes remove a man out of it; or where that is not to be done, we may provide him *a proper integument,* i.e. a paper cap."[62] What of concussion, another possible cause of madness? Battie commented, without elaboration, that "the ill effects of concussion are not easily prevented or removed, though concussion itself may be sometimes prevented." Monro's riposte was merciless: ". . . if this gentleman has any receipt for that purpose, it would be of such universal use, that it is not quite fair to keep it a secret; for it can scarce be imagined that he meant, it might be prevented by it's not happening."[63] After more in this vein, Monro summed up: "Upon the whole, I cannot help thinking, that this section has been expressly written [by Dr. Battie], to prove the truth of what was asserted by the *eminent practitioner* [i.e., James Monro] . . . *that management did much more than medicine in this disease.*"[64]

JUDGING A DEBATE

Monro's *Remarks* can and has been characterized as substantially out of tune with future trends in mental medicine and with significant intellectual currents often associated with the Enlightenment. In denying the importance of causation and of any nosology of madness (which, for Monro, was merely one disease with many symptoms), in rejecting the place of anxiety within the spectrum of mental maladies, and in dismissing the utility of theorizing on the nature of insanity, Monro, in many ways, stood resolutely against the tide of change or advancement in the study and treatment of insanity.[65] His conservative stance was equally evident in other respects. Therapeutically, for example, Battie gave evidence of being more innovative than Monro. While Battie stressed the dangers of "rougher cathartics, emetics," and other evacuants, impeached "vomits" in particular as "shocking" and often harmful, recommended that violent evacuations should be employed only in "chronical" cases, and advised a period of respite between each course of medicines, Monro, on the contrary, sided with the more interventionist and orthodox medical position that cures were often protracted or defeated by physicians' timidity in applying the necessary, strong dosages.[66] He insisted that evacuation could have ill effects only if "injudiciously administered; or . . . given too strong," or if, contrariwise, practitioners were "too afraid of the lancet." [67] Monro was particularly resolute in his advocacy of vomiting. His approval for Bryan Robinson, who used vomits "for a whole year together, sometimes once a day, sometimes twice with the greatest success," and for another colleague who prescribed sixty-one vomits for a patient during just seven months (including one a night for eighteen nights), emphasizes that he was far from hesitant in dispensing strong doses and marathon courses of treatment.[68] Whereas Battie made much of the variety of causes that could produce insanity, arguing for this very reason that "madness . . . rejects all general methods" and requires a greater focus on the individual case, Monro dismissed the very question of etiology as an imponderable mystery and insignificant for the practitioner in comparison to a focus upon the symptoms one could observe.[69]

That said, the dividing line between the praxis of Battie and Monro is not so marked as has sometimes been asserted. The two men were firmly united in their conviction that evacuation and depletion were frequently salutary if "repeated in proportion to the strength of the patient." [70] Medical authorities at Bethlem had long excluded from admission patients who were considered "too weak to take medicine," and Battie adopted the same practice at St. Luke's. In asserting that Monro's view of madness as "vitiated judgment" made "violent treatments" a prerequisite for its cure, historians such as Hunter and Macalpine have somewhat uncritically accepted Battie's assessment of the antiphlogistic remedies advocated by many other practitioners. Yet Monro denied that vomits were either "shocking" or violent (as Battie had termed them), and many contemporaries would have agreed with him. In continuing to espouse vomiting as "infinitely preferable to any other [evacuation]" if prudently dispensed, for example, Monro was not as far removed from the milder prescriptions for nervous and mental diseases prescribed by physicians like George Cheyne as has sometimes been assumed. Cheyne, after all, had explicitly argued that there was "no more universal and effectual Remedy . . . than gentle Vomits suited to the Strength and Constitution of the Patient." [71]

Monro's *Remarks* was a good deal more than the purblind defense of his father that some historians have dismissed it as being, just as Battie's *Treatise* was a good deal less than the radical anticipation of Tuke's moral treatment others have claimed it to be. It is often forgotten that

Monro gave quite clear outlines on the "management" of the insane, many of which represent a considerable softening of the uncompromisingly fierce prescriptions recommended by Thomas Willis and his epigones. Although emphasizing the need for obedience from the insane and the importance of gaining authority over them, Monro also stressed that such patients should be "talked to kindly," "used with the greatest tenderness and affection," and preserved from that which might add "to the misery of the unhappy patient." He further stated that "we should endeavour in every instance to gain their good opinion."[72] And he was also thoroughly appreciative of the maxim that "some are to be commanded, others . . . soothed into compliance."[73]

Nor are these the only respects in which it turns out that Monro and Battie were in substantial agreement about the nature of madness and how to approach it. Both, for example, denounced the use of the whip and the cudgel upon the insane. Monro confidently declared antique theories concerning the salutary effects of "beating" to be "deservedly exploded . . . as unnecessary, cruel, and pernicious,"[74] and, like Battie, he emphasized the importance of gentleness in managing the insane, to that limited degree anticipating the spirit of the "moral managers" of the 1790s and beyond.[75] More generally, both can be linked, in part, with the growing Enlightenment critique of traditional authority, including the medical and other theories of antiquity, as also with the Enlightenment moral and utilitarian exposure of certain cruelties and barbarities of the age.

Those disposed to view Battie as a progressive and Monro as an arch-conservative could point to the former's propensity to cite such modern authors as Locke, Sydenham, Willis, Stahl, and Mead, whereas Monro harped back repeatedly to the antique wisdom of classical authors to prove his points. However, the contrast can easily be overdrawn, and could lead to further anachronisms. Both authors looked to their own empirical experience as a primary source of authority for their claims, while Monro sporadically appealed as well to such contemporary figures as Mead and Robinson.[76] Moreover, despite his regular display of classical learning, Monro was selectively critical of Greco-Roman medicine. Indeed, keen to establish his claim that "I will never subscribe to the errors of antiquity," Monro turned the tables and attacked Battie for doing just that. He regularly responded to certain of Battie's passages, for example, by stating that he had found "nothing new" in them, and indeed much of what Battie said was thoroughly traditional.[77] Few physicians would have disputed, for instance, that "the stomach, intestines, and uterus, are frequently the real seats of Madness"; that madness could be caused by passions provoking a rush of blood to the brain, by overstudying, and venery and its concomitants; that it "frequently succeeds or accompanies Fever, Epilepsy, Child-birth, and the like"; or that alcohol was a particularly common provocation of "the crowds of wretches that infest our streets and fill our hospitals."[78] More directly, Monro sharply criticized Battie for having taken on board the antique therapeutic doctrine of substituting one extreme sensation for its opposite, especially of employing fear to cast out irrational anger. On similar grounds, Monro also contradicted Battie's assertion of the utility of "bodily pain" in the treatment of the insane.[79] Likewise, he attacked Battie for accepting the doctrine that the insane were insensible and immune to bodily disease or the extremes of temperature, although this was a belief repeated by numerous authorities on madness throughout the eighteenth and into the nineteenth centuries.[80]

However much he espoused a view of madness as deluded imagination, Battie was a long way from throwing vitiation theories out of court. His notions concerning "laxity," "obstructions," and "congestion" meant that, fundamentally, it was through degrees of vitiation that the "nervous substance" was so affected as to induce madness, while he conceded that "Consequential Madness" would become "Original Madness," once the "nervous substance" was "essentially vitiated."[81] The four principles of his medicinal therapeutics—"Depletion," "Revulsion," "Removal," and "Expulsion"—had long been applied by contemporary practitioners.[82]

While, in general, Battie adopted a more optimistic stance than Monro toward the cure of madness, his attitude toward madness as misassociation of ideas brought him to a pessimistic view of the imagination. He admonished his readers that the madman's attribution of his own disease could not be trusted, and declared that "chimaeras . . . exist no where except in the brain of a Madman" and that their causes were unknowable.[83] For all his positivity, at best Battie hoped "that the peculiar antidote of Madness is reserved in Nature's store," although he doubted it.[84] Whereas Battie pronounced "hereditary" and "Original Madness . . . incurable by art," Monro claimed that "*hereditary* complaints . . . are often treated with success" and accused Battie of extending the boundaries of incurability with such definitions.[85]

At the very least, Monro's *Remarks* constitutes both an amusing and an effective polemic, one that succeeds in puncturing many of his rival's pretensions, in pointing to some gaping holes in his arguments, and in demonstrating how insubstantial many of his claims to originality were. It is by no means clear, we suggest, that the book is inferior to Battie's *Treatise*. Nor is this simply a retrospective judgment from the distance of nearly 250 years.

Albrecht von Haller (1708–77), for example, the continental physiologist whose work on the nervous system Battie had leaned heavily upon in constructing his account of the etiology of madness, was as convinced as Monro that Battie's *Treatise* contained nothing of value. As he wrote to Tissot, "j'ai commencé à lire mes livres anglais. J'ai peu profité de Battie on Madness, c'est théorie toute pure, sans ombre d'expérience."[86] [I've begun to read my English books. I've gained little from Battie on Madness, it's purely conjecture, without a trace of empirical reality.] The novelist Tobias Smollett, himself of course an M.D., reviewed both volumes at length in the pages of the *Literary Review* almost as soon as they appeared.[87] Despite objecting to some overstatements and polemical excesses,[88] for the most part Smollett judged Monro's critique to be both powerful and effective.[89] A half-century later, a number of prominent early-nineteenth-century mad-doctors voiced similar sentiments. Both John Haslam, Bethlem's apothecary, and Bryan Crowther, Bethlem's surgeon, tendered posthumous praise to their predecessor in their published works. Crowther was particularly impressed by Monro's advice on the management of the insane, and quoted his views on vomiting at approving length, although his attempts to draw close parallels between Monro's and Pinel's rather differing versions of moral management may have been slightly overcooking the goose.[90] Haslam's praise is perhaps more surprising, for he was someone with a suitably low opinion of the clinical acumen of John Monro's son Thomas. Nonetheless he spoke approvingly of the elder Monro's book as the only English "work on the subject of mental alienation [before his own, of course!] which has been delivered on the authority of extensive observation and practice."[91]

If a certain amount of loyalty from Monro's former (and his son's present) colleagues and successors is to be expected, beyond Bedlam, too, Monro and his *Remarks* continued to win plaudits. Significantly, it was Monro, rather than Battie, who was distinguished as a "truly celebrated," "late famous and humane" physician by William Pargeter (1760–1810), the mad-doctor divine whose *Observations on Maniacal Disorders* (1792) has generally been seen as part of a wider trend in mental medicine in which management was beginning to be stressed beside, if not above, medicine. Pargeter even mentioned attending a patient with Monro and quoted a passage from John's *Remarks* directly as to the curative effect of a fever succeeding on a bout of mania. However, he evidently cribbed his fundamental maxim—that "the chief reliance in the cure of insanity must be rather on management than medicine"—almost verbatim from both Monro and Battie.[92] (Sir) Alexander Crichton (1763–1856) assessed Monro's *Remarks* warmly (if rather condescendingly) as a "sensible and elegant little essay," and quoted the Bethlem doctor's account of the symptoms of approaching phrenzy, "so faithfully and well" did he find them "described." Battie's work, by contrast, was curtly dismissed as a "wild romance."[93] Twenty years later, George Man Burrows, prominent metropolitan mad-doctor and proprietor of the Clapham Retreat, provided a similar encomium, commenting that Monro's *Remarks* was a more enduringly useful contribution to the medical literature than Battie's *Treatise*. Indeed, despite having wondered whether the pessimism of physicians like Monro and Mead about the prospects for discovering "the immediate cause of insanity" might be one reason for the profession's neglect of post-mortem dissection as an avenue of inquiry into mental pathology, he nevertheless termed Monro's "reply" to Battie "admirable." Antipathetic to metaphysical theories of mind of the kind Battie had espoused, he made only a passing dismissive reference to the "visionary opinions" expressed in that doctor's *Treatise*.[94] Contemporaneously, Francis Willis junior, the grandson of Reverend Francis Willis who treated George III, voiced his admiration for John Monro, distinguishing him as a "celebrated" physician "whose fame was established by the superiority of his skill and success in disorders of the mind."[95] Whereas Willis quoted repeatedly and predominantly approvingly from Monro's *Remarks*,[96] alongside the later writings of others at Bethlem, including both John's son Thomas and John Haslam, he virtually ignored Battie's work. Finally, writing in the 1860s, Munk bluntly (if somewhat hyperbolically) remarked that Monro's *Remarks* had "covered Dr. Battie with well-merited ridicule."[97]

While specific portions of Monro's work were criticized or simply ignored, others stood the considerable passage of time. For example, Burrows cited with approval Monro's "very judicious advice" (in agreement with Mead) as to the need to continue medical prescriptions "for a considerable time after recovery" to guard against the high risk of relapse in mental cases (although Battie also seems to have customarily recommended a month's observation before he would confidently quit an apparently recovered patient).[98] Burrows was rather more censorious of Monro's enthusiastic espousal of evacuation, arguing that vomiting was more effective on the circulation than as a simple evacuant, and that the time taken by Monro and Robinson to effect cures via emetics was well above the average and could have been equally well procured naturally, or else with "diet, management, or other remedies." [99] However, medical opinion was still sorely divided, even at this late juncture, as to the virtues of vomits. While authors like Haslam and William Saunders Hallaran (1765–1825) had voiced severe misgivings about the "violent" and "mischievous" effects of emetics, other authors continued to defend these remedies and to pay deference to Monro's earlier extensive experience. Joseph Mason Cox (1763–1818) cited his own experience as having "convinced" him that vomiting "takes precedence of every other curative means," rejecting Haslam's standpoint as theoretical twaddle and claiming that "every [specialist] physician . . . must differ from him when he treats of vomiting." [100] Similarly citing his own experience, as well as the backing of more recent authors such as Cox and George Nesse Hill (1766–1831), as late as 1823 Francis Willis junior was still advocating the use of vomits, firmly endorsing "their advantage and safety," and averring that "some cases . . . could not be cured without them." His first cited supporting source was Monro's opinion that depletion was the best remedy, and that "vomiting is infinitely preferable to any other [method], if repeated experience is to be depended upon." [101] Even if the passage of time was beginning to erode belief in depletion, authors like Burrows were careful not to condemn its former advocates, conceding that Monro's opinions were "certainly strengthened by the practice of many, before and since his day," and he still treated Monro's views with sufficient respect to give them detailed coverage and a thorough (if conclusively negative) trial over "several years" in his own practice.[102]

Battie's definition of madness as essentially a matter of false sensations also came under fire from authorities other than Monro. For example, when Battie repeated the definition in his *Aphorisms,* published just five years after his *Treatise,* he was severely criticized by a correspondent to the *Gentleman's Magazine.* This man (writing under the initials T. I.) agreed with Monro that madness consisted in "wrong judgment," and that it was "impossible for the senses to correct either the judgment or fancy," for just "as intellect doth not hear, or see, or feel, so the senses do not know." [103] On the other hand, views of insanity that stressed its seat in sensation and imagination, and delusion as its virtual essence, retained considerable currency after mid-century. Battie's assertion that "deluded imagination is not only an indispensable, but an essential feature of madness" certainly continued to win its sympathizers and adherents. Even Francis Willis junior seems to have taken this perspective firmly on board, his emphasis in his Gulstonian Lectures (1822) and *Treatise on Mental Derangement* (1823) on the roots of insanity in disorders of sensation being in relative accord with Battie's views (even if it did not cite them explicitly).[104] However, although formulations such as Battie's are certainly reflected to some extent in legal decisions over guardianship and insanity defenses from the mid-eighteenth century, it was not until after 1800 that delusions begin to achieve prominence in judicial rulings on insanity.[105] By the 1830s at the very latest, furthermore, a new generation of authorities on insanity, like Alexander Crichton and James Cowles Prichard (1786–1848), were voicing increasing disquiet and dissent at such definitions, emphasizing (as Monro had before them) the varieties of insanity where there was a complete absence of delusion.[106]

With scarcely an exception, twentieth-century historians have reversed the verdicts we have been discussing, and beatified Battie at Monro's expense.[107] This modern judgment has been rendered in remarkably similar terms by scholars ranged across an extraordinarily wide ideological spectrum. Writing during the 1950s and 1960s, the mother-and-son team of Ida Macalpine and Richard Hunter laid out and reiterated the basic elements of the contemporary view, presenting the fundamental contrast between the "progressive," pioneering Battie and the "conservative" Monro; the former opening up madness to psychological understanding and emphasizing "observation and management of the individual patient," and the latter benightedly insisting on viewing "madness as one uniform disease blindly and uniformly physicked."[108] Among other Whiggish clinician-historians who have selectively presented the history of psychiatry as an evolutionary progress toward modern knowledge, Denis Leigh distinguished Battie as "a man of great gifts" whose "position in the history of British psychiatry" was then "insufficiently acknowledged."[109] Devoting four pages of his 1961 study to Battie's *Treatise,* Leigh anachronistically and unfairly dismissed Monro's *Remarks* as "one of the poorest pieces of work ever written by a psychiatrist," the "reading" of which "today" showed it up to be "a singularly ineffective piece of work."[110] Klaus Doerner, whose revisionist text interprets the history of psychiatry from the perspective of neo-Marxism and German critical theory, is still more effusive, hailing Battie's book as "a revolutionary departure," "thorough and admirably brief

. . . exemplary and programmatic," and its author as the person who "supplied psychiatry as a science with its first 'paradigmatic' approach to its subject matter"—in the process launching "the 'moral management' movement for the total socialisation of all madmen." (Monro, meanwhile, is dismissed as a hidebound reactionary.)[111] Other historians have sung the same refrain, from George Rousseau's paean to the physician of St. Luke's[112] to the chorus led by Dora Weiner[113] and Stanley Jackson[114] that eulogizes him as the precursor of Pinel and the progenitor of psychological or moral treatment. Roy Porter, too, has added his own benediction, contrasting the enlightened and forward-looking optimism of Battie with the profound and largely pernicious pessimism of his Bethlem counterpart.[115] Capping the consensus, in a recent survey of the Battie-Monro debate strongly influenced by Doerner, and advancing a rather polarized model of "stances" toward madness that are either "endorsive" or "suppressive," Allan Ingram lauds Battie as the harbinger of a "new orthodoxy," bridging the gap between old Bedlam on the one side and moral therapy and the York Retreat (the Quaker asylum famously established by the Tukes in 1792) on the other. Battie's *Treatise* is hailed as a work of "openness and humane concern for the welfare of patients" and its "distinctions" detailed over several pages. By contrast, in around half a page, Ingram dismisses Monro's *Remarks* as "a document that should never have been, the manifestation in print of a silence that resents in every word the instigation that has compelled it to exist."[116] While alerting us to some of the ironies and deficiencies of Monro's text, this is surely a harsh and strikingly ahistorical assessment.

Only Akihito Suzuki has stood out against such an overly simple, Manichean perspective, urging us to avoid the teleology that infects these judgments and to view Monro and Battie within the clinical and philosophical context of their own times. This is salutary advice, and besides serving to remind us of the radically different assessment Monro and Battie's own contemporaries made of their debate, it helps us to avoid overstating the importance of Battie's innovations. Equally important, it allows us to see, as Suzuki demonstrates in detail, that Monro's views on the nature of madness had considerably more influence on late eighteenth-century mad-doctors than has customarily been recognized.[117] Monro's influence may also have something to do with the fact that his term at Bethlem extended over almost forty years, Battie's physicianship at St. Luke's, by contrast, lasting just twelve years.

There were exceptions to the consensus in support of Monro over

Battie, of course, for Battie and his *Treatise* certainly had their fans both inside and outside the profession in the late eighteenth and early nineteenth centuries. Perhaps Battie's most zealous devotee was the Kent madhouse-keeper William Perfect (1739–1809), whose 1778 *Methods of Cure* was heavily reliant on the example of "the late learned Dr. Battie" and "his most excellent *Treatise* on madness" and pointedly and totally ignored Monro's response.[118] Perfect swallowed hook-line-and-sinker Battie's basic understanding of madness as original and consequential, as well as his stress on anxiety as a constituent of the disorder and his conviction that "laxity" (or tautness) of nervous membranes was one of its major physiological causes. Inspired by Battie's upbeat faith in the potential curability of consequential types of madness, Perfect likewise believed that medical aid could not be summoned too soon. Discussing cases he had seen in his private practice and treated in his own house in West Malling, Kent, during ca. 1770–76, Perfect also followed "the ingenious Dr. Battie" in isolating his patients and strictly banning friends and family from visiting them, quoting Battie's dictum that "the visits of affecting friends as well as enemies ought strictly to be forbidden."[119] Like Battie too, Perfect was appreciative of the need to let nature work its magic, and to suspend or abandon the use of some of the harsher and "more painful" evacuative and counter-irritant remedies, especially when they had proved ineffective in a case, in preference for a milder regimen of tonics, relaxants, and medical elixirs.

Others also were more generous to Battie, even if few of them could muster Perfect's enthusiastic plaudits. Sir George Baker (1722–1809), one of George III's physicians, was a former pupil of Battie's and remained an admirer of his mentor.[120] Andrew Harper (d. 1790) was another aficionado, and he joined Perfect in adopting Battie's distinction between original and consequential madness, and between mental and physical causes of madness in his own work (*A Treatise on the Real Cause and Cure of Insanity* [1789]).[121] Other specialists too, such as the prominent provincial mad-doctor Thomas Arnold (1742–1816), were more respectful to Battie. Despite a general disposition to criticize primarily metaphysical notions of insanity, Arnold cited Battie's *Treatise,* but ignored Monro's *Remarks,* when listing the principal works on the subject in his *Observations on the Nature, Kinds, Causes, and Prevention, of Insanity* (1806).[122] Among the laity, the lawyer and literator George Hardinge (1743–1816), writing as late as 1814, was also lavish in his praise of Battie, remembering him as one of his "heroes," a "particularly gifted" mad-doctor with a thorough "experimental knowledge" and a "scrupulous" if not "romantic integrity." [123]

Nevertheless, as Suzuki has pointed out, such men were mostly exceptions to the rule. In Perfect's case, furthermore, it seems significant that in later editions of his text he was to abandon the somewhat naïve theoretical underpinning for his case discussions that he had cribbed so uncritically from Battie, including the relevance of any distinction between original and consequential madness. [124] One wonders whether this was in response to criticisms from colleagues and a growing consensus that Battie's musings were somewhat fanciful and inferior in their grounding and utility to Monro's *Remarks*.

As the nineteenth century unfolded, however, both Battie's and Monro's reputations and influence proved evanescent. Significantly, comparatively few of the nineteenth-century writers on insanity on the continent were to pay much attention to the work of either mad-doctor. There is scant reference to their work, for example, in classic treatises by men like Philippe Pinel (1745–1826), Jean E. D. Esquirol (1772–1840), Etienne-Jean Georget (1795–1828), Maximilian Jacobi (1775–1858), and Joseph Guislain (1797–1860). [125] Even in Britain, a number of prominent late eighteenth- and early nineteenth-century writers on madness (e.g., William Cullen [1710–90], Cox, and Hallaran) [126] were to pass rapidly by the contributions of Monro and Battie, which had little explicit role in providing the conceptual framework for notions of moral treatment and moral insanity that were so prominent in the new generation of writings produced by men like Samuel Tuke (1784–1857), John Ferriar (1761–1815), and James Cowles Prichard (1786–1848). [127]

When we move from the theoretical level on which their debate was conducted to the level of practice, still another irony surfaces. For all the noisy public differences between Monro and Battie, the mundane reality is that the plan, administrative procedures, and therapeutic régime of St. Luke's still had much in common with Bethlem. Indeed, the unspoken truth of the matter was that St. Luke's owed as much to Bethlem's example as it was a reaction to it, and practices at the two institutions were to come more and more to resemble each other as the eighteenth century wore on. By the 1780s, it was difficult to tell even the promotional literature of one institution apart from the other. [128] The determination of the governors of St. Luke's to admit medical students to the hospital's wards did not endure long, ending soon after Battie's departure and not being revived until 1842. [129] Pupils were common on the wards of London's general hospitals and infirmaries after 1750, but Bethlem and most public asylums were not to admit medical students to their wards until the mid-nineteenth century and beyond.[130]

A CAUTIOUS RAPPROCHEMENT

Despite the evident tension between Battie and Monro in the 1750s, relations between London's two most prominent mad-doctors seem to have improved as time went on. Not infrequently, Battie and Monro were called to attend on the same cases (although not always at the same time), as in the 1750s and 1770s, respectively, in the cases of Sir Charles Hanbury Williams and Lord Orford.[131] Where they did attend in consort, more often than not they seem to have reached a modus vivendi. Likewise, when summoned before the 1763 Madhouses Enquiry, both men gave very similar testimony, presenting a united front in this very public setting.[132] One aside in Monro's 1766 case book, made at Battie's expense, does seem to suggest that some rancor may have continued to nestle under the surface, Monro observing that one of his patients had been formerly attended by Battie "to little purpose";[133] and Monro's case book for 1766 also records another joint consultation that must have been a rather less than comfortable encounter for both men. In the latter instance, Monro was summoned alongside Battie before the Court of King's Bench in Mrs. Hannah Mackenzie's lawsuit, one of a number of cases in which false confinement was alleged.[134] Battie appeared as the physician who had previously certified the patient, but, like Monro, he was also asked to examine her present condition. Monro's testimony that he could find no marks of insanity in her would hardly have served to validate Battie's original assessment of the patient (though Monro confessed he was unhappy with the thoroughness of the examination he was permitted to make). Whatever ill-feeling this episode might have created, however, was averted because Battie concurred that she now seemed sane.[135]

In a more overt sign of their rapprochement, Battie crucially came to Monro's aid in the case of a Mr. Wood, a merchant from Philpot Lane, London, who had indicted the Bethlem doctor before Lord Mansfield in the King's Bench Court for imprisoning or falsely confining him as a lunatic, evidently in Miles's Hoxton House. This court hearing was one occasion when Monro may have had reason to be grateful to Battie for his emphasis on misassociation of ideas and deluded imagination as the essence of madness, despite their differences in print on precisely this issue. According to a retrospective account recorded by the famous law-yer (and subsequent Lord Chancellor) Thomas Erskine (allegedly taken directly from the mouth of Lord Mansfield), Battie's cross-examination and successful exposure of Wood's prevailing "morbid imagination" got Monro out of a rather tight corner:

> [Mr. Wood] . . . underwent the most severe examination by the defendant's counsel without exposing his complaint; but Dr Battye [*sic*], having come upon the bench by me, and having desired me to ask him what had become of the Princess who he had corresponded with in cherry-juice, he showed me in a moment what he was. He answered that there was nothing at all in that, because having been (as everybody knew) imprisoned in a high tower, and being debarred the use of ink, he had no other means of correspondence but by writing his letters in cherry-juice and throwing them into the river which surrounded the tower, where the Princess received them in a boat. There ex-isted of course, no tower, no imprisonment, no writing in cherry juice, no river, no boat; but the whole was the inveterate phantom of a morbid imag-ination. I immediately [continued Lord Mansfield,] directed Dr Munro to be acquitted.[136]

If Monro thought he had thereby freed himself from the coils of this troublesome individual, he was immediately disabused. Wood simply re-fused to accept the verdict. Describing what happened next, Mansfield commented that his actions revealed the craftiness of the mad and the rather difficult situation the courts—to say nothing of mad-doctors!—might find themselves in:

> . . . having been carried through the city on his way to the madhouse, he in-dicted Dr Munro over again, for the trespass and imprisonment in London, knowing that he had lost the cause by speaking of the Princess at Westmin-ster. And such, said Lord Mansfield, is the extraordinary subtlety and cun-ning of madmen that, when he was cross-examined on the trial in London, as he had successfully been before, in order to expose his madness, all the in-genuity of the bar, and all the authority of the court could not make him say a syllable upon the topic which had put an end to the indictment before, al-though he still had the same indelible impressions upon his mind, as he signified to those who were near him; but, conscious of his defeat at West-minster, he obstinately persisted in holding it back.[137]

As we can see, a relationship that had begun in animosity and rancor eventually subsided into a peaceable and even mutually supportive as-sociation. Yet significant differences remained beneath this veneer of ci-vility and cooperation. Monro's conservative and defensive reaction to the very real challenges presented by the foundation of St. Luke's and by Battie's *Treatise* never really abated. Practically speaking, his obduracy

only went to consolidate retrenchment at Bethlem itself, which imple-
mented barely a single reform in response to the example set at St. Luke's.
Monro and Bethlem's governors resisted a further twelve years after
St. Luke's foundation before following its example and proscribing the
indiscriminate admission of visitors. Even more tellingly, while Monro
clung to the Bethlem physicianship until his death,[138] his erstwhile rival
gracefully resigned his office in 1764 with a view to improving "medical
Knowledge." Medical progress, Battie characteristically remarked in his
own resignation letter, could only be hindered by "Men growing old in
confirmed Habits and Opinions," and failing to make way for "some
younger Physician." [139]

CHAPTER 3

Madness in Their Methodism

Religious Enthusiasm, the Mad-Doctors,
and the Case of Alexander Cruden

Many by Priestcraft, lose their Reason quite,
And always take the wrong Side for the right:
Thus Reason's hoodwink'd by the crafty Priest,
Who for himself does think it all a Jest.
So modern *Whitefields* with Diabolick Arts,
Do spread their Venom into all our Parts,
And teach pernicious Doctrines thro' the Land:
As a Reward, each Pastor should be hang'd.
　　　　　Anon., *Bethlem A Poem* (1744)[1]

If one of my Cloth should begin a Discourse of Heaven in the Scenes
of Business or Pleasure; in the *Court of Requests,* at *Garaway's* or
at *White's,* would he gain a Hearing, unless perhaps of some sorry
Jester who would desire to ridicule him? Would he not presently
acquire the Name of the mad Parson, and be thought by all Men
worthy of *Bedlam?*
　　　　　Henry Fielding, *Amelia* (1752)[2]

Methodists . . . have been looked upon as mad (on account of their
wild and frantic actions) by friends and relatives, by indifferent persons, by regular physicians (the most proper judges), by the world
in general, and have been sent to Bedlam, and adjudged there to be
persons distracted.
　　　　　Theophilus Evans, *A History*
　　　　　of Modern Enthusiasm (1757)[3]

Ridicule is the only antidote against this pernicious poison. Methodism is a madness that arguments can never cure; and, should a little
wholesome severity be applied, persecution would be the immediate
cry. Where then can we have recourse but to the comic muse? Perhaps the archness and severity of her smile may redress an evil, that
the laws cannot reach, or reason reclaim.
　　　　　Samuel Foote, *The Minor, A Comedy* (1760)[4]

. . . *Fanaticism* is a very common cause of Madness. Most of the
Maniacal cases that ever came under my observation, proceeded from
a religious *enthusiasm;* and I have heard it remarked by an eminent
physician, that almost all the insane patients, which occurred to him
at one of the largest hospitals in the *metropolis,* had been deprived

of their reason, by such strange infatuation. The *doctrines of the Methodists* have a greater tendency than those of any other sect, to produce the most deplorable effects on the human understanding. The brain is perplexed in the mazes of mystery, and the imagination overpowered by the tremendous description of future torments.

William Pargeter, *Observations on Maniacal Disorders* (1792)[5]

Enthusiasm and insanity bear such a close affinity, that the shades are often too indistinct to define which is one and which the other. Exuberance of zeal on any subject, in some constitutions, soon ripens into madness: but excess of religious enthusiasm, unless tempered by an habitual command over the affective passions, usually and readily degenerates into fanaticism; thence to superstition . . . and permanent delirium too often closes the scene.

George Man Burrows, *An Inquiry into Certain Errors Relative to Insanity* (1820)[6]

OPPOSING "SPIRITUAL PHYSICK":
THE MONROS AND "METHODICAL" MADNESS

The eighteenth century, or more accurately the century or so following the Restoration, is often seen as a period of profound change in the relationship between religion and madness.[7] In reaction against the chaos and madness of the Civil War (which had seemed to many worried observers to threaten the very nation becoming one great Bedlam), fear of the consequences of civil unrest and sectarian divisions had encouraged a heightened stress on the virtues of rational, reserved religion, polite restraint, and moral sobriety. From the excesses of Puritan piety, and the rebelliousness of Levellers and Ranters on the one side, to the querulousness of Fifth Monarchists, Quakers, and French Prophets on the other, the seventeenth century had seemed peopled with politico-religious radicals and revivalists creating havoc and uproar in the affairs of church and state. Leading Restoration Anglicans, such as Henry More (1586–1661) and Meric Casaubon (1599–1671), pictured a world that had been turned upside-down and a state that had literally lost its head, a civil society in which "enthusiasm"[8] had become and remained a threatening politico-social force.[9] In fact, according to such orthodox figures, enthusiasm was neither divinely nor diabolically inspired, as many proposed, but was a naturally explicable phenomenon, a dangerous madness, albeit one that could be prevented and sometimes, at least, cured. However, it was actually a force in a triumphant phase, and one that needed to be vigorously resisted and prosecuted. To some extent, perhaps, the stage-managed coup that was the Glorious Revolution furthered a sense that politico-religious differences were better settled via more tolerant, politically circumscribed means. New oaths of allegiance tended, more often than not, to be accepted as superficial observances, and non-juring nonconformists (with the notable exception of Catholics) found a relatively comfortable modus vivendi within the reformed post-1688 polity.[10] Yet for the ruling oligarchy, the threat posed by unbridled religious fervor remained a potent and ever-present source of anxiety.

The harsh but sporadically maintained religious intolerance of the earlier seventeenth century had formerly (and especially under Archbishop Laud) seen a number of politico-religious radicals and self-declared prophets carted off to jail and the Tower, or to Bridewell and Bedlam. After 1660, however, such responses gave way to a new, more subtle, form of repression, a discourse of stigma within which excessive shows of religious passion, pride, and vanity were increasingly identified with and discredited as mere madness and folly.

To be sure, the tendency to assail religious enthusiasts long antedated the excesses of Cromwell's Commonwealth. Yet it was not until the last third of the seventeenth century that madness began to be inextricably identified with enthusiasm. Early in the century, for example, Burton's anatomizing of melancholy had thrown a large measure of vitriol at the religious enthusiast, while the melancholic suffering, according to humoral medical theory, from an excess of black bile had oft been characterized as misanthropic and prone to dark and exaggerated fears and suspicions.[11] Simultaneously, though, the Burtonian tradition had also embraced a more sympathetic attitude toward the religious melancholic. It was a tradition that had partially endorsed the distinction and legitimacy of sensibilities of sinfulness and manifestations of emotional piety, and that had underlined the significant place for consolation, prayer, and spiritual physic in ministering to the troubled conscience and the diseased mind.[12] Elizabethan and Jacobean poets and playwrights, meanwhile, had turned melancholy into something of a cult, so that gloomy looks, dark clothes, and black moods appeared virtually à la mode, badges of distinction for the genteel, the intellectually sharp, and the artistic.[13]

In post-Restoration England, however, the Elizabethan cult that had made religious melancholy almost fashionable (for certain sections, at least, of the educated elite) receded, or rather was reformulated. This development occurred in the wake of an amplified focus, not so much on the low-spirited or spiritually dejected, as on the religious enthusiast, the mad religious fanatic, and (albeit somewhat later) the maniacal Methodist. Meanwhile, the rationalistic overtones of the Scientific Revolution and the mechanistic, materialistic underpinnings of the new philosophy (represented in particular by Newtonianism and Cartesianism) encouraged a more removed view of divine immanence and a closer concern with the earthly principles and axioms of physics, mechanics, the mind, and the body. Deists, endorsing toleration but disavowing the doctrines of divine revelation, espoused a Christianity wholly in accordance with rational principles. They posited a God whose laws governed the world from a distance, a divine architect discernible to the rational mind and therefore not mysterious, and yet not, perhaps, fully knowable.[14] Meanwhile, a reformed, legislatively endorsed Protestant polity, strongly anti-Catholic but less immediately threatened by (or implicated in) political-sectarian plots, allowed and encouraged a more concerted critique of belief systems that smacked of superstition, idolatry, and irrationality. Prophesy had been a vexed and contested, but also legitimate (or, at least, customary), tradition of religious activity—such that folly might have a special claim to praise, holiness, or insight. Now, claims of this sort became increasingly questionable. Careful scrutiny and skepticism, if not incredulity and mockery, were often seen as the appropriate responses to the spiritual transports of the visionary, while fanaticism was more easily attributable to ignorance and credulity, and pitiably or laughably ascribable to hubris and self-delusion, or else to physical and mental disease.[15] Of course, significant numbers of seventeenth- and early eighteenth-century clergymen and their flocks continued to experience dreams and visions, and also to provide a cultural space for their interpretation and propagation—although not always strictly within the framework of their own religious worship and proselytizing.[16] Yet among a growing and cohesive body of elite, university-educated Anglicans, the religious and sociocultural legitimacy afforded to such phenomena appears to have been narrowing. For Augustan satirical writers like Swift (himself an Anglican dean) and Pope, visions and nightmares were in essence the hobbyhorses and afflictions of the credulous, the vain, and the mad.[17]

By the early eighteenth century, a new-found appreciation of Stoic values and virtues, most particularly among the educated middling and upper classes, recommended restraint, resilience, and self-possession in the face of even the worst adversities. Concurrently, passion seemed drawn into a closer relationship than ever with delirium, underlining the age-old lesson of classical philosophy and medicine that failure to control the one was a certain route to the other. There emerged a new culture of right and reasonable religion, mandated and modulated by rational doubt and collective congregational consensus, and a more coherently unified relationship between church and state. In such a changed climate of opinion, claims to individual religious inspiration became suspect and subject to public criticism and ridicule—perhaps as never before. Latitudinarianism preached sobriety and moderation in all things and recommended a faith expressed through charitable and moral works rather than adversarial or grandiose expressions of belief.[18] Institutionally, and on the ground level of religious practice, meanwhile, the ratcheting up of diocesan and parochial visitation on English churches and parishes during the Georgian era—extending Anglican authority over the duties, observances, and conduct of the clergy—further constricted the avenues of expression for unorthodox religious zeal.[19]

On still another, related front, if one accepts MacDonald's and Murphy's arguments, this was also a period in which the extremes of religious conviction and emotional agonizing were seen as more fundamentally intellectually suspect and medically implicated. Not least, the broad period 1660–1800 marked a time when suicide itself was secularized and medicalized.[20] In the process, suicide and the very impulse to self-harm were radically redefined as less a matter of sin and the devil's temptations—the appropriate response to which was strict religious counsel and admonishment, or else religious and legal sanction in this life that mirrored a certain unregenerative fate in the next—and more a sign of mental disturbance and disease. Those inclined toward self-murder thus required medical treatment and, if possible, preventive measures.

Against this backdrop, religious enthusiasm became increasingly identified with dangerous fanaticism and irrational beliefs of all kinds, and a number of historians have characterized the Augustan Age as the period when the campaign against religious enthusiasm appeared at its most powerful and pervasive. The main tool of this campaign was Augustan satire, which increasingly represented religious ardor as a threat to social order, and made radicals and evangelicals the butts of sophisticated parody, through the printed word and a variety of visual media. Regularly raiding Burton's *Anatomy* to fuel their assault on religious maniacs and crazy enthusiasts, Swift, Pope, and other eighteenth-century writers allowed little scope for the more consolatory and legitimating side of the Burtonian corpus, appropriating instead the concepts and language of the new science and mechanistic medicine to castigate all forms of vanity and self-deception.[21] Rather than being full of spirit, as far as these Augustan satirists were concerned, the religious radicals of eighteenth-century England were more likely affected by the bodily ills of vapors, wind, or afflatus, their visions merely the promptings of their disordered and diseased bowels, infected imaginations, and vitiated judgments. The religious visionary was placed on the same plane as the eccentric inventor and those who projected and concocted crazy schemes: all were guilty of a folly that was, at best, an overestimate of their own talents and, at worst, a symptom of an infected and irrational fancy.[22] It became a ready and popular jibe whenever an orthodox churchman disapproved of certain religious opinions—in particular, opinions of a radical nature—to declare the author of such heterodoxy a madman.[23]

As a result of the commercial boom in the printing industry of this period, satirists could bank on an ever wider dissemination of such critical discourse, their words and images perhaps serving as a substitute for large-scale institutions in which to confine or contain the fanatical. Additionally, the popularization of discursive means of confining the crazy and the fanatical may have provided more grounds for thinking that enlarged institutional and legal means were required to contain the legions of unconfined maniacs roaming the kingdom. A rudimentary machinery of confinement from gaols, bridewells, and houses of correction to lunatic hospitals and private madhouses was certainly developing apace in this period. Yet, as Porter has convincingly argued, in actual institutional and numerical terms, there was nothing like any Foucauldian "Great Confinement" in eighteenth-century England.[24] Furthermore, as far as the religiously orthodox were concerned, the trouble was that— with a largely free press—religious radicals themselves could employ the very same weapons and tactics to spread their own views. Indeed, so many odd and eccentric radicals appear to have remained at liberty to print and proselytize their beliefs that one must question conventional historical views about the strength and success of this so-called campaign against enthusiasm.

Prophesy and religious inspiration continued to find sympathetic proponents and adherents in the eighteenth century, and the very popularity of sects such as the Methodists in some quarters is testimony to the persisting space in Augustan England for spiritual understandings of mental distress. This was a century in which a number of clergymen continued to perform a dual role for their flocks, offering both consolation or "spiritual physic" and material medicine to mentally troubled parishioners who sought them out. Meanwhile, Methodists and other evangelicals, some of whom enthusiastically espoused new medical techniques such as electricity and shock therapies, were also actively seeking out those troubled individuals, seeing it as very much their responsibility to intercede in the lives of the imprisoned, the sick, and the afflicted.[25] Over time, however, this type of activity came to be viewed with increasing disapproval—both by a growing body of medically educated professionals, keen to establish their expertise as mad-doctors, and by orthodox laymen and leading members of the political and social elites. Methodism began increasingly, especially during the 1730s and 1740s, to be stigmatized by its opponents and critics as the alter ego of Catholicism,[26] while its proponents were accused (like Catholics) of propagating idolatory, superstition, misery, and despair. Through its emphasis on sin and the spirit world, on hellfire and damnation, it was said to be actually driving its adherents into madness.

During the course of the eighteenth century, religious gloom and despondency, along with enthusiasm and evangelism, came to seem a darker threat. Yet, from the 1740s or 1760s, it is also the case that there was a partial resurgence of sympathy in certain elite social arenas for revivalists and for religiously inspired mortification. In particular, as part of a new cult of sensibility, men and women of feeling allowed more scope for being emotionally overcome and spiritually transported by worldly sufferings and pathos. In the wake of a counter-Enlightenment critique of rationalistic classical philosophy, stoical responses to suffering began to be seen and censured by a widening group of the educated elite and middling classes as the pretext for potentially inhuman "insensibility."[27] Indeed, for people "neither [to] grieve with the unfortunate, nor rejoice with the fortunate" came to be regarded as an arrogant, if not absurd, attempt to deny the naturalness of emotions and passions, to "annihilate" those things "which they ought to moderate." Contrariwise, the virtues of grief, joy, and even (righteous) anger began to be emphasized as essential qualities in the cementing of social bonds.[28] In the process, a broader identification was forged with those wearing and donning the rags and weeds of distress or displaying piously philanthropic fellow feeling.[29] On the one hand, from behind the self-indulgent and affected afflictions of the splenetic and vaporish figures who peopled the salons and caverns of Pope's *Dunciad* emerged the rather unattractive, heavy torpor of Boswell's hypochondria and Johnson's melancholy. Yet, on the other hand, self-declared sufferers like Boswell, who penned magazines entitled *The Hypochondriak* and partook of the license provided by mortification, were also part and parcel of a self-regarding and self-parodying culture, a culture where succumbing to sickness and morbid sensibilities might even be fashionable.[30] In some circles, the graveyard contemplations and "Night-thoughts"[31] of poets and scribblers, and the moving (if sometimes artificial) tears of sensible souls, became especially popular means of engagement with this world and the next, and signs and signals of a self-consciously superior politeness, civility, and humanity.

Where, then, did England's premier family of mad-doctors stand in all this, and how did their patients fare? To what extent did the mad-houses and lunatic hospitals they served and supported become part of any campaign to police and confine the threat of religious enthusiasm? Were they among the principal protagonists or the more reluctant participants in the controversy? One thing is certain: like others in the emerging specialty of mad-doctoring, the Monro dynasty could not avoid the debates that swirled around these issues.

In all probability, John Monro shared the traditional hostility of Bridewell and Bethlem's largely Anglican board of governors to sectarian religions, the Methodists in particular. It must be said, however, that most of the available evidence on this point appears to derive from the period of James's physicianship rather than John's. For example, attempting to visit Joseph Periam and other Methodist patients in Bethlem during the second quarter of the century, George Whitefield (1714–70) and John Wesley (1703–91) both complained that they were refused entry. According to Wesley, recalling an interrupted visit of a year or so before John's election as joint physician, it had been decreed that "none of these preachers were to come there" (although there is no trace of such an order in Bethlem's records). Wesley was repeatedly to censure Bethlem's medical régime in print—for this and other reasons—and here he laid on the sardonic irony with a trowel, alleging that the prohibition on allowing him in was "for fear of making them [the patients] mad." [32]

Methodism was pilloried by its critics throughout this period for its alleged encouragement of "unseemly" forms of worship, spiritual transports, and morbidly pious, agonizing behavior that was often dismissed as "methodical madness," tending toward the incitement of civil and mental unrest. [33] While Wesley and Whitefield loudly proclaimed that Periam was sane, and had merely been suffering from a spiritual crisis, they castigated James Monro and his colleagues for giving him purges and vomits when what he needed was counsel and guidance. Nor was this the only occasion when Wesley and his followers complained in these terms. For example, Wesley's journal for 1740 records the case of a teenager, Peter Shaw, whose mother dismissed Monro and his apothecary after six weeks of confinement, bleeding, and blistering failed to put a stop to his "praying or singing, or giving thanks continually." She complained that the treatment had merely left him "so weak he could not stand alone." [34] In a similar vein, Susannah Wesley wrote in 1746 to her son John complaining about "that wretched Fellow [James] Monroe," who had sent a follower named MacCune to a Chelsea madhouse when what he really required was "a Spiritual . . . Physician." MacCune's guilt-ridden self-torments and cries "to God for mercy and pardon" had served only to "confirm the Dr in the opinion of his madness," though to her eyes such behavior was "proof of his being in a right Mind." [35]

Such viewpoints were bound to generate antipathy in the doctor and among his allies. Furthermore, the fact that Bethlem was both metaphorically and genuinely becoming the backdrop of Methodism's stage must have been far from palatable to the institution's medical staff and governors. Yet that was precisely what now materialized, both in dramatic and artistic representations like *The Human Barometer* (1743) or *Harlequin Methodist* (ca. 1750) and when Methodists elected to set up their bantering booths on open space abutting the hospital in Moorfields, or when they used Bethlem as a point of reference in their sermonizing.

The Human Barometer appears to have been one of the earliest contemporary works to recreate this literal juxtaposition in symbolic detail. The first verse describes the "melancholy edifice" of Bethlem and the "intellectual ruins" of its inmates, and the second sketches the synonymous scene of Whitefield preaching before his converts:

> Now to the adjacent Field direct thy way,
> This will the same in miniature display,
> There mounted on his tripod Whitefield stands,
> Silence and the canonick Garb commands,
> With arms extended see he apes St Paul,
> And counts his own an apostolick call,
> Gesture and voice betray the heated brain,
> In groans his converts echoe back again,
> And souls impressed with thoughts of grace, or sin,
> Expectorate their sense in solemn din,
> These of enthusiastic transports boast,
> But are to Argument and Reason lost.[36]

Quacks, too, set up their stalls in Moorfields,[37] and satirists often could not resist making the connection between the theatrical peddling of medicine and the equally theatrical quality of Methodists' ministrations. Harlequins were commonly associated with low forms of theater

that appealed to the "ignorant" masses, and sometimes also with foreign influences charged with corrupting the religion and morals of the
people. Thus Methodists were anathematized for preying in a low theatrical way upon the credulity of the poorest sort (both financially and
intellectually), literally making a "farce," or comedy, out of religion,
while frightening and maddening their followers with their melodramatic threats of hellfire and damnation. Not unlike constructions of the
mesmerists later in the century, their adherents were often represented
as women whose sobriety and chastity were held up to doubt and whose
putatively emotional susceptibility and weaker intellects were portrayed
as all the more vulnerable to the seductive powers of male Methodist
preachers.

The verses of *Harlequin Methodist*—a satirical song of ca. 1750 that
was sold for 6d. and was illustrated by a print depicting a Methodist
dressed as Harlequin—constitute one of a number of contemporary satires published on the dispute over the proprietorial rights to theater direction and the employment of actors in the city between John Rich
(1682?–1761), David Garrick (1717–79), and other actors and playwrights. Rich, playwright and manager of the Covent Garden Theatre,
was also satirized in *British Frenzy: Or, the Mock-Apollo* (1745),[38] and
had been famous since the 1720s for his leading role playing a harlequin
in his own dramas and for using harlequins as comic devices.[39] In subsequent years, he converted to Methodism after taking a devout Methodist for his second wife, and was criticized thereafter as a "Harlequin
Methodist" for lowering the tone of modern theater, while concurrently
selecting actors on the basis of their religio-moral standpoints.

In this particular print, the Harlequin Methodist is shown preaching
from a stool before a group of mostly female auditors, with Bedlam as
his stage set. The accompanying song included the following lines:

Then come all, good Folks, to my School,
Near *Bedlam* my Tripod I place,
And hear me hold forth from my Stool,[40]
Of Truth, and of Day-light and Grace.
Go no more to the Old House, I pray,
Where Satan has ta'en his Abode,
But come, if you please, ev'ry Day
To mine: It will soon be the Mode . . .
No Players I'll have but are Saints,
No rakebelly, swaggering Ballies,
No Whores that use Washes and Paints
To draw in their vile carnal Cullies

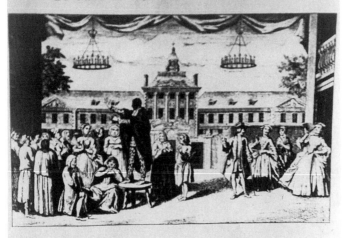

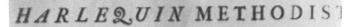

FIGURE 14. *Harlequin Methodist. To the Tune of, An Old Woman Cloathed [sic] in Grey* (London, 1750?). Engraving (accompanied by satirical song in verses) representing a Methodist in the theatrical guise of a cloaked and masked harlequin, preaching on a bantering stool before an appreciative audience in Moorfields, with Bethlem and madness itself as the symbolic stage backdrop. This song and print were produced by allies of the famous actor and theater director David Garrick (1717– 79) to satirize his rival John Rich (1682?– 1761), manager of the Covent Garden Theatre and writer of comedies (e.g., *The Necromancer; Or, Harlequin Doctor Faustus* [1723] and *The Spirit of Contradiction* [1760]), who had converted to Methodism. Madness is thus also linked with low theatrical entertainments and with pandering to the base passions of the masses. Reproduced by kind permission of The British Library. Shelfmark 1890.C 1 (10); 12403AA34(2); 7410A72(2).

My Women inspired shall be,
My Men fit for Martyrs to die
Most holy in ev'ry Degree,
And *chaste*, like MY DEARY and I.

Similarly, if rather more viciously, a three-penny broadside ballad, apparently sold to Bethlem visitors in the 1740s and fawningly loyal in tone to that institution, its governors, and staff, attacked Whitefield and the Methodists as practitioners of "Diabolick Arts" and peddlars of "pernicious Doctrines," whose "Priestcraft" caused "many" to "lose their Reason quite/And always take the wrong Side for the right," for which it recommended "each Pastor should be hanged." [41] In this way, as Methodists engaged with Bethlem, the ruse somewhat backfired on them, Methodism becoming inextricably linked with madness, and their Anglican and other opponents (including some of those connected with the hospital) jumping at the opportunity to associate them with popery, superstition, and unreason. [42]

Interestingly enough, not only Bethlem, but its rival St. Luke's, became identified as a backdrop and receptacle for the "Methodically mad." The successful application by its founders to lease the Windmill Hill Foundry—a headquarters for Wesley and the Methodists since 1739 [43]—as their site for the lunatic hospital had provided an immediate and irresistible opportunity for further satire. Faced with possible eviction, Wesley had appealed to a relatively sympathetic committee at St. Luke's, [44] eventually securing an agreement to carry on renting the premises from the hospital (as the new leasee) at £9 per annum. While this ensured the continuing role of the foundry as a Methodist meeting house, with Wesley and the Methodists having become tenants to St. Luke's, and the foundry directly contiguous to what became the north side of the hospital, it was also ensured that St. Luke's was for sometime after linked with mad Methodists: indeed, it was explicitly lampooned as "the Foundry Hospital." [45] The irony certainly did not escape the *London Evening Post,* which commented mischievously in 1750 that "a great Number of rational People think that the Foundry has been a religious Madhouse for some Years past; and now, very probably, it may be converted into an Hospital for Lunaticks." [46]

The propensity of Methodists to visit, or—as far as orthodox Anglicans and more secularly minded rationalists were concerned—to interfere with, the incarcerated and a wide range of sick, lunatic, and criminal cases made them difficult to ignore both within and beyond such arenas of social interaction. There was even, for example, Methodist in-

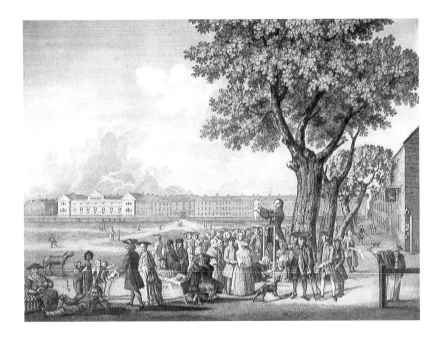

FIGURE 15. Robert Pranker after John Griffiths, *Enthusiasm Displayed* (ca. 1755). This etching and engraving depicts a Methodist, possibly George Whitefield, preaching a sermon on a bantering stool in Upper Moorfields, before a mixed crowd of listeners/adherents and passersby. In the background stands the plain and distinctive edifice of "St Luke's Hospital for Lunaticks," toward which he appears to be gesturing. While some are relatively attentive, and a couple of particularly rapt and humbly attired females are shown kneeling at the preacher's feet, perhaps associating Methodism with the seduction of poor, emotional, and intellectually frail women, most of the crowd's attention is elsewhere. Those who are in real need, such as a drunkard, a cripple, a blind man, fruit sellers, and a group of poor children (with an effigy of Guy Fawkes?), are totally oblivious to the preacher, and (presumably) vice versa. Anticipating Hogarth's later engraving (*Credulity, Superstition and Fanaticism* [1762]; see figure 17), two bearded Mohammedans (or Russian Orthodox priests?) are shown to posit a predictably skeptical eastern perspective on the bizarre, if not mad, social mores of "civilized" western religion. Reproduced by kind permission of The British Library. Shelfmark 1890.C 1 (10); 12403AA34(2); 7410A72(2).

volvement in the aftermath of the notorious case of Lord Ferrers (discussed in detail in chapter 6). One of Ferrers's cousins was the countess of Huntingdon, Lady Selina [Shirley] Hastings (1707–91), derogatively dismissed by Walpole as "the Saint Theresa of the Methodists." Visiting the earl in the last days of his confinement in the Tower, prior to his public execution, she was less concerned with either her cousin's mental state or his forthcoming earthly fate than with the dangers to the condemned man's immortal soul.[47] Her intervention in Ferrers's case (which allegedly involved her keeping him from seeing his mistress lest he should "die in adultery" and encouraging Whitefield, who served at one point as her chaplain, to "pray and preach about him"), was castigated by Walpole as rank enthusiasm and a sign of "how violent bigotry must be in such mad blood."[48] "With all his madness," he sneered, "Lord Ferrers was not mad enough to be struck with Lady Huntingdon's sermons."[49]

Many balked at the Methodists' meddling, yet active intercession through both prayer and consolation toward the plights of the sick, the distressed, and the distracted was a core tenet of their evangelical faith, Whitefield and Wesley preaching again and again as to the Christian's duty to "Intercede for all that are any Ways afflicted in Mind, Body, or Estate."[50] Almost as often as they were pilloried as mad enthusiasts, Methodists sought solace in the retelling and reinventing of traditional Christian parables as to the inevitability of the fearful, the ignorant, and the wicked taking the wise and pious for fools and mad. As Whitefield preached often in his sermons: "These were looked upon by them as Enthusiasts and madmen, as Persons that were Righteous over-much, and who intended to turn the World upside down."[51]

What must have made matters worse, from the mad-doctor's point of view, was that Methodists, like other "enthusiastic" Protestants, invested mental turmoil with profound spiritual significance.[52] Anxiety and despair, the tortures provoked by the acknowledgment of guilt and sin, the perils of damnation and the promise of salvation, the literal struggle between the divine and the temptations of the Evil One for the possession of an individual's soul: these were central elements of passionate forms of Evangelical Christianity that steadily gained adherents—although only, as the Anglican elite liked to represent it, among the unlettered and the unwashed. In such circles, scriptural discussions of demons and witches served to reinforce popular belief in an almost palpable spiritual world of supernatural malevolence and satanic temptation, one of whose most visible manifestations was maladies of the mind.[53] Religious revivalists thus helped secure the survival of earlier perspectives on madness that mixed together religious and magical causation with naturalistic forms of explanation, and saw divine retribution, demoniacal possession, witchcraft, or the misalignment of one's astrological signs as being as (or more) plausible an explanation of distraction as an account pitched in terms of bodily indisposition.[54]

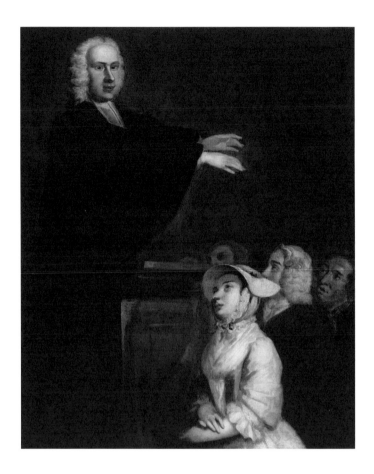

FIGURE 16. *George Whitefield,* by John Wollaston (1742). Oil painting showing George Whitefield preaching from a lectern. Whitefield's face is possessed by an intent but rather distracted stare, while his arms are outstretched as if he is trying to mesmerize his congregation, who are represented with rather bewitched aspects, with a particularly entranced woman directly beneath Whitefield's hands. Her form remarkably anticipates that of the woman beneath the lectern in William Hogarth's later *A Medley: Credulity, Superstition and Fanaticism* (1762) engraving (see figure 17). The congregation are evidently in their Sunday best, but one (far right) has a vacant expression and wears a rather rude-looking garb that probably would have identified him to an eighteenth-century audience as a member of the ignorant lower classes. Reproduced by courtesy of the National Portrait Gallery, London, ID No. 131.

Meanwhile, proponents of "enthusiastic" Protestantism proffered not merely explanations of mental disturbance that were consonant with these long-standing popular beliefs, but also alternative forms of spiritual healing and religious therapy. For the Methodists, vigil was just as, if not more, appropriate a response to mental tribulations as medicine. (John Wesley himself fervently believed in demonomania and advocated spiritual healing through communal rituals of prayer and fasting.)[55]

By mid-century, the tensions not only between Methodism and the Anglican elite, but more specifically between some of the most prominent Methodists and the best-known mad-doctor of the age, James Monro, were already well entrenched. Itinerant sermonizers preaching hellfire and damnation were routinely accused of scrambling the wits of the too credulous who flocked to their revival meetings:

> Struck with puritan looks, and bare fac'd assertion,
> They stake their all below, for the skys in reversion,
> 'Till politic Satan cuts off the entail,
> And sends them to Bedlam, to Box, or to Jail.[56]

It seems highly likely that a similar attitude to piously emotional evangelicals was bequeathed to John. His library certainly included a wide range of literature on the subject of enthusiasm and Methodism, including a number of Whitefield's publications, as well as texts both critical and supportive of the Methodists and demonology.[57] The *London Evening Post,* a reliable source for the Bethlem party line, continued to attack the Methodists after mid-century, relating in an edition of 1766, for example, how

> a Methodist Clergyman, at the recommendation of one of the parishioners, imposed himself upon the Lecturer of a parish at the west end of the town, to give him a sermon, where he ranted and raved an hour and a quarter, till several of the congregation left the church. It were to be wished, that a list of Methodist Preachers were published in all the papers, that the Clergy of London and Westminster be upon their guard against them.[58]

The hospital's staff claimed that, throughout John Monro's physicianship, Bethlem continued to receive a substantial proportion of patients from the ranks of the Methodists. Sophie von la Roche observed in 1786—evidently on the authority of John Gozna, the Bethlem apothecary from 1772 to 1795—that "the greatest number of older women come from the Methodists' ranks, usually from child-bed, which gradually gives way to a quiet kind of lunacy; but these cases are mostly

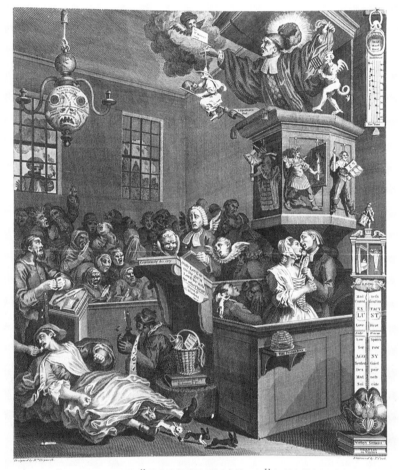

CREDULITY, SUPERSTITION and FANATICISM.

A MEDLEY.

Believe not every spirit, but try the spirits whether they are of God because many false Prophets are gone out into the World.

Published by ... J. Robinson, Paternoster Row October ... 1768

FIGURE 17. *A Medley: Credulity, Superstition and Fanaticism,* by William Hogarth (1762). A reworking of Hogarth's earlier engraving *Enthusiasm Delineated* (1761), a satire on the folly and perils of Enthusiasm. A ranting figure in an orthodox preacher's gown, underneath which he sports a harlequin's suit, addresses his ecstatic and hysterical flock from his literal and appropriately chosen text, "I speak as a fool," in a savage commentary on sectarian religion, popery, superstition, and the extent of popular gullibility. Elaborating on his text, as his toppling wig reveals the tonsured pate of a papist priest, the preacher's declamations crack the sounding board above his head. From his outstretched hands he dangles puppets of a

cured."[59] Statistical evidence was also employed to back up such assertions: the figures concerning Bethlem's admissions during 1772–87 (with which Gozna had furnished William Black for his *Dissertation on Insanity* of 1810) purported to show that over 10 percent of the patients had been disordered as a result of religion and Methodism.[60] Continuing in this tradition, Gozna's successor as apothecary, John Haslam, did not mince words in castigating Methodism for its ill effects on the weak

---

witch hovering on her broomstick and the Devil, emphasizing the Methodists' and Catholics' much disparaged beliefs in magic and possession and their alleged tendencies to employ stories of hellfire and damnation to terrify their flock as to the consequences of sinning. (In the 1761 *Enthusiasm Delineated,* which contains a number of significant variants on these themes, the preacher holds a puppet of the Trinity, identifying trinitarian beliefs with diabolism.) The preacher's vociferations rouse the rabble to a pathological pitch of excitement, throwing many into hysterical ecstasies and cataleptic trances. Members of the congregation are shown gnawing on icons of the body of Christ, equating transubstantiation (and, therefore, Catholicism) with cannibalism, bestiality, and madness. Gazing at the preacher, a Jew destroys lice between his thumbs, while the Bible in front of him lies open at the "bloody" pages of the Old Testament. Whitefield, or "Dr Squintum," himself (identifiable through the by now customary depiction of his cross-eyed looks) is portrayed, flanked by cherubs, as a clerk with a stricken face and duck's wings, mocking his pretensions to angelic piety. Lower still, the text of a hymn by Whitefield spills over the lectern. High above, Whitefield's suggestion that he wanted his Tabernacle to be "a soul trap" is parodied in a sign held by another cherub that reads "St. Money Trap." Elsewhere in the picture various superstitions and pious frauds perpetuated by religious enthusiasts are on view. In the foreground is a representation of Mary Toft, an especially notorious fraud (as exposed by medical men) who alleged that she had given birth to six-

teen rabbits and a tabby cat in 1726. To her left, a crouched figure vomiting nails and staples represents the "Boy of Bilston," another well-known contemporary fraud, or false miracle. By their side, a basket filled with Whitefield's journals stands atop an edition of King James I's *Demonologia.* John Wesley stands to the left rear of the picture, pointing up to the "New and Correct Globe of Hell" that lights the proceedings, a sphere marked with the locations of the Molten Lead Lake, Pitch and Tar River, the Bottomless Pit, the Horrid Zone, Brimstone Ocean, and Eternal Damnation Gulf. In the right foreground, a thermometer registering the passions emerges from an overheated brain, piled on top of two books, "Wesley's Sermons" and "Glanvil on Witches" (i.e., Joseph Glanvill's *Saducismus Triumphatus* [1726]). Upon the thermometer rests an icon of the "Drummer of Tedworth," a famous ghost—credence in whom was fostered by Glanvill and Wesley. The scale registers lust as (with hot blood performing the function of mercury) it rapidly rises toward madness and raving. To the left, a randy and well-dressed aristocrat is shoving a religious icon down the dress of a swooning servant girl distracted by visions of hellfire, recalling the common accusation that Methodists used religion to seduce their female adherents. Outside the church, at the very back of the picture, a Mohammedan sporting a turban gazes through the window calmly smoking his hookah, implying that even heathen religions seem rational and sagacious by comparison with this medley of sectarian and Catholic enthusiasms and superstitions. Reproduced by kind permission of The Wellcome Trust.

and impressionable minds and consciences of its adherents. Such views were widely held among specialists in insanity, Haslam, for example, being loudly applauded in the *Annual Medical Register* (for the year 1809) for his robust opinions.[61]

The Anglican divine and specialist in mad-doctoring William Pargeter (1760–1810) (who had been a student with Haslam at St. Bartholomew's Hospital and mentioned attending a case with John Monro[62]) was equally damning of the influence of Methodism and fanaticism in general on the mental faculties. He commented at enormous length in his *Observations on Maniacal Disorders* (1792) on Methodists as enthusiasts and "*deluded people*" who had literally "infested" various parishes, blaming them for turning numerous people mad with their stories of "Hell flames" and augmenting "the number of suicides in the nation."[63] Pargeter declared himself mystified that the instances "of their hearers or penitents being sent to Bedlam or to the grave" had not "convinced them of the . . . evil and absurdity of their conduct"; his ire had perhaps much to do with the fact that these people had "seceded from the Church."[64] He expressed particular outrage at the advantage he believed Methodist "fanatics" were accustomed to take of "ignorance and indisposition," especially of female parishioners, comparing it to looters "who avail themselves of the confusion at a fire, to plunder the sufferers."

Where the mentally frail were concerned, not only Methodism, but religious devotion in general was viewed over an extended period as being highly suspect by medical practitioners. Whereas for a limited time during the last decades of the seventeenth century the Bethlem governors had deemed religious consolation for "capable Lunaticks" a beneficial and appropriate duty of the Bridewell chaplain, this practice fell into disuse thereafter, and for the duration of the century that followed patients were largely isolated from pious offices. On the other hand, it was at the very period when Haslam was writing—at the turn of the century, and more than accidentally coincident with the growing prominence of moral management—that specialists such as Joseph Mason Cox began to afford Methodism and religious consolation a more sympathetic reading. Partly reflecting the prominence of Evangelicals in the movement for "lunacy reform," there occurred a gradual reassimilation of divine service into a new generation of hospitals and asylums for the insane.[65] Likewise, in contrast to Haslam, Bryan Crowther—writing in 1811, toward the end of his period of office as Bethlem surgeon and expressing gratification at having recently learned about Bethlem's earlier religious traditions—took a decidedly non-sectarian view of the relationship between insanity and religion. Demanding "proof, in place of bold and bare assertion" of "the [alleged] prevalent effect of methodism in producing insanity," he warmly supported the introduction of "a devotional system of worship" to hospitals for the insane "of every religious persuasion." [66] This was despite his concern and conviction that "enthusiasm and madness" were near "relatives," and that any lunatic hospital chaplain would need to be chosen with extreme caution and should himself be required to "avoid every controversial point connected with religious subjects." [67]

Sources of this sort tell us a great deal about the divergent and changing attitudes of mad-doctors in general toward the world of the spirit over the course of the long eighteenth century. Yet they can be only indirect and partial guides to the more specific question of John Monro's views about evangelicals and religion. If many possible sources that might have revealed his opinions tell us frustratingly little, one of John's particularly colorful patients, an odd character who was also treated by John's father James, provides some rather more conclusive evidence concerning this particular mad-doctor's somewhat skeptical, if not antipathetic, attitude toward spiritual transports and individual claims to divine inspiration.

PROVIDENCE VERSUS THE MAD-DOCTORS: ALEXANDER THE CORRECTOR AND THE MONROS

Alexander Cruden (1701–70),[68] who was later to style himself "Alexander the Corrector," first encountered the Monro family in 1738, when James was called upon to treat him at Matthew Wright's madhouse in Bethnal Green. For the elder Monro, the case must at first have seemed an utterly routine one, and for the first week, he was content, following his standard practice, to prescribe the administration of purges and vomits without setting eyes on his patient. Nor would his first encounter with the eccentric Scot have caused him much alarm, for Cruden was a slight, physically unimpressive man, afflicted with a stammer and stutter. Moreover, the patient's expostulations about the injustice of his confinement, and the "barbarous Usage" he had been subjected to, were the sort of complaints James had doubtless heard many times before. The eminent mad-doctor's response to this apparently hapless creature was simply to "order him to be blooded in the left foot" by the apothecary.[69]

But appearances were deceptive. Cruden, like the tar baby, proved to

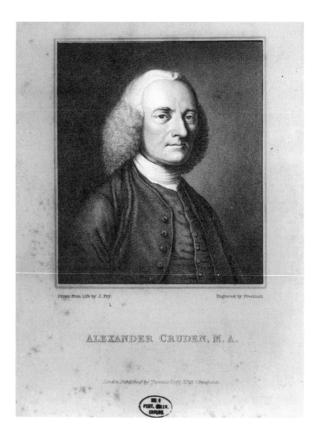

Drawn from Life by J. Fry.   Engraved by Freeman.

ALEXANDER CRUDEN, M.A.

London Published by Thomas Tegg Nº73 Cheapside.

FIGURE 18. Portrait of Alexander Cruden, M.A., engraved by Freeman from a drawing from life by J. Fry (undated; early nineteenth century?). Reproduced by kind permission of the Ashmolean Museum, Oxford, Hope Collection.

be someone who could not be shaken off once touched.[70] Others to their horror would discover (or had already discovered) the same thing. As a young man in Aberdeen (where he been educated rigidly in the principles of Presbyterianism and had taken his degree at Marischal College ca. 1720), Cruden had pursued a local belle so importunately that his parents had been obliged to confine him as a madman in the "tolbooth" or town gaol. Following his release, he had emigrated (around 1726) to London, finding an outlet for his obsessiveness by working as a proof-

reader, or "corrector of the press," in Wild Court. His career in the print
world was interrupted for a time when, in 1729, he obtained employment in the household of James Stanley, the tenth earl of Derby (1664–
1736)—a retired regimental colonel and Lord Lieutenant of Lancaster,
and a former Whig MP under Queen Anne.[71] The job—as a reader in
French to his Lordship—did not last long, though the connection to the
unfortunate aristocrat certainly did. Cruden began badly on the day he
arrived at Halnaker Castle (near Chichester, in Sussex) by mistaking the
butler for his lordship. He then made matters worse by discoursing at
interminable length on the evils of the episcopacy to this butler, an un-
swerving High Churchman. Finally, he ensured his dismissal in July by
exhibiting his purely theoretical knowledge of French—a language that
he had learned only as a by-product of his proofreading, and one that he
had never heard spoken! His lordship, by contrast, had spent part of his
early years in Flanders fighting the French, and had made many friends
among the French aristocracy. His own failing eyesight, and not any
lack of fluency in the language, had led to the engagement of Cruden to
read to him. One can only imagine Lord Derby's feelings when he heard
the pronunciation of his new employee, though with characteristically
aristocratic sangfroid, he behaved as though nothing whatsoever was
amiss.

Cruden's bizarre pronunciation may have proved a source of some
amusement to the household, but if so, the mirth must have proved
short-lived, because for months after his dismissal, he bombarded his
poor employer with demands for reinstatement and unwanted details of
his personal travails.[72] Obdurate and persistent as always, Cruden invested much time and effort in learning to pronounce French in a more
conventional fashion. He even took up residence and lessons at the
house of a Madame Boulanger in Crown Street, St. Anne's Soho (a quarter of London well populated by French Protestants), and wrote repeatedly to the earl throughout the summer and autumn of 1729 in an attempt to win back his job. In a manner not dissimilar to the one he later
adopted when protesting about his confinements at the hands of the
Monros, Cruden became fixated on the notion that his dismissal from
his position at Halnaker was unfair and a profound slight on his character. He strove uneasily to bridge his evident feelings of inadequacy and
failure, modulating his frequent appeals to Derby and to a higher justice
by a determination to submit to the designs of Providence and a conviction that his latest tribulations were merely God's way of trying him. In

his desperation to win the earl over, he even made veiled threats to Lord Derby, insisting that he would indeed obtain "justice" and speaking of his plans to print "an account of his treatment."[73]

All, nonetheless, was for naught. Even a personal visit to the earl's Lancashire house at Knowsley, so that he could demonstrate his progress in person, failed to produce the necessary change of heart: Lord Derby peremptorily declined to have anything more to do with him, and that was more or less that.[74]

Soon, however, he took aim at a still more powerful patron—the Hanoverian court found itself in receipt of his attentions. After unrelenting petitions and approaches to men of influence such as the renowned Royal Society president and Oxford physician (Sir) Hans Sloane (1660–1753), Cruden obtained in 1735 the Royal Warrant for the then vacant, but unremunerative, office of "Queen's Bookseller." During this year and the first part of the next, Cruden, a devout Presbyterian and strict Sabbatarian, married his religious zeal and his personal punctiliousness to produce *Cruden's Complete Concordance to the Old and New Testaments* (1737)—an exhaustive work of reference that remains in print to this day.[75] Strategically, he dedicated his *Concordance* to the queen and, book in hand, he began to haunt the royals, whom he saw as Britain's bastions against the perils of "Popery and Slavery."[76] His indefatigable persistence seemed rewarded when Queen Caroline (wife of George II and a considerable patroness of religious radicals) personally accepted a copy of the book from his hands on 3 November 1737.[77] But the promise of continuing royal favor was cruelly dashed barely a week later when the queen was taken fatally ill. Although Cruden thereafter proudly styled himself "Bookseller to the late Queen" and dedicated his two 1739 publications to the king and to Lord Harrington (William Stanhope, ca. 1690–1756), the secretary of state for the north, any real hope he had of further royal patronage or preferment vanished with Caroline's death late in 1737.

Within a few years, so too did Cruden, at least for the historian attempting to reconstruct the details of his life. We know that in the period from 1740 onward, Cruden spent some time occupied as a private usher in an Enfield boarding school, writing to Sir Hans Sloane about his employment.[78] Around the same time, he made use of the scholarly skills he had developed through his work on his *Concordance* by constructing a universal index to Milton's *Paradise Lost,*[79] a work published in 1741 and a labor of love that must have further fueled his fertile eschatological imagination. During subsequent years there is evidence that he was primarily employed in the city as corrector of the press, working on editions of books such as Matthew Henry's (1662–1714) *Exposition of the Old and New Testaments* (1708–10) and on his own *Compendium of the Holy Bible* (1750).[80] Occasionally this strange and truculent man provoked further trouble and briefly reemerged from urban anonymity. In 1748, for instance, Cruden's obstreperousness and incorrigible propensity to interfere with swearers and Sabbath-breakers saw him in difficulty again with the authorities. Having rebuked a foul-mouthed captain and started an altercation in Green Park, he was arrested and "confined about an hour in a darkish place" near the gate of St. James's Palace, and was only released when a friend provided surety of four or five shillings to an officer of the Board of Green Cloth.[81] Yet, apart from these fragmentary glimpses of Cruden's movements during the years between 1740 and 1752, there is a curious and conspicuous silence about this period in his own accounts (otherwise replete with minute details of his activities), and the surviving records have hitherto left these years shrouded in mystery. Cruden, it turns out, had something he regarded as so deeply discrediting that he sought by every means possible to conceal it: not confinement in an ordinary madhouse, for so far from covering up his incarceration in this sort of establishment, Cruden repeatedly did everything he possibly could to publicize these episodes; but something closely related that he saw as decidedly more stigmatizing. We shall defer revealing for the moment the source of his secret shame.

As the preceding recital has begun to suggest, Cruden was a person incapable of taking no for an answer, and in the months following the completion of his *Concordance,* his importunate and unwelcome attentions to a Mrs. Payne, "a Gentlewoman of a great fortune,"[82] had eventually led a Mr. Robert Wightman (possibly a financially interested protector, or a rival for her affections) to cart him off to confinement as a lunatic.[83] Shut up in every sense in the madhouse, he complained he was "Chained, Hand-Cuffed, Strait-Wastecoated . . . Imprisoned" and periodically abused by his keepers and routinely bled, vomited, and purged at the elder Monro's direction. At last, on 31 May, which was his birthday (and Cruden took omens of this sort very seriously), he made a dramatic escape. In the small hours of the morning, having sawed through a bed-leg with a table knife he had acquired, he scaled the madhouse wall (losing a slipper in the process). A strange kind of Cinderella, he

hobbled off barefoot and still in chains back to London, where he refused to shed his shackles till he had secured a legal order to do so from
the Lord Mayor of London![84]

Cruden considered his escape (like most momentous events in his life)
"Providential,"[85] and according to his own account had borne his
confinement and its associated beatings and mistreatment in "great
Serenity in his Mind, and trusted that God would bring him out of all
his Troubles."[86] Never one to be reticent about his religion, Cruden had
made no effort to disguise his expectations from those confining him,
and before long, his "enthusiasm" had prompted an extended interrogation from James Monro. Dramatizing this interview (to Monro's discredit) in his writings, Cruden portrayed the mad-doctor asking him to
explain

> how he expected to get out of this dismal place? The Prisoner answered, That
> he came thither with submission to the Will of God, and he waited God's
> time for his Deliverance. *Monro* said, Do you expect that a Miracle will be
> wrought for your Deliverance? The Prisoner replied, That he had writ to
> some persons of the first Rank, and if they did not assist him, he would write
> to others, in order to be sound in the use of Means. *Monro* was so unman-
> nerly as to enquire, To whom had he written? But the Prisoner told him, He
> knew that best himself.[87]

For James, the profession of such beliefs was itself a clear sign of mental disturbance, and he promptly informed Robert Wightman, the Edinburgh merchant who was responsible for Cruden's confinement, "that
the Prisoner was a Man of Sense and Learning, and of a good Education,
but that he was a great *Enthusiast;* and he believed that he thought that
God would send an Angel from Heaven, or would work some Miracle
for his Deliverance."[88]

Not long after, evidently worried by Cruden's threats to commence
a prosecution against him and his associates, Wightman allegedly attempted to get Alexander to sign an undertaking that he would absolve
and indemnify him of any wrongdoing, keep the peace, and remain at
his lodgings. Not surprisingly, Cruden refused the request, only to find
that considerable efforts were being made to get him removed to Bethlem. Indeed, the Corrector claimed that, during the months before and
even after his escape, Wightman, James Monro, and others were deter-
minedly discussing and attempting to negotiate his conveyance to that
hospital—efforts that were, he was convinced, part of the general plot
to get rid of him and silence his plans to prosecute his "tormentors." Just
as likely, however, the attempt to remove him to Bedlam was provoked

by a desire to make his confinement more secure and by doubts as to the ability, or willingness, of those who committed him to continue to pay to support him. In any event, Cruden made equally strenuous efforts to avoid this fate, writing letters both to the Bethlem governors and to his own parochial officers.[89]

Just how involved James Monro himself was in the initiatives to move Cruden to Bethlem is unclear. When the case came to court, he denied under oath that he was part of what Cruden referred to as the "BLIND-BENCH." Cruden, though, was convinced that Monro was a key member, if not "Chairman," of the "confederacy."[90] He also alleged that Monro had been present at a meeting in June or July of 1738, when he had attempted to establish that Cruden was still insane and had openly discussed sending him to Bethlem.[91] Whatever the truth of the matter, Monro must have been concerned to discover that, both before and after his escape, Cruden had secured the services of other physicians to testify to his sanity. These practitioners included the well-known Scottish doctor Alexander Stuart F.R.S. (d. 1742), who was a London private practitioner, Royal College of Physicians censor (1732 and 1741), and former physician to St. George's Hospital; a Dr. Robert Innes;[92] a Dr. Rogers;[93] and the eminent antiquary and London specialist on gout and the spleen, William Stukeley (1687–1765).[94]

The mounting contentiousness of Cruden's confinement may explain why Monro seems to have lost patience with his charge and become increasingly concerned to distance himself from the case. According to Cruden, on coming to Bethnal Green "as usual to visit his Patients" about a fortnight before the former's escape, Monro had told him that "he had nothing to say . . . nor anything to do with him."[95] Nevertheless, Monro evidently prescribed for Cruden on at least one subsequent occasion,[96] and his apparent desire and belief that he could be easily quit of the troublesome Corrector would prove to be wishful thinking.

Once he escaped, Cruden attempted to be as good as his word in carrying out his previous threats. The very public response to Monro's role in his confinement from the newly delivered Alexander was condemnation of James as corruptly in league with his captors. Rounding on his mad-doctor, Cruden hurled a whole series of personal insults at him.[97] More disturbing than verbal abuse from a discharged madman, Monro next found himself a joint defendant in a lawsuit in the King's Bench.[98] Cruden sought £10,000 in damages for "false imprisonment for nine weeks and six days at five pounds an hour, being £8280, and the assault and other damages at £1720."[99] James may have been exasperated—

and was certainly displeased—at being sued by his former patient. However, Cruden's claim that "Monro threatened to make his Servants beat the Person who served him with the Writ"[100] seems distinctly unlikely.[101]

The suit, not surprisingly, was unsuccessful. A herd of witnesses was mobilized and substantial quantities of evidence were introduced to prove that Cruden had indeed been insane. Characteristically, Alexander responded by condemning the whole proceedings as corrupt, denouncing the witnesses as liars and accusing his own attorney (Henry Jenkins) of being incompetent. Lest this had not sufficed to explain his defeat, he alleged that it had been Monro's friendship and "interest" with the judge that was ultimately decisive.[102]

John Monro had had some slight involvement in the aftermath of Cruden's 1738 confinement,[103] so one suspects that, when he was once again drawn into the Scot's affairs, he approached the case with more than a little ambivalence. He would not have been alone: Michael Duffield, the first madhouse-keeper asked to confine Alexander in 1753, declined the honor (and potential profits), expressly alarmed by his prospective patient's prior litigiousness. On this latest occasion, it was Alexander's own sister, Mrs. Isabella Wild, who sought his confinement, and his religious enthusiasms were even more directly implicated in his alleged madness.

By now convinced that God had called upon him to take the lead in suppressing licentiousness and immorality, the Corrector was "much affected by the many sins being committed in the public streets of London, particularly by the crying sin of profane swearing . . . and also . . . the great sin and evil of Sabbath-breaking." He "often rebuked in a meek manner those were openly guilty of that unprofitable sin." On "Monday the 10th of September 1753," however, in the neighborhood of Southampton Buildings, the fearless Cruden took matters much further: his censure of a group of young men fell upon deaf ears, and one of their number,

> with a shovel or spade in his hand, . . . was guilty of swearing in the presence of Alexander, which so greatly offended him that, contrary to his usual custom, he took his shovel and corrected him with some severity . . . [launching] an emblematical or typical battle . . . which was thought to have continued about an hour [leaving the Corrector somewhat the worse for wear].[104]

His sister being informed of the fight, and convinced that it signaled a revival of her brother's madness, promptly decided he required a new period of confinement. Despite the demurral of Duffield, the first person to whom she applied, his nephew Peter Inskip proved only too willing to welcome Alexander into his madhouse, "two doors beyond The three jolly Butchers in Little-Chelsea," where his new lodger professed himself to be "in great calmness and tranquillity of spirit, being intirely resigned to divine providence." [105]

Within a few days of his confinement, Cruden's complaints about inadequate observance of the Sabbath and his ostentatious bouts of public praying led his captors to view him as "extremely religious, which was judged by Inskip and some poor creatures round him to be a great sign of insanity" and in consequence, "the barbarous Inskip bound him very closely in the Strait-Wastecoat." [106] John Monro, called in for the first time on the fourth day of his confinement, listened gravely to Cruden's account of "the battle of Southampton," and then departed, apparently without prescribing for his patient, but taking the time to inform "Inskip that the Corrector had had an action at law against his father." [107] Every three or four days thereafter, Monro returned, occasionally prescribing the removal of some twelve ounces of blood and "some purging medicine" [108] and generally conversing

> in a very friendly manner: The Corrector thinks him a very valuable gentleman, of good capacity and genteel behaviour; but he perceived he has not studied deep in divinity. He would therefore advise him and other gentlemen of the profession to study the scriptures, to mind the concerns of their souls, and to pray for and earnestly to seek salvation through Jesus Christ. . . . [109]

On a number of his visits, we know that John questioned Cruden in considerable detail about his religious beliefs and their connections to his famous "battle," focusing particularly on Cruden's claim that his intervention had been in some sense "emblematical." Such language was associated with hints that the proofreader's actions had been symbolic of his personification of Christian virtue and his role as God's chosen instrument. [110] However, perhaps because of Cruden's prior confinement and treatment by Monro senior, he seems to have been well aware that such views were likely to be perceived as evidence of insanity, and when the younger Monro sought to explore this territory anew, his peculiar patient seems to have fenced and dissembled as best he could. When Monro asked, for instance, what he meant by terming himself a "Corrector," Cruden politely indicated that he was "declining conversation on that head" and sought to change the subject; [111] and on another occasion, questioned about his conviction in being Providentially chosen,

"Alexander told him that he would suspend his thoughts about these things."[112]

Not unreasonably, Cruden suspected that Monro's questions were a form of entrapment, designed "to intangle him." However, he was rather in a Catch-22 situation, for his refusal to answer Monro's "insnaring questions" almost certainly served only to confirm the mad-doctor's convictions about his delusive thinking.[113] The major difference between doctor and patient, as far as Cruden was concerned, was about religious matters. Monro, evidently, was firmly disposed to see Alexander's religious beliefs as delusions of grandeur and to doubt the very possibility of divine revelation and mission. Cruden, on the other hand, attempted to prove in conversation (as he strove latterly to do in his publications) that the mad-doctor was simply untutored in spiritual matters:

> In conversation the Corrector had sometimes the better of the argument with him, particularly in religious matters, and if the Corrector was his tutor he would teach him the very catechism or first principles of religion, the doctor not seeming to understand the chief design of the gospel and of divine revelation, namely, that it is a gracious constitution of God for the recovery of fallen sinful man thro' a mediator.[114]

Alexander, as usual, was oblivious to the fact that the effort to win this particular battle almost ensured that he would lose the war.

For Cruden's own recital of the case strongly suggests, though of course it cannot definitively show, that John was disposed to see Alexander's "enthusiasm"—the barely suppressed conviction that one had been specially singled out and specifically chosen to perform divine work—as prima facie evidence of mental imbalance. Essentially, on the basis of the information he elicited about these eccentric beliefs, Monro continued to uphold Cruden's confinement and to treat him for his "madness." Yet in the end, John seems to have seen him as basically harmless, and thus did not object when, on 29 September, Mrs. Isabella Wild abruptly decided to acquiesce to Cruden's release from custody.[115] Cruden, for his part, diplomatically still swallowed Monro's prescriptions for a few days following his liberation.[116]

For once, Cruden seems to have appreciated the younger Monro's forbearance, and on this occasion, when the proofreader sued for false confinement, the eminent mad-doctor did not find himself among the defendants. Rather, it was his sister Isabella Wild whom Cruden took to task, once, that is, she had rejected his initial proposal for a settlement (namely, acknowledging her "wickedness" in arranging his confinement). Cruden proposed by way of penance that she should spend two days in Newgate Prison, during which time, "I shall not omit praying that the confinement may be greatly sanctified to her, and may be a means of grace being bright'ned in her soul." [117] He had admonished his sister in similarly imperious terms "that he was like *Alexander the great* who used to set up a piece of a candle before a town; and if they submitted before it went out, then they had safety and protection; if not, they were put to the sword." [118] His warning going unheeded, he again brought suit for £10,000 in damages in the King's Bench, alleging against his sister and her husband, and Inskip and his "Chelsea-myrmidons,"

> that they did make an assault upon the Corrector and violently seize him in his bed at five o'clock in the morning, and him did evilly treat and imprison; and him contrary to the laws and customs of England against his will did detain; his letters and messages did stop and intercept and him from the assistance comfort and conversation of his friends and acquaintances did keep obstruct and hinder and cords and strait-wastecoat [*sic*] did put upon him, and for a long time did confine the plaintif, namely for the space of seventeen days and six hours from the 12th to the 29th of September 1753. By reason of which the plaintif is much injured in his reputation, calling and business and his constitution and health were [so] much weakened, that his life was in great danger. . . . [119]

The suit was heard in Westminster Hall on 20 February 1754.[120] To Cruden's dismay, however, still another campaign of "war at law" proved no more successful than its predecessor, notwithstanding his reiterated conviction that "God in his wise and wonderful Providence . . . designs that *Alexander* shall be a *Joseph* and after his humiliation a prosperous man." [121] Although John Monro was not himself summonsed to defend his conduct, he was nonetheless to appear as a key witness for the defense. Cruden's sister's lawyer, Goodwin (whom Alexander preferred to call "Bad-wine"), called only four witnesses and Monro was the last of these. He wasted little time in informing the court and offering substantive proof that, in his judgment, Cruden's confinement had been appropriate and necessary, and had exerted a beneficial effect on the eccentric Scot.

Cruden's account of Monro's testimony provides further evidence that John was something of a doubting Thomas toward his patients in religious matters. Alexander's general reports of previous conversations with Monro alluded to the mad-doctor's suspicions "that Alexander entertained some [insane] ideas of the Southampton-battle being only emblematical or typical, and that he gave way a little to the notion of emblems," [122] and this was very much the burden of the mad-doctor's remarks at the trial. Monro testified, for example, that he had asked "about him being a General" (an additional title Alexander had adopted as befitting his sense of being engaged in "the battle of Southampton" and other metaphorical campaigns against the enemies of his spiritual mission), and reported that "the Corrector [had] replied, that was to be as God pleased. The doctor and the Corrector differed about religion." [123] Taken as a whole, Monro's evidence demonstrates that he had paid particular attention to Cruden's faith in emblematic or symbolic happenings, and saw these as symptomatic of a settled mental disorder—an interpretation that very much accorded with a growing stress in contemporary medical writings on insanity as being characterized by a dominant delusion, a delusive subject, idées fixes, or the persistence of desultory and disordered ideas. At the trial, Monro also indicated that he regarded Cruden's speech as revealing a disturbed state of mind. His talk about religion, in particular, replete as it was with evasions, was characterized as fragmentary and disconnected. Cruden was particularly keen to contradict Monro on this point, insisting that "the Corrector's conversation [was] not broken, but connected." [124] These and other expostulations, however, failed to sway those listening to the proceedings. Having heard from Monro, the judge promptly ordered the jury to return a directed verdict for the defense, "which they did without going out of Court." [125]

Renewed rejection did not deter the relentless Cruden, who now became convinced that the Almighty had yet larger designs for him. His "darling scheme" involved the appointment of a "Corrector" or censor of the morals of the whole British nation—a people who, in his eyes, were clearly much in need of moral reformation. [126] With his new scheme lending urgency to his lobbying, Alexander began to haunt St. James's and other royal palaces. He dedicated one of his peculiar pamphlets (published in 1754 to protest his treatment as a madman) to the queen's son, "his Royal Highness William, Duke of Cumberland," God's instrument in preserving Protestantism and administering "the Death-stroke . . . to the cause of Jacobitism." [127] Convinced that his various "Afflictions are designed by Providence to be an Introduction and Preparation to his being a Joseph and an useful prosperous Man," [128] he made repeated, but vain, attempts to present this work to the king in person. When that failed, he sought to hand his precious papers to the courtiers, hoping they would intercede for him. Lord Poulet was apparently one of the few to receive a pamphlet, "for being goutish in his feet he could not run away from the Corrector, as others were afterwards apt to do." [129]

Undeterred, as always, Cruden now set out a rather more elaborate program for correcting Britain's morals, which he outlined in a further "memorial to king and parliament." Lamentably, he reminded them, "for many years, infidelity and impiety have greatly prevailed among his *Majesty's* subjects . . . [and] it is generally observed that atheism and vice increase more and more, if effectual means are not taken to stem the torrent of those two dreadful evils." [130] As it was, in the absence of a "Corrector," the country was awash with "profane swearers, Sabbath-breakers, lewd men and women, and other notorious sinners [and] a general want of a sense of religion among the People." [131] "And if we continue in our sins," he warned, "and provoke God to be against us, all our *ships of war* cannot protect us and deliver us from the power and tyranny of *France.*" [132]

Supposing that one accepted the need to re-moralize a nation wallowing in sin, a crucial issue arose: "Who shall be the *Corrector of the People?*" [133] It must, quite naturally, be someone of

> great integrity . . . of great meekness and a lover of peace . . . and he ought to act in a just and compassionate manner imitating the tenderness of a father to his children, and to have such a temper and conduct as may convince the People that his principal aim is their real happiness. [134]

Fortunately, just such a candidate was to hand: Alexander himself!

With what for him was unusual insight, Cruden acknowledged that some might immediately object to his appointment. After all,

> Alexander has been in the academies [madhouses] of Bethnal Green and Chelsea; and is he to be chosen Corrector of the People? To this it may be replied, That it is the ordinary method of Divine Providence to humble before he exalts, to cast down before he raises up; and the inspired Solomon says, Before honour is humility. [135]

It would not take but a moment's reflection for the unbiased observer to see that Alexander's tribulations fit precisely this pattern. He was, he assured both king and parliament, "an *extraordinary man*, whose history is hardly to be parallel'd for uncommon afflictions, and Providence's most graciously delivering him out of them." [136] And lest there be any remaining skeptics, he insisted that "Alexander is of the opinion that *Divine Providence* purposes to make him *Corrector of the People*" [137]— indeed, "I have been convinced since *September* 8, 1753, that God in his sovereign and gracious *Providence* hath [already] appointed me *Correc-*

tor of the People." He awaited only official confirmation through the passage of legislation by parliament and its endorsement by the king.[138] It would be a long wait.

Despite his apparent lack of progress, Cruden convinced himself also that he was predestined for a knighthood, an honor that he expected would come his way at any moment. Indeed, so sure was he of becoming Sir Alexander that, before his appearances at the king's levée, he took the precaution of hiding a £100 bill on his person so that he could promptly pay the associated fees.[139] A little later, with an eye to furthering his self-appointed crusade as the Corrector, he sought nomination for election as an MP for London, being convinced that his success on this front, or as a candidate—Dick Wittington-like—for Lord Mayor, had likewise been "foretold."[140] In the event, his candidacy was greeted with mirth and ridicule, and Cruden elected not to attend the poll.

In the months that followed, he took the opportunity presented by the case of Elizabeth Canning to once again sue (rather shamelessly) for "some token of honour and respect" and "even an yearly reward" from royalty, penning a memorial on the case to the king in his guise as the Corrector in June 1754.[141] Canning's arrest and Old Bailey trial for perjury, after she had been attacked, injured, and robbed in Moorfields and then falsely imprisoned on meager rations, had won widespread sympathy from eighteenth-century society, but must have struck a particularly resonant chord with Cruden. His memorial on her behalf not only appealed for a royal pardon for Canning, as other contemporary pamphlets had done, and for preferment for himself, but—with Cruden's typical audacity on sensitive politico-religious matters—lectured the king on his responsibilities as the divinely ordained ruler and head of England's Protestants.[142]

Contemporaneously with his intervention in the Canning affair, Cruden was once again making unwelcome advances to a woman of high birth. On this occasion, he ambitiously courted the attentions of the late Sir Thomas Abney's (1640–1722) daughter, and he gave an account of his rejection in still another pamphlet that formed the third part of his *Adventures*.[143]

Perhaps, on another occasion, the far from eligible Cruden's endless harassment of gentlewomen and his lobbying of the influential in support of his various schemes might have provoked still another involuntary sojourn in a madhouse. Certainly, he made a regular nuisance of himself in the corridors of power, and word of his eccentricities and escapades must certainly have reached Monro. Yet there is no sign that the eminent mad-doctor (or Cruden's sister, Mrs. Isabella Wild, come to that) was tempted in the least to be drawn back into the case by this renewed evidence of his one-time patient's "enthusiasms." One suspects that Monro may finally have learned his lesson from his family's prior encounters with this provoking, thoroughly tiresome, and maddeningly obsessive character.

THE "MADMAN" AND HIS MAD-DOCTORS

Previous accounts of Cruden have tended to concentrate on his first rather than his second private confinement in London, and have failed to provide any systematic comparison of the two events. These confinements at once resemble and differ from each other in some rather significant ways. Cruden's detention at Chelsea lasted just seventeen days (from 12 to 29 September 1753), and John Monro cooperated in his release. By contrast, his incarceration at Bethnal Green was prolonged over sixty-nine days (from 23 March to 31 May 1738), was only curtailed by his escape, and would have been extended even longer if James Monro had had his way. Whereas Cruden alleged that the Bethnal Green servants stole and extorted money from him, there is no evidence (or claim) of him being robbed in Inskip's house, when he was under John's care.[144]

At both madhouses, Cruden was placed under similar degrees of restraint and seclusion, including being strait-jacketed, chained, or strapped tightly to his bed. Likewise, many (though not all) of Cruden's letters were stopped at both Bethnal Green and Chelsea.[145] Nonetheless, while Cruden alleged that Inskip would treat not only himself, but the most sober member of the College of Physicians as "a Tom of Bedlam, by tormenting him with the Strait-Wastecoat and severe usage," during his stay at Bethnal Green he was apparently restrained more constantly (sometimes being chained to his bedstead through the whole "night and day"). In addition, he implied that James was being duped as to the severity of restraint being used by the servants, as it was always removed on the doctor's visits.[146] At Bethnal Green, Cruden incurred a ban on visitors, without ticketed authorization from his doctors and "captors," and went for weeks on end without being visited by anyone except those associated with the madhouse. One presumes that similar restrictions were imposed at Chelsea. Yet Cruden's own account makes it clear that neither ban was uniformly maintained. At times, he was visited quite frequently by friends and relations, with whom he was permitted to take tea. The implication is that his seclusion was not always as severe as he made out.[147] At Inskip's, in Chelsea, instances of visitors being turned away appear to have been less conspicuous, and ironically, one of the only individuals mentioned who did experience problems was the surgeon whom John Monro himself had sent to bleed Cruden. (The man with the lancet complained he had had "much difficulty" getting "access to the prisoner.")[148]

Again, his own account shows plainly that Cruden was allowed out on walks in the garden at both establishments, something that he did in company with John Monro at Chelsea, and that was instigated on his behalf at Bethnal Green on James Monro's explicit advice. While at Inskip's, Cruden was even permitted a temporary visit to Great Chelsea, under the watchful eye of his keepers. At Bethnal Green, by contrast, he was merely granted the occasional freedom of the parlor, and fears of him escaping meant that even these small liberties were usually compromised by his being placed under some form of mechanical restraint.[149]

Both doctors prescribed similar doses of purges, vomits, and bleeding, and Cruden alleged that both doctors dosed and bled him routinely and excessively, the bleeding James ordered from his foot leaving it "for some months after benumn'd," and John once ordering twelve ounces of blood to be taken.[150] Both Monros were also attacked as the prime representatives of a profession that Cruden had little respect for. The Corrector queried in 1739: ". . . is there so great Merit and Dexterity in being a mad Doctor? The common Prescriptions of a Bethlemetical Doctor are a Purge and a Vomit and a Purge over again, and sometimes Bleeding, which is no great Mystery."[151] And in 1754 he similarly observed:

> . . . tho' a person be not a conjuror he may set up to be a mad-doctor, the chief prescriptions being bleeding, purging, vomiting, and sometimes bathing: And if these are not effectual . . . the patient is incurable. . . . What is Dr. Monro? A mad-doctor; and pray what great matter is that? What can mad-doctors do? prescribe purging physic, letting of blood, a vomit, cold bath, and a regular diet? How many incurables are there? . . . physicians . . . are often poor helps; and if they mistake the distemper, which is not seldom the case, they do a deal of mischief.[152]

What John thought reciprocally of his odd patient is, unfortunately, only partially recorded, and then by Cruden rather than Monro himself.

Cruden claimed that during his time at Bethnal Green, he was the victim of "Blows and Wounds" from a keeper named Davis, whom he disdained as a "ruffian" and a yeoman. He subsequently complained of similar abuse while at Chelsea at the hands of a "brutal" and "bullying" ostler and keeper called Hare. The failure of either Monro to look deeply into, or remedy, such abuses was highlighted by Cruden as typifying their negligence.[153] In John's case, the alleged neglect was even more brazen, as he was said to have been unresponsive to his patient's explicit request to have the keeper "removed," seeming to believe that Cruden was simply complaining for the sake of it and that, if conceded to, "would soon want another change."[154] Despite Cruden's appeals and protests, the only alteration Monro recommended was for his patient to be bled and purged—although, being prescribed for did not displease the patient, who believed that cooperation in this area was the only way of getting "out of their clutches."[155]

Cruden's objections to his yeoman and ostler keepers seem very much about the offense they presented to his own self-perception and his opinion as to the kind of attendance a man of his station deserved—as much, in other words, about the perceived gap between his own and his keepers' social and educational status, as about the latter's actual character and competence. He referred to Hare, for example, as "an ignorant and country clown, fitter to take care of horses than men."[156] Yet one should not push the distinction too far, since the class and quality of attendance were matters apt to have been quite closely connected. Furthermore, Cruden was far from the only contemporary patient to object to the lowly nature of madhouse attendants, many of whom seem to have been recruited from the lower reaches of the social hierarchy, beneath even the rank of their patients' household servants.

As for medical attendance, according to Cruden, James "did not visit him till a Week after his Confinement" at Bethnal Green, and in total attended him just four times, while his "short visits" were "like a bird upon the wing."[157] One suspects, though, that the claim that James had "not so much Concern for them [his patients] as a Farrier hath for his Horses" is an exaggeration.[158] Certainly, Cruden was willing to acknowledge in print that John had been substantially more attentive than his father. His objections to the "impertinent" and "unmannerly" interrogations James carried out on him in 1738, which bordered on simply denying the appropriateness of a medical consultation, suggest how difficult the role of the mad-doctor was in such cases, even if Cruden was hardly alone among contemporary patients in feeling that his privacy and genteel status were not adequately respected by the mad-doctor's diagnostic probing. Cruden's decision to make James Monro a defendant in his 1739 lawsuit had evidently attracted criticism, both because it might be thought to have damaged his chances of success and presumably out of some sort of deference to the physician's social position and professional role. While this was something that Cruden was at pains to justify, his subsequent decision not to prosecute John may imply a more balanced assessment of the events of 1753.

Cruden's portrait of John's moral character was also, in some respects, significantly more sympathetic than what he had to say about James. In one of his 1739 publications, the devout Sabbatarian alleged that James Monro was "a common Swearer and an irreligious Man, who doth not cohabite with his Wife, and [is] of bad report as to his Chastity and Loyalty." [159] By contrast, Cruden "liked" John Monro "the better," "because he had heard that he was not a jacobite nor an adulterer, as was reported of a certain maddoctor [i.e., James Monro]." [160] Significantly, both here and in general, rather than seeking common ground with the Monros in their mutual Scottish ancestry, Cruden was at pains to assert his own orthodox national and social identity as a "British" or a "London Citizen" (by contrast with the Monros' Jacobite-tainted ancestry).[161]

Although Cruden pretended to be merely attacking James Monro's "character" and "Integrity," and "not [to] accuse him of want of Ability," perversely and emphatically he did both, dismissing the lawyers who had spoken "so well of" him in court and their claims that he had been "very useful in curing Lunaticks" as incompetent "judges of his business." [162] Cruden criticized James for being arrogant and rude toward him, and had said to James's face, putatively quoting another "eminent Physician . . . 'That Monro had been always on the severe side with his poor patients' . . . and . . . if he wanted a Physician, Monro should be the last man he would choose"; but he never seems to have charged John with harshness.[163] Whereas James was accused of prescribing medicine six days before actually seeing him and of failing to "enquire about its Operation," or at least always to ask the patient himself,[164] John was somewhat perversely criticized for not prescribing frequently enough and was actually "begged . . . to prescribe" by his contradictory patient—Cruden somewhat improbably suspecting that failure to do so would suit the mad-doctor and his other captors' interests in prolonging his confinement.[165]

In most respects, however, there was little to choose between Cruden's verdict on the performance of father and son, as indeed between his treatment at the different madhouses of an uncle and nephew. Cruden portrayed James Monro as "intirely Wightman's Creature" or

"Tool." [166] Meanwhile, although he spared John such severe accusations of conspiratorial prejudice, he still accused him of having "a natural bias to encourage his own business and to favour Mr. Duffield and his relations," and abused him as one of a number of "blind wrong headed creatures." [167] The fact that John had nevertheless declared him insane more or less obliged Cruden to convince himself that the doctor paid too much attention to "what Inskip told him" and that it was "interest" that "inclined him to wish his patients in disorder whether or not [they actually were]." [168] Cruden also accused both Monros of being more concerned with their profits than their patients, although allegedly John had trouble actually getting paid by Mrs. Wild and co. in 1753. [169]

CRUDEN'S FINAL CALL FROM GOD

Cruden continued, in the years that followed the public spectacle he had made of himself in the mid-1750s, to be entertained and indulged in high academic and social circles in Oxford, Cambridge, and London, partly on the strength of the fame of his *Concordance*. Yet he had become a figure of fun and entertainment for many of his dining companions, also finding himself the butt of some rather cruel practical jokes. On one notorious occasion, for instance, Cruden finally received his long-expected knighthood at Cambridge, in a mock ceremony performed by a "Miss Vertue"—a prank that the self-deluding Cruden allegedly took seriously.[170] Though some, like J. Neville of Emmanuel College, Cambridge, judged him "an extraordinary man," this was clearly a minority view. His erratic and grandiose behavior led most to a very different conclusion: "poor man (I pity him heartily) . . . [for he is] not . . . quite in his right mind." [171] Nevertheless, for all the teasing and mockery to which he was subjected, what seems just as remarkable as his relatively brief periods of confinement as a lunatic is the forgiving sympathy and free rein he was afforded in eighteenth-century society. Reactions to this most peculiar man provide striking evidence of the tolerance that existed at the time for quite extreme forms of eccentricity.

When the American mad-doctor Benjamin Rush saw Cruden in the 1760s, he certainly accepted that Cruden "had been deranged," as Rush understood it, "from hard study." By this time, however, Cruden seemed to be "in good health" and his philosophical reflections on what he now saw as the rather more occasional earthly operation of Providence plainly impressed Rush and suggest that Alexander had acquired a degree of objective distance as to the trials and tribulations of his life:

"God (said he) permits a great deal of the sin that is committed in this world to pass with impunity, to convince us that there is a day of Judgement, but he now and then punishes it, to convince us that he governs the world by his Providence." [172]

Others also remembered Cruden affectionately, but for rather different reasons, the Reverend E. Jones vividly recalling his "person, *full* dress, or *ad*-dress," and in self-deprecating fashion comparing his own vanity to that of "an old *Alexander the Corrector.*" Describing "the time that Dr Ashton brought him to dine in our College-hall at Eton," Jones also spoke of having in his possession some of Cruden's "*crazy Talvs* [*sic*—tales?] and querulous pages, with his offers to represent the *Laity* in Parliament," which he had purchased at the time, apparently by way of payment for Cruden's traveling expenses, "before I knew how much we should be indebted to him for his *Concordance.*" [173]

Even as he aged, Cruden continued to find new outlets for his enthusiasm. Six years on, recalling his earlier involvement with Canning and consistent with his unremitting identification with the plights of the incarcerated, Cruden took his mission to Newgate. After visiting and praying with a sailor called Richard Potter, condemned to be hanged for apparently unwitting involvement in forgery, Cruden successfully secured Potter's contrition and conversion, and the commutation of his sentence to transportation, triumphantly trumpeting the whole proceedings in yet another of his pamphlets, this one dated 1763.[174] At the same time, Cruden continued to pursue a number of further publication projects, including a second and third edition (in 1761 and 1769) of his *Concordance.*

Perhaps sensing that he was approaching the twilight of his life, in 1769 Alexander extended or diverted his mission as corrector back to his own origins, visiting his native Aberdeen to preach and promulgate his writings and publishing a last pamphlet urging his "deputy correctors" to redouble their efforts to reform the people.[175] Shortly after his return to London, on 1 November 1770, Cruden was to meet the final call from his maker. Unswervingly zealous to the end, he was found on his knees in the closet he had transformed into an altar, his corpse melodramatically frozen in the wholly characteristic act of praying.

A LAST JUDGMENT OF CRUDEN'S CASE

The trouble with Cruden's various accounts of his confinement and of his treatment at the hands of the Monros and others is that, by and large (in the apparent absence of surviving trial transcripts), we have no alternative version of those events and can largely only surmise the attitudes of his doctors from what he saw fit to say about them. Cruden was far from an unbiased or straightforwardly reliable witness, keen as he was to establish that his confinement had been unjust and his usage barbarous. His evidently obsessive tendencies, his rather inflated regard for his own importance, divinely mandated as he felt it to be, and his tendency to portray those who confined him as conspiratorial persecutors, might simply be put down, as they certainly were by the Monros and other contemporaries, to pathological (if not paranoid) suspicion and delusionary mental disorder.

Yet not only contemporary judgments but also modern verdicts on Cruden, by both psychiatrists and psychiatric historians, have been harsh and dismissive. It is not just that he has been portrayed as an unreliable narrator of the events of his own life because of his mental affliction, but that the content of his writings has been viewed (or rather disregarded) by some commentators solely through the prism of his presumed pathology. Parry-Jones, for example, accorded him little attention, contenting himself with the opinion that "the whole picture suggests an eccentric, grandiose, paranoid personality";[176] and Hunter and Macalpine similarly regarded him as a clear-cut case of paranoid mental derangement.[177] As we hope we have shown, however, there is much more than this to the Corrector. Cruden's mental disturbance (however evident and coloring of his experiences it seemed, or seems, to some) did not deprive him of his acute powers of perception and eloquence in reporting what had happened to him, gifts that he displayed in his writings in abundance. Nor should the supposed effects of his illness and subjectivity be permitted to negate the tremendous insights his writings offer, from the special vantage of the patient, into the mad-trade and into the practice of contemporary mad-doctors like John Monro and his father. Here is one of the few accounts we possess of a patient's view of the experience of being designated and confined as mad. Peterson criticized Cruden for his "biased" and "extreme" views, but nevertheless concluded that he "was treated arbitrarily, unfairly, and cruelly."[178] Porter's recent and fuller treatment represents a more nuanced picture, carefully examining both the excesses and the resonances in Cruden's often credible accounts of the Monros and the mad-trade.[179] Substantially following Porter, Ingram's recent analyses give Cruden credit for being "a genuinely pious, if fractious and showy man," and point to the ultimate irrelevance or unanswerability of questions as to just how mad

Cruden really was. More pertinent, Ingram suggests, are such questions as to what extent and why he was regarded as crazy by contemporaries, and how Cruden presented his case in an effort to refute such claims.[180]

In examining these questions, any attempt at a balanced assessment must recognize that Cruden's writings patently distort and exaggerate (if not invent) the record in places, and fail ever to concede a fault on his own part. They also avoid emphasizing, or even mentioning, events that are at odds with Cruden's presentation of himself as injured victim, or those that he himself saw as undermining his claim to be a trustworthy witness to his own persecution. Here we return, at last, to the substantial hiatus during the 1740s in Cruden's narration of his life story, the mysterious and discrediting secret that we mentioned earlier.

For there is one ironic fact in particular that Cruden was evidently determined to suppress: namely, that—despite and in realization of his earlier fears on this front—he was indeed admitted to Bethlem during the period between his confinements at Bethnal Green and Chelsea. To be Bedlam mad was, in Cruden's eyes (and not his alone!), the ultimate defacement of one's social identity, the clearest signal to others of the loss of all social respectability and trustworthiness. Small wonder that this episode of incarceration never merited a mention in his relentless pamphleteering! Nonetheless, quietly testifying to the conspicuousness of Cruden's ellipsis of narrative, the Bethlem Admission Registers record his reception on 17 December 1743, under the treasurer's warrant, his parish of residence as Enfield, Middlesex, and his discharge on 3 March the following year, his condition (as usual) going unrecorded.[181]

Given that Cruden had been working as a private usher in the Enfield district (which he described to Hans Sloane as thoroughly à la mode, boasting almost fifty private coaches), there seems little doubt of the accuracy of this record.[182] Cruden's silence about this period is plainly a significant omission. It provides, as we have suggested, wordless but eloquent testimony to his profound anxiety about the stigma of public lunatic hospitals, and it demonstrates convincingly the selectivity of his published accounts of his life as a lunatic. As early as 1738, Cruden had expressed his terror of such a fate (of which he had portrayed James Monro as a major proponent): "for he was perhaps more afraid of Bethlehem than of death," believing that it would render him and his works "despicable" and signal the end to his reputation and "Usefulness."[183] However, we can only speculate about whether Cruden was right or wrong in this belief. For the closed character of Bethlem's records (and James and John Monro's decisions not to broadcast this discrediting fact about their tormenting sometime patient) kept the relevant information safely hidden for more than 250 years.

Cruden's fears, even if they came partially true, were perhaps rather melodramatic and extreme, though many contemporaries of genteel sensibilities expressed similar dread at the prospect of Bedlam. Cruden had entertained virtually indistinguishable concerns about being sent to private madhouses, and likewise was to report almost identical fears of plans afoot five weeks after his release from Inskip's in 1753 to send him to St. Luke's. The day before his discharge from Chelsea, Cruden had debated this question with John Monro at some length, denouncing the madhouse as "a place of humiliation" and his presence there "a dishonour for one of his character." Monro's attempts to convince him otherwise, when, as Cruden declared, "the world generally judged so," were predictably unavailing.[184] Cruden, not surprisingly, insisted that he would have preferred to take what medical advice he chose at his own lodgings. After his release, Cruden likewise referred to St. Luke's as a "dishonourable" and "dreadful place," allegedly informing the hospital's own secretary "that he would rather give all he was worth than be carried [there]." [185] As with many people from the "respectable" classes, part of what had bothered Cruden about Bethnal Green, as also about the prospect of going to Bethlem or St. Luke's, had been fear of being degraded and losing his social identity as a result of being associated with other patients of a lowly or pauper grade. (Inskip's Chelsea madhouse was a much smaller establishment, without a distinct pauper block, so that there was less occasion for this eventuality or anxiety.)

It would be a mistake, obviously, to underestimate the strength of the stigma attached to most forms of confinement in a madhouse in this period. Yet it would be equally wrong to focus only on its symbolic effects, for confinement had consequences beyond those to a person's character. Indeed, every bit as significant as the impact on one's social standing and identity could be the damage thus inflicted on one's health and employability. After his discharge from Bethnal Green, for example, Cruden complained that he had been "much injured," not only in "Reputation," but "in his Calling . . . and Business; and his Constitution, Health and Strength were, and still are very much weaken'd and impair'd." [186] Such claims are difficult to dispute. The description Cruden provides of his physical mistreatment is sufficiently vivid and substantiated with circumstantial detail, and the debilitating effect of a régime of heroic bleeding and purging so abundantly obvious, as to leave little doubt of the repercussions on anyone's health and stamina. Although Cruden seems to have exaggerated the point in additionally alleging that "his Body [was] so much wounded that his Life was in great danger," in fact he was merely repeating a standard legal formulation of words that one finds in a number of other contemporary cases claiming damages for personal injuries.[187]

Cruden's suggestions, more generally, that the Monros were unappreciative to the point of "prejudice" against his spiritual mission and sensibilities, and that they were negligent in their scrutiny and treatment of his case and the way he was cared for by the madhouse-keepers, carry more conviction than some of his other allegations. They coincide with what we may gather about the style of the Monros' attendance on the insane from other contemporary sources. Horace Walpole jocularly observed in 1794 that he "would be sorry to have it thought hereafter that I had ever been under the care of Dr [John] Monro."[188] Cruden's case demonstrates that, at least on some occasions, patients had more than reasons of reputation to regret the mad-doctor's attendance.

Mad as a Lord

*Monro and the Case
of the Earl of Orford*

Patty, I like this doctor don't you? We will have him next time. . . .

> Lord Orford to his mistress, speaking
> of John Monro (1778)[1]

. . . both the physicians were good, but their medicines would signify
nothing: . . . he [Orford] did not know what was the matter with
him, but he himself must struggle with it. . . .

> Lord Orford, as paraphrased
> by Horace Walpole (1777)[2]

While they sit a picking Straws
Let them rave of making Laws;
While they never hold their Tongue,
Let them dabble in their Dung . . .
Let them with their gosling Quills
Scribble senseless Heads of Bills;
. . . Let Sir T— that rampant Ass,
Stuff his Guts with Flax and Grass;
But before the Priest he fleeces
Tear the Bible all to Pieces . . .
Those are A—s, Jack and Bob,
First in every wicked Jobb,
Son and Brother to a Queer,
Brainsick Brute, they call a Peer . . .

> Jonathan Swift,
> *The Legion Club* (1736)[3]

LUNACY AND THE MONEYED CLASSES

Physicians who catered to the whims and welfare of the wealthy had long found themselves consulted about the problems associated with the presence of lunacy in the families from whom they made their livings. The moneyed classes were, of course, no more exempt from the travails madness brought in its train than any other segment of society, though they could afford levels of assistance and ways of providing for their disturbed relations that were self-evidently out of the reach of the masses. As with all forms of illness, their preference was for treatment at home or some close facsimile thereof, where they could maintain a semblance of control over the proceedings. Where madness was concerned, however, the dishonor and stigma it brought in its train provided families with a powerful additional motive for sequestering the sufferer within a situation that approximated the domestic circle, helping to control gossip and publicity about the source of their shame. Throughout the eighteenth century and into the nineteenth, therefore, general physicians found themselves consulted about insanity and its treatment in the regular course of their ministrations to their aristocratic and upper middle class clientele. As late as the 1820s and 1830s, even in the face of growing social and legal disapproval, society physicians like Halford, Seymour, Baillie, Hue, and Tierney continued to participate in this long-established tradition of home care. Their private practices incorporated a good deal of contact with the insane, and as a matter of routine, they derived some of their fees from the provision of discreet advice and treatment for such mad folk.[4]

In affluent circles, as one would therefore expect, the gradual emergence over the course of the eighteenth century of a small coterie of physicians specializing in lunacy modified, but did not fundamentally alter, these traditional patterns of practice. Over time, it simply became increasingly common, as and when prominent metropolitan medical men were summoned to the households of worthy, but distracted, citizens, or to assist their provincial brethren in the diagnosis and management of the mad, for one of the more celebrated mad-doctors to be brought in on the consultation and asked for his advice. As the most prominent among such specialists in Georgian London, John Monro and William Battie derived much of their income from their involvement in cases of this sort. Of course, if the lunatic proved unusually troublesome, recalcitrant, or dangerous, even the very wealthy might be tempted to avail themselves of the services of one of the new madhouses that, since the late seventeenth century in particular, had sprung up like wildfire in and around the city. In these circumstances, Monro and Battie profited by referring the patient to the madhouse with which they had established connections. More usually, however, ministering to affluent patients in their own homes provided the mad-doctors with highly lucrative opportunities to peddle their wares, sometimes attending individual cases for months or even years at a time.

Of course, this was not merely a matter of making a medical living and plying a trade, for the mad-doctor and the madhouse offered families a distinctive and desirable service at a time when irrational behavior appeared—perhaps, as never before—to be a threat to the integrity, status, and financial security of the household. Most practitioners claimed—to be sure, at a price—to be able to offer a cure, and the restoration of a distressed family member to his or her place in society. At the very least, they offered genteel families a certain degree of assurance that they were (and would be perceived to be) doing the right thing, and taking the finest available advice. (After all, good advice was something that cost, and was best bought from practitioners of superior social standing and education.) The emerging group of specialist practitioners thus promised to provide, if not the restoration of the sufferer to sanity, then some sort of relief and respite from the burden, anxiety, and embarrassment such deranged and difficult individuals might cause.

Fortunately, we have particularly detailed information on Monro's and Battie's involvement with one such patient, George Walpole (1730–91), the third earl of Orford and the grandson of the Whig grandee Sir Robert Walpole, England's longest serving prime minister. To be sure, what we know of Lord Orford's madness and its treatment comes very largely from a single source, his uncle, Horace Walpole (1717–97) (later the fourth earl), and his immediate circle of correspondents, includ-

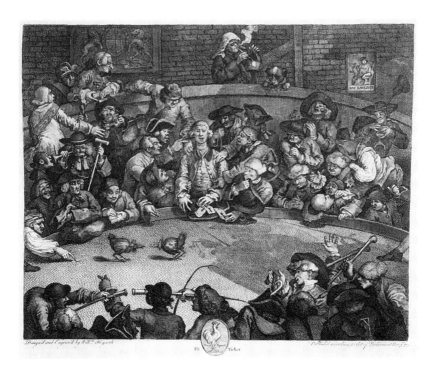

FIGURE 19. Hogarth's *The Cockpit* (1759). The blind Lord Albermarle Bertie is shown betting away his fortune on a contest whose likely outcome he can neither see nor (therefore) forecast, surrounded by a predatory gang of commoners who deride his disability and lack of judgment while exploiting his frailties in order to fleece him of his money. His lordship is thus represented as being dragged down to the idiotic level of the masses, foolishly putting his faith in blind fortune. Reproduced by kind permission of The Wellcome Trust.

ing Orford's other uncle (and Horace's brother), Sir Edward Walpole (1706–84). We have no immediate access to Monro's own views (or, for that matter, the views of any other practitioner), nor are we able to be sure precisely how Orford felt about his treatment at Monro's and his uncles' hands. We are forced, therefore, to reconstruct Monro's and Orford's attitudes and actions indirectly, via accounts that are inevitably prejudiced toward justifying the circumstances surrounding the confinements. Nonetheless, as the most famous and prodigious letter writer of his age, Horace could be relied upon to comment at revealing length (however subjectively), on matters both great and small, and the de-

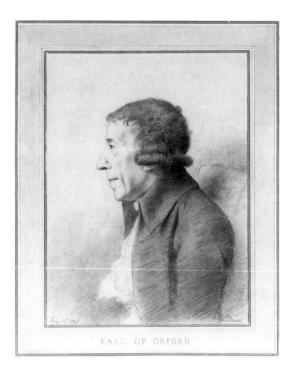

EARL OF ORFORD

FIGURE 20. Portrait of Horace Walpole (1717–97), the fourth Earl Orford, in old age, drawn in pencil by George Dance the Younger (1741–1825) in 1793. Reproduced by kind permission of the National Portrait Gallery, London, Heinz Library and Archive.

rangement of his own nephew is naturally something he discussed in intimate detail.

From any available vantage point, there is scant evidence that Monro ever substantially disagreed with Walpole as to his nephew's care. Indeed, Monro appears to have been thoroughly and rather unquestioningly prepared to put himself at Walpole's disposal, his style of practice seeming to exemplify the relationship Jewson posited as so characteristic of eighteenth-century medicine, by which doctors were heavily dependent on their patrons.[5] Orford's case thus provides us with a privileged view of mad-doctoring and of the domestic handling of insanity among the rich and powerful—albeit one that (because of its authorship) substantially deprives both the mad-doctor and the patient of agency.

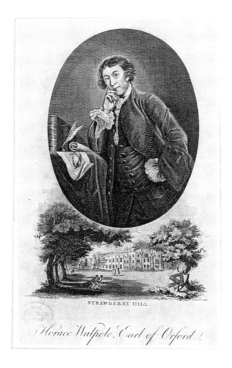

FIGURE 21. Another portrait of Horace Walpole, drawn in pencil by W. Evans (either William Evans of Bristol [1809–58] or William Evans of Eton [1798–1877]), showing Walpole in his later years, and beneath him the family home at Strawberry Hill. The inclusion of the family shield and crest emphasizes the importance of family identity to him. Reproduced by kind permission of the Ashmolean Museum, Oxford.

THE MADNESS OF A WHIG GRANDEE

Lord Orford's illness appears to have had three more or less distinct phases. It first manifested itself at the beginning of 1773, when he was treated by Robert Glynn, a Cambridge physician (later Clobery) (1719–1800), and Russell Plumptre (1709–93), the Cambridge Regius Professor of Medicine.[6] Once he was diagnosed as suffering from "insanity," however, these doctors were soon joined by Monro's rival in mad-doctoring, William Battie, and by another well-known London private practitioner (a former Cambridge theologian and rector of Ovington), John Jebb (1736–86).[7] It was apparently not until a second bout of

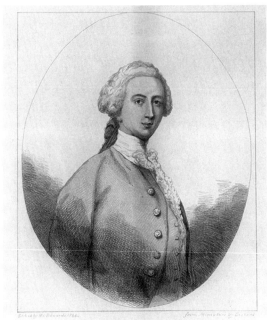

THE RIGHT HON. GEORGE WALPOLE, THIRD EARL OF ORFORD.
LORD LIEUTENANT OF NORFOLK 1756.

FIGURE 22. *The Right Hon. George Walpole, Third Earl of Orford. Lord Lieutenant of Norfolk 1756* (1844), engraving etched by W. C. Edwards, after miniature by Liotard. Reproduced here by kind permission of the National Portrait Gallery, London, Heinz Archive and Library, NPG Engravings Reserve, No. 40635.

mental derangement in 1777–78 that Monro was eventually called in (Battie having died the year before).[8] He jointly attended with Jebb. By the time of Orford's third attack in 1791, Monro was evidently too old and ill to attend, and his son Thomas replaced him.

The surviving evidence suggests that there was little significant difference between Orford's treatment by Battie and his cohorts and the approach adopted by Monro and Jebb at the time of the second attack. If anything, notwithstanding Battie's gestures about "mildness" in his *Treatise,* the methods employed during 1773–74 were somewhat harsher than those Monro adopted. Battie and Jebb (as Monro and Jebb were

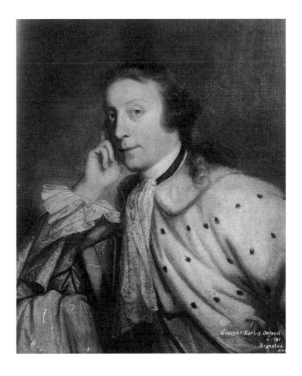

FIGURE 23. Portrait (framed) of George Walpole, third earl of Orford, by Sir Joshua Reynolds (ca. 1751). Oil on canvas. Reproduced by kind permission of the National Portrait Gallery, London, Heinz Archive and Library, NPG No. 384/10.

later to do) recommended a close domicilary confinement in London, isolation from friends and social gatherings, and the imposition of the rod of restraint and coercion whenever those in attendance felt it was necessary.

At the time of his first breakdown in 1773, Orford's illness clearly manifested itself to Walpole in the traditional style of the lunatic wasting his estate. Hurrying to Houghton, Orford's country seat, in the immediate aftermath of the crisis, Horace was dismayed to find

> a scene infinitely more mortifying than I expected; though I certainly did not go with a prospect of finding a land flowing with milk and honey. Except the pictures, which are in the finest preservation, and the woods, which are become forests, all the rest is ruin, desolation, confusion, disorder, debts,

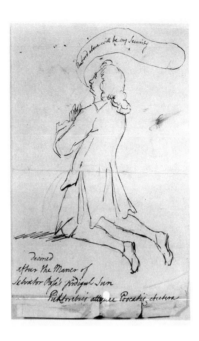

FIGURE 24. Caricature of Orford, drawn by George Townshend (mid-eighteenth century, ca. 1751–58). Pen and ink, by one of the most renowned caricaturists of the day, the MP, Lieutenant General and General Governor of Ireland and later Earl of Leicester, George, Fourth Viscount and First Marquess Townshend (1724–1807). Townshend is regularly (and rather acidly) referred to in Horace Walpole's correspondence. He was also formerly a leader of the Norfolk Militia, and Orford's odd conduct as Lord Lieutenant of Norfolk and colonel of the Norwich Militia must have been only too familiar to him (see, e.g., Colonel William Windham and George Townshend, *A Plan of Discipline, Composed for the Use of the Militia of the County of Norfolk* [London: 1759 and 1760]). His drawing depicts Orford as a mad enthusiast on his knees in prayer, exclaiming, "The Lord above will be my Security," possibly satirically implying that nobody else could be found who would. It was "desined [*sic*] after the Maner [*sic*] of Salvator Rosa's prodigal Sun [*sic*] Pictorebiis attquee Poeatis, etcetera." This Latin motto, meaning "Pictures as Poetry, etc.," seems to derive from Horace ("*Ut Pictura Poesis erit, similisque Poesi, Sit Pictura*"—As a picture is a poem, similarly poetry is a picture) and from the view "that a Poem should be a *Speaking Picture,* and . . . a Picture should be a *Living Poem*" ("Of Painting," *London Magazine* [June 1732], pp. 788–89). Rosa (1615–73) was himself renowned as a frenzied artist and dabbler in black magic, so that anything modeled on his work, or literally "Salvatorean," was jocularly regarded as crazy or diabolical (see, e.g., Lady Sydney Morgan, *The Life and Times of Salvator Rosa* [London: Colburn, 1824]; Jonathan Scott, *Salvator Rosa: His Life and Times* [New Haven and London: Yale University Press, 1995]; Salvator Rosa [pseud.], *The Group; Composed of the Most Shocking Figures, Though the Greatest in the Nation: Painted in an Elegy on the Saddest Subjects, the Living, Dead, and Damned . . .* [London: For the author, 1763]. For an example of a number of similarly framed contemporary literary skits on the prodigal son parable, see Joseph Flower, *The Prodigal Son: a Poem . . . ,* 2nd ed., with additions [Bath: 1750]). Reproduced here by the kind permission of the National Portrait Gallery, London, Heinz Archive and Library, NPG No. 4855 (66).

mortgages, sales, pillage, villainy, waste, folly, and madness. I do not believe that five thousand pounds would put the house and buildings into good repair. The nettles and brambles in the park are up to your shoulders; horses have been turned into the garden, and banditti lodged in every cottage. The perpetuity of livings that come up to the park-pales have been sold—and every farm let for half its value.[9]

Orford was confined at his uncle's command in a Hampstead house (Hampstead being generally perceived, at that time, to have all the advantages of a pure country environment in easy reach of the city). When at his worst, or in "his fit" (as those who attended him called it), Orford was "forced to be confined in his bed at night, and pinioned in the day" in order to prevent him escaping or harming himself "as he incessantly tries [to do]."[10] His refusal to eat was countered by force-feeding with broth. Only later, when he was perceived to be convalescing, was this management somewhat relaxed, being replaced by a regimen chiefly distinguished by persuasive means designed to secure isolation, a suspension of communication with others, calm, and dietary moderation. The doctors made Orford promise to keep "himself cool and quiet for some time, neither writing letters nor seeing company."[11]

Yet, even on this occasion, neither Horace Walpole's, nor the physicians', control over his treatment was complete. During this period, for example, some of Orford's friends visited and insisted on taking him "into company, extremely with the disapprobation of his physicians," following which the medical men agitated for "authority to use more restraint."[12] Walpole himself blamed Orford's mental disease on his nephew's rash self-dosing with quack remedies and his disregard for orthodox medical advice. Equally salient, as Walpole saw it, were Orford's exposure to the cold of the country air, and the overindulgence of his appetites and whims (encouraged, he thought, by Orford's dubious acquaintances).[13] Clearly he was partially echoing Battie and the other physicians here, and Walpole was to continue to censure his nephew's stubborn, if intermittent, propensity to ignore medical advice, to observe "no regimen," and to eat and drink "intemperately" as time went on.[14]

Battie and Jebb declared Orford successfully recovered at the end of December 1773, although Battie took the precautionary measure of waiting a month for signs of relapse before quitting the case. Yet Walpole was not convinced, even at the outset, that the "recovery" was permanent. On being informed that his unstable nephew was fit to be at large, concerned with his own and his brother, Sir Edward's, reputation, Walpole bemoaned the "frightful," or no-win, "situation" he felt himself in. He could not continue to insist on Orford's confinement, no matter his own conviction that the earl would neither recover nor get well, "for nobody can restrain him, if the physicians pronounce him in his senses; and if he does mischief to himself or others, there will not be wanting kind friends to blame me for setting him free." [15] Recalling this same predicament a few years later when his nephew fell ill once more, Walpole stressed how they "threw open his [Orford's] doors," and had been obliged to do so, despite believing him still insane. As proof of his deranged mental state at that time, Walpole related a catalogue of Orford's eccentricities once he was set at large. The rather mild nature of these excesses may suggest that Walpole was prone to overstate the case. One should note, however, his rapier-like wit, here employed to make fun of his nephew's infirmities. Ever the clever correspondent, Walpole sought almost by reflex to divert and entertain.

> I attended him to Houghton, and saw nothing but evidence of distraction. The gentlemen of the country came to congratulate his recovery; yet, for more than six weeks, he would do nothing but speak in the lowest voice, and would whisper to them at the length of the table, when the person next to him could not distinguish what he said. Every evening, precisely at the same hour, sitting round a table, he would join his forehead to his mistress's (who is forty, red-faced, and with black teeth, and with whom he has slept every night these twenty years), and there they would sit for a quarter of an hour, like two paroquets, without speaking. Every night, from seven to nine, he regularly, for the whole fortnight, made his secretary of militia, an old drunken, broken tradesman, read Statius to the whole company, though the man could not hiccup the right quantity of syllables. [16]

Speaking once again of this first attack in the 1790s in conversation with Joseph Farington, Walpole claimed that he was "not surprised when he first heard of his [Orford's] madness in 1773, as many singularities had prepared him for it." [17] This conversation alerts us to a vital fact that helps further to contextualize the attitude of Orford's uncles to his illness. For, according to Farington, Horace Walpole confessed that he was "well convinced" that Orford was not even related to him by blood, and that, rather than being "the Son of my Brother [Sir Robert Walpole]," Orford was the bastard son of an adulterous affair between Sir Henry Oxenden and Lady Orford. [18] Indeed, Horace reckoned that his father (the elder Sir Robert), likewise, did not "believe his *nominal grandson* to be *really His descendant.*" [19] These circumstances provide an essential means of accounting for Walpole's tendency toward negative assessments of his nephew's behavior and mental powers, which verged at times on doubly disowning him. On the one hand, Orford's

dubious birth rights made it possible and desirable for the other Walpoles to see his madness as a constitutional matter. On the other hand,
his madness provided them with a further reason for dissociating themselves from him in private, while careful in public to display a fastidious
regard for him. Contemporary mad-doctors seem to have been becoming more concerned about the transmission of hereditary taint as the
eighteenth century progressed, William Pargeter, for example, emphasizing the dangers "when Madness exists in the blood of families, and
shews itself regularly in the several branches of the pedigree" and "denouncing those who engage in" or "encourage . . . alliances" and "matrimonial contracts" with such families as "enemies to their country." [20]
Rather than some kind of runt in the litter impugning the integrity of
the household, however, Orford could, to some extent, be discreetly dismissed as neither in blood nor in nature a true Walpole. In related fashion, Horace was similarly censorious of Orford's mother, whom he referred to as an "extremely vicious" person who "solicited men." [21]

Nevertheless, Horace's experience of his nephew's earlier illness and
continuing odd behavior probably made him all the more prepared for
a renewed bout in 1777, and (even if he suspected that Orford was
related to him only in name) he was far from being disposed to eschew
responsibility for his relative's conduct and health. When the second
breakdown came to light, however, Orford was residing with friends in
the country at the Eriswell parsonage, near Mildenhall, in Suffolk, and
the greater distance decidedly complicated his uncle's attempt to manage the case. From Walpole's point of view, there were a variety of reasons to be concerned about the situation. At first blush, rural residence
might seem preferable, a means of restricting the scope of society gossip;
but in reality, being in the provinces provided no guarantee of avoiding
scandal. The country was still a very public place, with established nobility and gentry—those Walpole called "the gentlemen of the country" [22]—abounding in their country seats. (Even the continent provided
no safe haven from society gossip, when half the gentry was there during the summer.)

Orford's country residence placed him in an environment that allowed freer rein for eccentric conduct, and Walpole made it plain that
he was distinctly uncomfortable about the amount of freedom of movement his nephew was being allowed in the Eriswell setting. He worried
that the patient might escape or commit some sort of violence, and he
was adamant that little had been or could be done for him there in the
way of specialist medical treatment. Walpole complained vehemently,

furthermore, that his nephew's intimates and servants, whom he described as "low wretches," had hidden the relapse from himself and from London society, and that the delay in seeking care had worsened his "symptoms till they were terrifying." [23]

When he summoned Monro and others to examine and minister to Orford, Walpole clearly considered himself to be making an appropriate effort to secure "the best physical [i.e., medical] advice" for his nephew.[24] Now that Battie was dead, Monro was evidently perceived as the next most obvious and appropriate choice within a small range of leading contemporary mad-doctors in the metropolis. Yet Walpole's enlistment of the services of such elite London physicians was not merely a matter of doing what was in the best interests of his sick relation. His appeal to Horace Mann to "imagine [not Orford's plight but] what I suffered!" is one of many indications that Walpole was inclined to put his own feelings before those of his nephew.[25] Throughout the weeks that followed, as he deployed financial and professional muscle to restrict his nephew's movements, Walpole was attempting to wrest control of Orford away from friends and relatives whose management of the case he disapproved of. He was mortified by the thought of the potential and actual embarrassment his mad nephew's conduct could bring in its train were Orford insufficiently restrained.[26] His letters to friends like Horace Mann repeatedly emphasize his efforts to "preserve" or "save" the family "from ruin"—motives that his correspondents undoubtedly would have found understandable, even admirable, given the weight men of their class placed on family integrity and reputation.[27]

Walpole's decision to hire Monro and get the "best" doctors to attend his nephew's bedside was a more or less self-conscious sociocultural strategy, serving to demonstrate to elite society that he was behaving responsibly, judiciously, and as a gentleman, not resorting to the quackish alternatives that might be favored by the ignorant, the poor, and the low-bred. Throughout his nephew's periods of confinement, Walpole heard the rumors that he and his brother were financially motivated, and Orford himself at times voiced suspicions that his uncles were "looking to reversions." [28] Such concerns arose almost inevitably in cases of mental derangement among the wealthy and famous, and the Walpole brothers did what they could to defuse them, stressing how "unwilling" they were "to take direction of his affairs" as early as April 1773—a gentlemanly reluctance Horace reemphasized several times in the months and years that followed.[29] Walpole was certainly tempted to seek legal advice and obtain a commission of lunacy, the

complicated Chancery procedure for declaring someone mentally incompetent. However the trouble he anticipated and had already encountered, together with Orford's intermittent hostility toward him,
ultimately persuaded him to drop the idea—a decision that, he subsequently claimed, was motivated by consideration rather than prudence:
"my brother and I have too much tenderness and delicacy to take out
the statute of lunacy." [30]

Even without the legal authority an inquisition would have granted
him, for a brief period during his nephew's first illness Walpole played
a hand in his financial affairs. At the time of the second breakdown, he
was insisting that, during his earlier assumption of control, he "had
greatly improved his [nephew's] fortune, and should have effected more,
had [Orford] not instantly taken everything out of my hands" once the
doctors pronounced him sane. [31] Yet neither his scrupulous management
of the estate nor his protestations about the reluctance with which he
had intervened to confine his relation could deflect suspicion. Evidently
stung by society gossip about his conduct and motives, Walpole conceived that he could still the wagging tongues by making a public display of his concern for his nephew—if need be, paradoxically enough,
by making a veritable public spectacle of him. Somewhat petulantly, he
declared that he "would place him in the face of the whole town, where
everybody might see or learn the care that was taken of him." [32] This
proposal, while fueled by his feelings of being unjustly misrepresented
in society, was made for the sake of his own standing in London and
hardly reflects well on Walpole's unselfishness. Whatever sympathy one
is tempted to muster for Walpole's anxieties concerning the table-talk
about himself, his family, and his mad nephew is substantially offset by
the evidence that litters his correspondence showing that he was as much
an author of gossip about the mad and the bad as he was a victim of it.

HOW TO TREAT A LORD

Evidently, as soon as he sought medical counsel about Orford's illness in
1777, Walpole was strongly advised by Drs. Monro and Jebb that his
"very mad" nephew should "be brought immediately to town"—advice
that, as we have seen, was in line with his own preferences in the matter. Such a recommendation appears orthodox and unsurprising in medical terms too: it was consistent with Monro's general stress in his practice on the need to confine the deranged, to assume authority over each
case and to maintain a relatively strict medical regimen if one was to

have any chance of effecting a recovery. On trying to implement this advice, however, Walpole encountered staunch opposition from Orford's mistress, Mrs. Martha Turk (ca. 1737–91), from one of Orford's stewards (probably a William Withers, described as a "rascal" by Walpole), and from an anonymous neighboring parson, who "cried out I should kill him if I conveyed him [to London] from that paradise."[33] Orford's other steward (who was also his attorney and accountant), Carlos Cony (ca. 1774–91), also joined the chorus.

Walpole's imperious response, that they had "concealed the illness to the last moment they could"; that he "had never heard of a madman being consulted on the place of his habitation";[34] and that the doctors he had consulted were "not to be doubted,"[35] is suggestive of his arrogant, rumbustious character. More than this, however, it reflects the common tendency to dismiss more or less out of hand the personal preferences of the mentally afflicted. Like many others, Walpole appears to have seen the mad as the most unreliable judges of their own best interests. When, for example, those at Eriswell justified not calling in a physician to Orford because he himself "has no [i.e., a bad] opinion of physicians," Walpole castigated their decision as preposterous, for to take seriously the view of "a lunatic" was ipso facto absurd.[36]

One should scarcely be surprised, of course, to discover that disputes erupted about how to deal with Orford's erratic and alarming behavior, for it was assuredly not atypical for both madness itself, and the interventions of medical specialists like Monro, to cause profound dislocations and strains in familial and interpersonal relations. On the one hand, this case illustrates the dangers with which removing the sick were, or were deemed to be, attended. On the other hand, it alerts us to how lodging a deranged individual with his friends in the country might appeal to some as a means of hiding the illness. The whole sequence of events accents the highly contested negotiations that often surrounded decisions to confine family members as insane in different arenas, and demonstrates how various factions might seek to deploy medical knowledge for their own purposes. Nor were the judgments the different parties reached necessarily stable ones over time: there is some evidence, for instance, that even Orford himself wavered in his objections to the methods and attendance of the physicians his uncle had summoned. Walpole reported him on one occasion in 1778—in conversation with the mistress his uncle sardonically termed "his Dalilah" [sic]—"speaking of Dr Monro" with evident approval. "Sensibly" (and rightly as it turned out), Orford anticipated a future need for the mad-doctor's services: "Patty, I like this doctor don't you? We will have him next time."[37]

Unable to get his way about moving the patient, Walpole visited Eriswell parsonage to see his nephew in April 1777. He found the latter "in bed" and "very mad," with only "momentary [lucid] intervals." Horace noted disapprovingly that while Orford was taking medicines that "operated sufficiently" and was attended by servants, he was under no apparent restraint.[38] Walpole clearly believed Eriswell (located "on the edge of the fens") was an unhealthy and inappropriate habitation for a sick man, censuring the parsonage's cold, smoky rooms and referring to it as

> that wretched hovel . . . one of the most improper places upon earth . . . being so out of the way of all help [it seems to have been forty miles from Beevor's, who was the nearest doctor] . . . built of lath and plaster [so that] . . . he might escape with the greatest ease . . . [with] not a decent lodging room, and . . . ponds close.[39]

As Walpole continued to try to use the authority of the London physicians to get Orford removed to his own custody in the city, he was highly disparaging of the behavior of others whom he perceived as apt to employ "every artifice to prolong the stay at Eriswell."[40] However, remaining in the country was clearly what Orford himself wanted. Notwithstanding Walpole's dismay and disapproval, Orford and his friends at Eriswell successfully prolonged his residence there, with the assistance of local medical advice. Dr. John Beevor (1727–1825) declared that "my Lord Orford has so considerable a degree of fever and flux . . . [that] he cannot be removed at present," and that, for now, was that.[41]

In Walpole's struggle to influence affairs at a distance as best he could—a predicament he found himself in so often that historians have tended to characterize him as a "great outsider"[42]—he relied upon his metropolitan medical consultants. Once he had been brought in on the case, Monro wasted little time in dispatching one of his own men to the scene to take charge. It is not clear precisely who this "man" of Monro's was, but more than likely he was one of the keepers or private attendants the mad-doctor seems to have used regularly to initiate a confinement. He may well have been the same "keeper" who was still at Eriswell in May, when Beevor thought Orford almost recovered, and Walpole had left. At this juncture, Orford's mistress appealed to Walpole to follow

Battie's precedent and "leave the keeper, at least for a month" in order to ensure "his life will be safe"—a clear enough indication that such forms of attendance were not going unappreciated even by Orford's closest circle.[43]

It may seem curious that Monro felt no need at this and other stages to attend Orford in person. Such judgments are, however, anachronistic, for Monro's behavior was by no means unusual for someone engaged in private medical practice in eighteenth-century England. Successful contemporary physicians had numerous patients to see, and medical men at least perceived nothing untoward in sending attendants and assistants to act as their proxies. Metropolitan practitioners were naturally not keen to traverse great distances to visit patients in less accessible portions of the countryside, and were frequently happy to prescribe from afar. Their very ability to practice in this fashion not only helped them to maintain a busy and lucrative business, but also served as a token of their professional and financial standing. To be sure, personal relations with clients were vital in the eighteenth-century medical world. Yet, in aping the aristocracy and gentry by retaining and building up small retinues of servants whom they employed in both business and domestic matters, physicians sought to give substance to their genteel status (or their social pretensions to it). Not the least of the virtues of such underlings was that they provided a measure of insulation against the contaminating effects of physicians getting their own hands too dirty—literally and metaphorically. Naturally enough, though, such self-interested tactics often failed to meet with the approval of patients and clients themselves.

From time to time, nevertheless, metropolitan mad-doctors and conventional physicians alike were persuaded to travel miles into the country to visit and attend certain patients—just as both Monro and Jebb did in Orford's case. Their need to retain custom and to maintain good relations with those who hired them more or less required it, and outweighed any reluctance they might have felt to venture out of town. Despite contemporary sociopolitical and cultural divisions, typified by those who referred to themselves as "country" Tories and Whigs in contrast to their counterparts in the city, there was no simple polarity in this period between town and provinces, and elite doctors themselves, like many of their gentrified and middling customers, maintained households and social bases in both places. Rarely, in fact, do physicians seem to have refused the requests and business of their more powerful and wealthy patrons—although the dangers to their reputations and pock-

ets that might attend a more contentious or wrongful confinement sometimes recommended such a course.

Once Monro's man "happily [as Walpole put it] arrived" on the
scene, Orford was restrained in a strait waistcoat and three men were assigned to watch him "constantly."[44] Soon after, on Orford attempting
to abscond through an open window and becoming "outrageous at being opposed," one of his "guards" was "forced to take him in his arms
and fling him on the bed." Arrangements were swiftly made for the installation of "bars for the window," and Orford was also rather primitively restrained with "a handkerchief around his legs."[45]

It would be misleading to exaggerate the amount of influence Monro,
or any doctor, was able to exert in such cases. Monro was one, and not
even the most prominently featured, of a number of medical practitioners in attendance on Orford. Indeed, he seems to have been in rather
remote attendance initially, and it was Jebb whose advice was preemi-
nently cited by Walpole. Walpole himself was clearly more influential
than any doctor in setting the terms of his nephew's management during 1777–78, as he had also been in 1773–74. It was Walpole, for example, who sometimes permitted, or even "ordered," new measures of
restraint, including the bars to Orford's windows after his attempted escape.[46] In the early stages of the 1777–78 attack, he primarily relied
upon Jebb's rather than Monro's advice, and throughout the period until Orford's recovery, it was Jebb who routinely kept the Walpoles ap-
prised of the progress of the case.[47]

From late April 1777, much of the day-to-day decision making was
in the hands of John Beevor, the aforementioned local Norwich physician who had been summoned to Eriswell by Orford's friends, though
on occasion, when Beevor grew doubtful of his ability to manage the
case, he appealed for Jebb (and presumably Monro) to be consulted.[48]
For the most part, however, it was Walpole who decided whether and
when to summon the city doctors.[49] Over time, he grew somewhat more
dependent on Monro's advice, especially after Beevor's hopes for Orford's recovery in May 1777 proved illusory and the patient's condition
began to worsen. By July, Monro was offering a firmer diagnosis to Walpole, although it is unclear whether he had actually seen Orford yet
(Walpole being himself, by this time, "excluded from my Lord's confidence" and keeping informed mostly via letters). Monro surmised that
as Orford had not grown "furious" in the current "sultry weather,"
"fixed madness" was indicated, underlining the emphasis he, Jebb, and
other contemporary doctors commonly gave to seasonal influences on

insanity. This is something that is also evident in his case book for 1766, and is a belief that was fully enshrined in the régime of seasonal evacuations for patients that prevailed at Bethlem under the Monros.[50]

Given a somewhat larger measure of authority, Monro attempted as best he could to impose a more restrictive régime on his patient. Orford's mail was vetted, for instance, and it seems that he was actively discouraged, if not prevented, from sending letters while he was still considered to be seriously deranged, just as he had been at the time of his previous attack. Significantly, Orford's "first act of sanity" in 1778, as Walpole characterized it, was to write a letter to "his rascally steward," which Monro carried unsealed to Walpole.[51]

The madhouses now emerging in this period were made notorious by their critics because they exercised precisely this sort of control over their inmates. Pamphleteers like Daniel Defoe (1661–1731) complained that, behind their barred doors and windows, the sane were shut up without means of redress or communication. Yet contemporary opinion varied from person to person, and case to case, as to the appropriateness of depriving the insane of pen, ink, and paper. Many seem to have regarded it, as Walpole himself put it, as "a wrong, uncharitable or prejudicial thing"[52] to permit the letters of the mad to go out into society. There were genuine fears among those who moved in superior social circles of plaguing, deceiving, and upsetting the recipients, and exposing the senders and their families to shame, trouble, and ridicule—a circumstance that, many believed, would be deeply regretted by the mad in the event of their recovery. Speaking, in another context, of the "railing epistles" that often appeared in the newspapers, Walpole actually made the opposite and typically Whig case for press freedom. Tongue in cheek, he used one of his own epistles sent to the *Public Advertiser* in 1767 to suggest that "some mad doctors" (possibly he was thinking of Monro himself) reckoned "venting our thoughts or abuse in print" helps "keep many a poor politician out of Bedlam." Further developing the medical analogy, he emphasized how "wholesome these evacuations" were.[53] However, this declared liberty for politicians and "incurable scribblers" (those whom, earlier, the Tory Dean Swift [1667–1745] had liked satirically to envisage confined in Bethlem's incurables wards, alongside himself as one of the worst cases) to rail and to publish their mad effusions was apparently not to be extended to real mad folk who, like Orford himself, were actually in confinement.

Despite their best efforts to control the situation, all was not smooth sailing during the months of Orford's confinement for Walpole and his medical minions. Orford's intermittent but growing resistance to his uncle and the physicians, and his ability to get his own way with his "crew" of dependants (as Walpole called them), rendered the balance of power a shifting and highly negotiable one, in which Monro was often only a marginal player, and even Walpole was gradually ousted from his central position of authority. Frequently obliged to keep tabs on his nephew by letter from afar, Walpole bemoaned the fact that he lacked the power to implement his own and the physicians' advice, and he voiced increasing complaints about the uncooperative attitude of Orford and his companions.[54]

At first, for example, it was Jebb's and (less frequently) Beevor's prescriptions that governed Orford's treatment, and the patient found himself subjected to bleeding and "cooling medicines." Subsequently, however, Orford refused to submit to them, preferring to take quack remedies of his own liking, such as "tar water." Indeed, he was able much of the time to enjoy a surprisingly free rein in his conduct and regimen. Walpole complained that "he takes violent exercise, eats voraciously, drinks a good deal of wine, and goes to bed at nine, where he lies till eight the next day," something which Jebb regarded as calculated to "throw the blood to his head."[55] Understandably, this sort of laxity and indiscipline left Walpole and the doctors frustrated, and yet Orford's own point of view that "both the physicians were good, but their medicines would signify nothing: that he did not know what was the matter with him, but he himself must struggle with it . . ." puts the alternative case rather well.[56]

Although Walpole was to accuse some of Orford's acquaintances of sowing "distrust" for his motives in taking charge of his nephew,[57] a further source of the resistance from the patient and his dependents was the apparent harshness of the methods that his uncle and his London doctors advocated and employed. There seems little reason to doubt that Walpole, John Monro, and the other doctors who attended Orford were convinced that they had his best interests at heart. Walpole protested regularly to his family and others as to his "care and tenderness" for his nephew and insisted that he was thinking "of nothing but my Lord's health and safety."[58] Indeed, he claimed that "if ever I had merit in any part of my life it has been in my care of Lord Orford."[59] Not everyone accepted such claims, however: Orford himself plainly resented being confined and physically restrained, and many of those in his immediate household took their cue from him. Nonetheless, even though Orford's management at the hands of his uncles and his physicians appeared overly harsh to some of his friends (as it indubitably does to modern eyes), it seems fair to say that the disquiet and suspicions of Orford's dependents themselves seem a little exaggerated. Furthermore, Orford's "crew" may have had their own financial reasons for ensuring that the lord's estate (on which they themselves were being supported) was kept intact.

On balance, nevertheless, Walpole appears to have been prone to protest his good intentions too much to be completely believed. To be sure, when Orford fell ill for a third and final time, in 1791, it was evident that his uncle was much concerned and distressed by the news. Yet there is abundant evidence that his views of his nephew's misfortunes extended beyond simple sympathy, and that the motivations of this complicated man were rather more complex and distinctly muddier than he himself willingly conceded. As the 1777–78 attack unfolded, and Walpole came to feel that he had insufficient control of the case, he increasingly lost patience with those who had Orford's confidence, and voiced his dismay with his nephew's own "ingratitude" and "distrust." By 1778, Walpole was denying that he had ever "pretended to tenderness" toward him, "for which in his life he never gave me cause."[60] Repeatedly complaining of the damage to his own "constitution" the "anxiety" about Orford had caused him, Walpole sometimes appears to have been more sorry for himself than for his wayward and deranged nephew. His assertions of his noble "suffering" in these and ensuing years, of having only "pique[d] myself" by "treating him with far greater tenderness than ever [a] lunatic was treated" (which Walpole claimed to have done "not only for his sake, but as a precedent for others in that unhappy condition"),[61] cannot help but seem exaggerated and self-regarding. Perhaps they are also symptomatic of his tendency toward rational intolerance for loss of control over a situation (however difficult and chaotic)— indeed for irrationality in general. Walpole, as a man who always sought to exercise a meticulous control over all aspects of his own life, had been hurt and affronted by being, in his own view, "cast off [by his nephew] in so outrageous a manner." Resentfully and peevishly, he refused to involve himself subsequently: "I cannot stoop to be only a tool," nor "stoop to flatter a madman."[62] This, in turn, suggests much about the limits to his tenderness and his darker reasons for having enlisted the aid of the mad-doctors—although, as good time would tell, Walpole could never fully stand aside from the affairs of so close and conspicuous a deranged relative.

LORD ORFORD RECOVERS HIS WITS—
AND LOSES THEM AGAIN

Ultimately, it was Monro who brought Walpole the news, at the end of March 1778, that his nephew had finally "come to himself."[63] How much Monro's own ministrations had to do with Orford's recovery in 1778 is doubtful. In retrospect, one suspects that most recoveries in this period may be best understood as spontaneous, or unrelated to the therapies deployed. Having engaged in a more personal attendance on Orford during the preceding months (though never acting entirely alone), Monro may have been eager to claim credit for the "cure." Yet, there is no explicit evidence of this, and the phrase "come to himself" (if a direct quote from Monro) implies an acknowledgment of a process that was partly, at least, out of the doctor's own hands.[64] What seems more significant is that, among his contemporaries, Monro does appear to have received some credit. The most immediate cause ascribed for Orford's recovery at the time, as far as Walpole related it, was held to be an apothecary's draught he had been given by his keeper.[65] Very possibly this was the keeper originally installed at Eriswell by Monro, and the draught one actually prescribed by Monro. Whatever the truth of the matter, the London physician's strict management of the case had plainly met with Walpole's almost unreserved satisfaction.

Walpole initially professed himself delighted at the news of his nephew's return to reason, writing to "all" his relations about this great, if not "marvellous," "deliverance," and his intention of "making the recovery as public as I can."[66] Even in retrospect, Walpole could refer to Orford's 1778 recovery as "perfect." However, at other times he looked upon his nephew's sobriety in rather more ambivalent and negative terms. Orford's condition, he believed, was constitutionally inveterate: he had "always been distracted," or at least "not perfectly in his senses from his youth," and he "ought to be" in a madhouse.[67] While such an interpretation might, under other circumstances, have threatened to taint the family name and Horace himself with hereditary madness, as mentioned earlier, Walpole had good reason to doubt his biological connection with his so-called nephew.

Both Horace and his brother had previously lamented the speed with which Monro and the other doctors were prepared to pronounce Orford sane, the Walpoles believing emphatically (and not without grounds) that mad-doctors' diagnoses tended toward prematurity. The month of convalescence that Battie had stipulated in 1773 as a measure for the security of Orford's restitution was something that neither Walpole thought quite adequate—and soon Horace was expressing similar reservations about the latest "cure." He gave colorful and melodramatic vent to such feelings in a letter written within days of Orford's putative recovery, lamenting that he had too soon "resumed the entire dominion of himself . . . is gone into the country, and intends to command the militia," and exclaiming "what a humiliation, to know he is thus exposing himself." [68] Walpole's rather judgmental attitude toward the case and tendency to believe that his nephew's confinement should be considerably more severe and prolonged flew somewhat in the face of the more indulgent alternatives that had substantially won the day. Privately, he acknowledged that he had resisted the temptation to confine Orford for longer only because of his belief that "my character and Sir Edward's are at stake." [69]

Yet for all of Walpole's professed skepticism, neither he nor Monro, nor for that matter any other of his nephew's doctors, was prepared to insist on Orford's continued detention. The contentiousness of the case, the pressure being exerted in support of Orford's liberty by his dependents, and the evident financial, social, and political influence that he could still command, made all parties less keen to detain him and unwilling to take the risk of keeping him confined as soon as he was no longer legally certifiable. Consequently, once Monro had declared Orford sane in 1778, Walpole immediately enjoined him to quit the case "as soon as he possibly can with safety." [70] Monro, meanwhile, can have had little impulse or financial inducement, let alone sufficient legal and familial mandate, to interfere in the case any longer.

More than a decade later, in 1791, Orford succumbed to a third "fit of frenzy." By this late date, John Monro was in semi-retirement and approaching death. His son Thomas had begun to take on his father's business and inherit his former clients, and it was Thomas whom Walpole now "sent down" to Orford. [71] Once more, Walpole became a hive of activity around his nephew: "I have been entirely shut up with my own family since Lord O's illness, receiving and writing letters, etc." [72] Walpole spoke of dispatching Monro to Orford's residence at Brandon, in Suffolk, "on the first notice of my nephew's disorder," but that notice had been slow in coming. Since 1778—and this is something that surely provides an unambiguous measure of the unhappiness of Orford and his intimates with his uncle's management of his madness—Walpole and his physicians had mostly been kept at bay. Walpole ruefully acknowl-

edged that he would not even have heard about his nephew's latest disorder "had not Lord Cadogan, who lives in the neighbourhood, sent me
word of it."[73] In view of this attempt to keep him on the sidelines, and
given all the hostility and suspicion that had swirled around his involvement in his nephew's illness for almost two decades, there is more than
a touch of irony in the final resolution of the case. For the younger
Monro's ministrations proved unavailing, and Orford rapidly succumbed to his frenzy. Ultimately, as the twist of fate would have it, with
the premature death of his nephew, Walpole succeeded to his estate and
title, remaining the fourth earl of Orford until his own death some six
years later.[74]

CHAPTER 5

Mansions of Misery

Mad-Doctors and the Mad-Trade

I have been bound and tortured in a strait waistcoat, fettered, crammed with physic with a bullock's horn, and knocked down, and at length declared a lunatic by a Jury that never saw me; and, what would make a man tear his flesh from his bones, all through affected kindness . . . [in] a mad-house, that premature coffin of the mind. . . . A trade to which seventeen years of the prime of my life has been sacrificed . . . on the 8th of October, 1778, I was overwhelmed with astonishment at being carried away to Hackney, to take my abode with idiots and real or supposed madmen, some of them just as mad as myself.

William Belcher, *An Address to Humanity* (1796)[1]

The idea of a *mad-house* is apt to excite, in the breasts of most people, the strongest emotions of horror and alarm; upon a supposition, not altogether ill-founded, that when once a patient is doomed to take up his abode in these places, he will not only be exposed to very great cruelty; but it is a great chance, whether he recovers or not, if he ever more sees the outside of the walls.

William Pargeter, *Observations on Maniacal Disorders* (1792)[2]

Dr. Battie visited and attended [Dame Cartwright] . . . he desired the nurse and the deponent and her other servants to prevent her from reading or writing, as he gave it as his opinion that reading and writing might disturb and hurt her head . . . she grew very importunate for the use of pen and ink, and frequently asked for it in a very clamorous manner. . . . Dr Battie endeavoured to dissuade and pacify her, and told her that whatever she wrote he must appear as a witness against, but that if she would wait till she got well he would be a witness for her. . . . Dr Battie in order to quiet and gratify her consented that she should have them . . . her hands which had been for some time before kept constantly tied were let loose . . . and they to humour her went into the adjoining room. . . .

Cartwright v Cartwright (1793)[3]

GREAT BRITAIN A GREAT BEDLAM:
THE WIDER MARKET FOR THE MAD-BUSINESS

Monro and his rival Battie were at once the most visible and the most respectable faces of one of the least reputable of the many new service industries that, taken together, formed so vital a part of the birth of a consumer society in eighteenth-century Britain.[4] Increasing affluence and the growing commercialization of existence brought in their train new wants and desires, new ways of satisfying old needs, new professions, and new institutions all vying for the public's purse. Madness had always been a frightening and puzzling disorder. Wild ravings, disturbances of the senses and the intellect, deep depressions—all the most serious manifestations of mental disturbance and disarray: these are profoundly threatening and troublesome aspects of the human experience with which every society must somehow cope. Existing coping mechanisms, however, were undergoing a gradual but fundamental reorganization in the eighteenth century. One of the central features of this novel machinery was the emergence of the mad-business—a "trade in lunacy" whose key elements included a growing reliance on institutionalization (particularly in profit-making "madhouses") and on an increasingly visible cadre of mad-doctors.

The attendance of Monro and Battie (at separate junctures) on cases like Sir Charles Hanbury Williams (ca. 1708–59), the verse-writer, diplomatist, and MP (and another of Horace Walpole's many correspondents), emphasizes that as much as such mad-doctors were competitors, they were also able to share in and benefit from a large and ever-expanding pie of profits from the private mad-trade. Indeed, they were able to cream off some of the most well-heeled and best-connected clients.[5] Affluent families anxious to minimize gossip and scandal, but also eager (if not desperate) for some advice about and relief from the fear-some troubles, traumas, and travails madness made manifest, increas-ingly sought assistance from those who advertised their expertise in the management of these disorders. Such a clientele was in a position to pay handsomely for discreet aid, advice, and reassurance. Lucrative opportu-nities thus existed to profit from their plight, provided that mad-doctors could somehow convince them that they could contain (if not remedy) the practical problems the lunatic posed and, perhaps as important, that they could help to maintain a degree of confidentiality about the shame and stigma that threatened them. Adapting the standard therapeutics of the age (with its emphasis on bleeding and purging, diet and regimen, and the mutual interpenetration of mind and body) to prevailing social and familial needs and concerns undoubtedly formed a *part* of many physi-cians' practice.[6] Yet, stressing their specific familiarity with the diagno-sis and treatment of the mad (a clinical expertise whose possession was invaluably confirmed by their prominent hospital appointments), Monro and Battie were especially well placed to build upon such opportunities for medical intervention and to demonstrate how one might transform them into a full-time, specialized career. In the process, they were be-ginning to construct the basis for a new profession and commerce and to constitute a market others were not slow to join them in exploiting. And, in accordance with the preference in genteel circles for treating all forms of illness at home, where they could maintain some semblance of control over the proceedings (for all save the most dangerous and incor-rigible lunatics), the ministrations of these mad-doctors emphasized care in domestic surroundings, rather than in the madhouse or asylum.

The poorer classes had, of necessity, long relied upon extra-institu-tional forms of care in coping with the deranged and mentally dis-abled—though, for them, this usually meant only that the family (at times with the help of cash doles, nursing assistance, or means of re-straint provided by the parish) was compelled to make whatever ar-rangements it could.[7] Such patterns of domestic and private care for the insane remained the dominant form of provision all through the long eighteenth century, for England's "Great Confinement" of the mad was unambiguously a nineteenth-century phenomenon.[8] In stressing these historical continuities, nonetheless, we must not neglect the crucial changes that were now under way.

England's growing affluence and the advent of a thoroughgoing reor-ganization of society along market principles inexorably, as we have suggested, prompted and made possible the emergence of very different patterns of care. For rich and poor alike, what had once been exclusively a domestic burden was increasingly handed over to strangers, entrepreneurial outsiders who offered alternative forms of management and care—madhouse-keepers, lay and medically qualified alike, who made increasingly vocal claims to expertise in the management of the mad. John Monro's career, and the pattern of activities revealed in his 1766 case book, only make sense when placed in this larger context.

The mad and the mopish, the distracted and the deranged, the delusional and the troubled in mind, were (and are) not merely disturbed, but profoundly disturbing. They were often themselves in great distress and simultaneously the source of great stress on the lives of those forced to interact and cope with them. Unquestionably, they constituted a threat, both symbolic and practical, to the social fabric; and a profound burden and source of worry to others as they sought to conduct the business of daily life. Whether ranting and raving or melancholy and withdrawn, the insane provoked upheaval and uncertainty at every turn, arousing a kaleidoscope of emotions and a host of practical problems for relatives and the community at large. They were the source and the harbingers of commotion and disarray in the family; social embarrassment and exclusion; fear of violence to people and property; the threat of suicide; and the looming financial disasters that flow from the inability to work or the unwise expenditure of material resources. The problems were scarcely novel, but the increased affluence of many segments of Hanoverian England and the entrepreneurial character of a civil society in which people eagerly sought new opportunities to gain a living prompted families with means to be willing to pay others to assume some portion of these troubles for them, and provided no shortage of volunteers for the task. Madhouses for the well-to-do thus arose, as Roy Porter has indicated, "from the same soil which generated demand for general practitioners, dancing masters, man-midwives, face painters, drawing tutors, estate managers, landscape painters, architects, journalists, and that host of other white collar, service, and quasi-professional occupations which a society with increased economic surplus and pretensions to civilisation first found it could afford, and soon found it could not do without." [9]

At the other end of the social spectrum, changes in the social structure and associated changes in mentalités contributed both directly and indirectly to heightened difficulties in coping with the mad within a family setting. These changes included such factors as the spread of wage labor, increased geographical mobility, London's proliferating attractions and opportunities for rural migrants who were then highly vulnerable to economic misfortune (especially if they were members of the rapidly expanding servant class now dependent on contract, not custom),[10] and perhaps a weakening of emotional and kinship solidarities in the face of the spread of a more calculative outlook on daily life. Furthermore, all these myriad transformations (those we have in mind when we speak of the advent of a full-blown capitalist market economy and the concomitant commercialization of existence) inevitably threatened to increase "the number of lunatics who failed to be contained in their families" and consequently fell "out of their domestic realms and [became] public problems."[11] Once such pauper (or poorer) lunatics could no longer be dealt with by self-sufficient family units (or their families began to refuse to contain and maintain them), the problems they posed for the larger community multiplied accordingly, heightening the interest of parish Poor Law officers in finding some alternative means of disposing of them and the threat they represented.[12] Again, this situation effectively augmented the demand for the emerging trade in lunacy. The process undoubtedly fed upon itself: that is, the more visible the madhouse became as part of the cultural landscape, the more all segments of society were drawn to take advantage of its services.

Like much else in a fluid and extraordinarily innovative social order, the arrangements that emerged for handling the insane were ad hoc and unsystematic. Those entering the mad-business were drawn from a wide array of backgrounds—clergymen, both orthodox and non-conformist, businessmen, widows, surgeons, speculators, and physicians: any and all were free to enter the trade. In the absence of any official regulations or oversight, an open marketplace produced a predictably heterogeneous set of arrangements, with institutions varying widely in size, clientele, organization, and therapeutic régime. Here was a social space that allowed for considerable experimentation, and in the process contributed to the development of craft skills in the management of the mad.

The very nature of the mad-business, however, with its attendant secrecy and physical isolation, almost inevitably created gothic fantasies about what transpired behind madhouse walls. Eighteenth-century writers were not slow to exploit the dramatic possibilities such settings represented, providing both fictional and polemical portraits of gaol-like establishments, presided over by unscrupulous ruffians exploiting the sinister and corrupt possibilities of their trade. In the process, the new literary discourse of the madhouse both played off and helped to cement the dubious reputation of the enterprise.

Eliza Haywood's narrative, *The Distress'd Orphan, or Love in a Madhouse,* which went into at least four editions between 1726 and 1790 (plus a number of unlicensed, pirated editions), was perhaps the classic early synthesis of the various themes associated with the iniquities of the madhouse and the false confinement of women. As was customary in such Grub Street productions, the confinement that structured the story arose from familial conflict over a romantic liaison and the control of a personal estate: Annilia, the daughter of an eminent city merchant, lost both parents at a young age and is heiress to a substantial fortune. She finds herself nefariously confined as insane by her uncle and guardian, Giraldo, after falling in love with a foreigner (Colonel Marathon). Her uncle is determined that she should marry his own son, Horatio, thus ensuring the passage of her estate as a dowry. The confinement (mimicking what was often the case in reality) is initiated in her own home by the uncle ordering her door locked and "one of the Footmen to bring a Smith, that her Windows may be barr'd." The uncle, meanwhile, acts under the pretense of protecting Annilia from her own mischievous and suicidal propensities: "for 'tis not Improbable but when she finds she is restrain'd in her Humour she may offer to throw herself out."[13]

Subsequently, finding her intractable and fearing that the authorities will discover that she is in fact sane, the uncle sends Annilia to a madhouse near to the city, whose master and keepers are portrayed as pliably corruptible: "for a good Gratification, the Doors would be open as well for those whom it was necessary, for the Interest of their Friends, to be made Mad, as for those who were so in reality."[14] The secrecy vital to such confinements is assured by another customary ruse: conveying Annilia in a hackney coach in the dead of night "under the Guard of two or three Men belonging to the Keeper of the Lunaticks," her protests literally silenced by "stopping her mouth."[15]

In stock narratives like this one, the confinement of the allegedly insane and the madhouse itself were portrayed as covert means of humbling the "pride" of women desirous of determining their own fates with respect to their marriage and their property. Simultaneously, being locked up in this fashion constituted a profound "offence" and unnatural disrespect to the "modesty" of the female sex. For both sexes, the madhouse was a place paradigmatically defined by its role in securing the deprivation of individual liberties while foreclosing all means of redress. For the female sex in particular, its bolts, bars, and chains symbolically mirrored the tyranny and constraints of social institutions that prevented women (or rather, free-born and genteel ladies) from exercis-

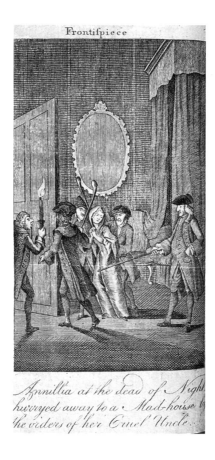

Frontispiece

Annillia at the dead of Night hurryed away to a · Mad-house by the orders of her Cruel Uncle.

FIGURE 25. Engraving from the frontispiece of the fourth edition of *The Distress'd Orphan, or Love in a Madhouse* (1790), with the description "Annillia at the dead of Night hurryed away to a Mad-house by . . . her Great Uncle," depicting a visit to the "distressed" Annilia during her confinement in a metropolitan madhouse. Reproduced by kind permission of The British Library. Shelfmark 1890.C 1 (10); 12403AA34(2); 7410A72(2).

ing free choice in love and from obtaining a reasonable degree of social and legal equality.

In her own home, Annilia's room is locked and "grated like a prison."[16] In the madhouse, her deprivations are still more severe: for example, its keepers "never Permit the Use to their Patients [of paper, pen, and ink]," and she is never supplied with any clothes beyond those she arrived in.[17] In what rapidly became a standard characterization, the keepers in charge of her confinement were represented as "inhuman

Creatures," "Ruffians," "pityless [*sic*] Monsters" and "ill-looked fellows," wedded to the terrific mode of instilling "awe" and dread in their patients via lashings, mechanical restraint, and neglect. On the pauper side of the house, the keepers

> never came to bring them fresh Straw, or that poor Pittance of Food allowed for the Support of their miserable Lives; but they saluted them with Stripes in a manner so cruel, as if they delighted in inflicting Pain, excusing themselves in this Barbarity, by saying that there was a necessity to keep them in awe; as if Chains, and Nakedness, and the small Portion of wretched Sustenance they suffer'd them to take, was not sufficient to humble their Fellow-Creatures.[18]

Their patients, meanwhile, were depicted as "helpless Objects of Compassion, who being Hand-cuffed, and the Fetters of their Legs fast bolted into the floor, can stir no farther than the length of their Chain."[19]

More fearsomely still, readers were titillated with the thought that the "horrors" of the interior of the madhouse were apt to make the sane—particularly those of a genteel and tender disposition—quite mad: "The rattling of Chains, the Shrieks of those severely treated by their barbarous Keepers, mingled with Curses, Oaths, and the most blasphemous Imprecations, did from one quarter of the House shock her tormented Ears; while from another, Howlings like that of Dogs, Shoutings, Roarings, Prayers, Preaching, Curses, Singing, Crying, promiscuously join'd to make a Chaos of the most horrible Confusion."[20]

The Distress'd Orphan employs yet another device that becomes standard in madhouse dramatizations: an emphasis on the ease of admission and difficulty of release from such establishments. Characteristically, too, it plays off the unreliability of appearances by having Marathon enter the madhouse disguised as a melancholy country gentleman appropriately named "Lovemore." Lacking any legal recourse, he effects Annilia's escape (a full fourteen weeks after her admission) by a clever ruse—making a wax copy of the cell keys—and then heroically scaling the high walls of the madhouse with his "trembling" sweetheart over his shoulder. In the end, virtue is rewarded, and the perpetrators of the false confinement punished by banishment and premature death. Yet this work made no direct appeal to the legislature, and legal redress is conspicuous by its absence, the achievement of moral justice depending instead on the actions of Annilia's beloved. The message is thus one of contempt for a judicial system that turns a blind eye to the fate of free-born English-[wo]men, and disdain for legal means that were anyway—or so the author alleged—biased according to ability to pay.

Such melodramatic renderings of the vulnerability of the female heir-ess bereft of parental protection should obviously be seen less as a bal-anced, or authentic, social commentary on conditions in private mad-houses, than as part of an Enlightenment and "age of sensibility" critique of contemporary barbarities and injustices—a critique that naturally tended to cast the miniature world it described in the worst possible light in order to further its cause. Yet factual false confinement contro-versies too, such as *Mrs Clerke's Case* (1718), demonstrate that women with fortunes (in this case, a widow) were genuinely vulnerable to incar-ceration as mad in just the ways that were exploited in these literary nar-ratives—all the more so, given the hazy boundaries of those disorders of mind and body being constituted by doctors and owned by sufferers as vapors, spleen, and nerves.[21] Recent research on King's Bench and other legal records by scholars such as Elizabeth Foyster is suggesting that women figured largely in cases involving false confinement in mad-houses, being locked away with the qualified support of laws designed to enforce rules of coverture governing the property of wives and to sanction their "reasonable" restraint and correction.[22] As she argues, in fact, the main contest in such areas may well have been between hus-bands and wives, rather than involving single women and widows.

Whereas emotionally and socially susceptible females predominated as the victims in this partly literary and partly literal construction of the madhouse, there were also a fair number of actual and fictional male equivalents suffering similar fates. James Newton (1670?–1750), the proprietor of a madhouse in Islington, was one of few to be convicted (and the many to be lambasted) for a false confinement, or, as an anon-ymous 1715 pamphlet put it, for "violently keeping and misusing" William Rogers at the behest of his wife.[23] Calling upon a growing common knowledge and concern about such abuses, Tobias Smollett ar-ranged for Sir Launcelot Greaves, his mock-heroic English Don Quixote, to be seized and carried off to a madhouse run by the eponymous Bernard Shackle. This was deployed as an occasion for a warning that "in England, the most innocent person upon earth is liable to be im-mured for life under the pretext of lunacy, sequestered from his wife, children, and friends, robbed of his fortune, deprived even of neces-saries, and subjected to brutal treatment from a low-bred barbarian, who raises an ample fortune on the misery of his fellow-creatures, and may, during his whole life, practice this horrid oppression, without question or control."[24] Daniel Defoe had earlier raised similar fears,[25] which by the 1730s had become sufficiently universal to become the subject of an opera-burlesque.[26] Before the century's end, in the wake of further protests by pamphleteers and disaffected former patients,[27] the image of these "mansions of misery" could scarcely have been less salubrious. In the words of William Pargeter,

> The idea of a *mad-house* is apt to excite, in the breasts of most people, the strongest emotions of horror and alarm; upon a supposition, not altogether ill-founded, that when once a patient is doomed to take up his abode in these places, he will not only be exposed to very great cruelty; but it is a great chance, whether he recovers or not, if he ever more sees the outside of the walls.[28]

The exposés produced by nineteenth-century lunacy reformers would demonstrate that, at times, the madhouse lived up to and exceeded the darkest imaginings of its critics.[29] Yet modern research has shown how partial and unreliable the global indictments of these institutions as benighted and brutal were, for unquestionably there were some madhouses whose proprietors took a personal interest in their patients, and where the reality of daily existence was distinctly less grim.[30] More considerate approaches were, of course, more prevalent in places that chose to take in only the "more remissively Mad," and those with putatively more refined sensibilities, whose conditions had long been held to be "healed more often with flatteries, and with more gentle Physick."[31]

In London, where John Monro's practice was based, a handful of madhouses specializing in the poor and in handling military lunatics whose care was underwritten by the state grew extraordinarily large. In Hoxton and Bethnal Green, for example, there were three establishments containing between 250 and 500 patients apiece by the late eighteenth century: Hoxton House and Whitmore House in the former, and Wright's, later known as the White (and Red) House, in the latter. But these were exceptional, even in the metropolis. Most eighteenth-century madhouses were small, often ephemeral and informal family enterprises, containing fewer than ten patients, and were extremely diverse in their orientation and operations. Few were purpose-built, for it was obviously cheaper to adapt existing buildings to the purpose. (Besides, unlike the situation that was to develop in the nineteenth century, a limited connection was seen at this time between the characteristics of the physical space within which lunatics were confined and the possibilities of curing them.) In many establishments, carceral and security concerns tended to be paramount, with bolts and bars supplemented freely with gyves, chains, manacles, and straitjackets; but in others, an ordinary dwelling house might be adapted to accommodate a handful of less threatening inmates in a less overtly custodial setting.

Physicians did not need to own a madhouse directly in order to profit from this new line of business. On the contrary, many a society medical man preferred to avoid the socially contaminating effects of too close an association with this or any other form of trade, opting instead for fees generated by referrals, or for prescribing treatments, either with or without a visit to examine the alleged mad man or woman. Even John's father, James, had chosen this mode of practice, combining the visibility and modest demands of his Bethlem physicianship with a pattern of providing attendance and advice to remunerative aristocratic patients confined in domestic settings, bolstered by retainers and fees from independent madhouse-keepers who used his services. Benjamin Faulkner (d. 1799), the lay proprietor of a madhouse in Chelsea, went so far as to advocate this separation of medical and proprietorial functions as a general rule, which allowed patients (or more likely, their families) to select their own physician and helped allay (or so he thought) the already rampant fears of improper confinement for corrupt and mercenary motives.[32]

However, the rewards of speculating more directly in this variety of human misery could be considerable, and the temptation to do so correspondingly great. Anthony Addington's madhouse at Reading provided the foundation of the family fortune and yet did not preclude his subsequent ascent to the role of court physician—besides helping to underwrite his son's rise to be prime minister of Britain.[33] William Battie, John Monro's self-made rival, died in 1776 an exceedingly rich man. (According to Walpole, he was worth £100,000, although other sources put it at nearer £200,000,[34] and this vast sum was mostly attributable to the profits of his madhouses in Islington and Clerkenwell.)[35] Charlotte MacKenzie notes that "lunatic keeping was profitable enough for [Patrick] Colquhoun to list it in 1803 as one of the more lucrative middle class occupations: he estimated forty families derived an average income of five hundred pounds a year in this way, making it comparable to some of the church's more generous livings, or the income derived from teaching at one of the better schools."[36]

John Monro's surviving case book for 1766 shows him pursuing all these many ways of making a living from madness: providing advice and prescriptions to patients in private, domestic settings; referring patients to private madhouses run by others, as well as obtaining fees for his visits to and prescriptions for them; and (though the evidence on this point is indirect and inferential) taking patients into his own private mad-house, Brooke House in Hackney, an establishment he had been connected to since at least 1762.[37] Monro's will suggests that he was in command of a fortune similar to Battie's by the time he died.

The mid-eighteenth century saw a torrent of criticism of the unregulated state of private madhouses, fed by scandalous tales of alleged false confinement and intermittent, but influential, appeals for legislative intervention—all of which were met initially with official indifference. Eventually, however, the rising tide of complaints of corruption, cruelty, and malfeasance in the mad-trade provoked some feeble and flickering interest in parliament, and both Monro and Battie found themselves called upon to testify in the brief inquiry that was finally launched in 1763. The proceedings were cursory in the extreme, only four cases of alleged false confinement being considered, only two madhouses (Miles's at Hoxton, and Turlington's at Chelsea) being inquired into, and only eleven witnesses being named as having been summoned.[38] They culminated in a printed report of just eleven pages, even though the limited testimony that was taken seemed calculated to raise rather than mitigate public anxieties. Each case involved women (namely, Mrs. Hester Williams, Mrs. Hawley, Mrs. Smith, and Mrs. Durant) who had allegedly been falsely confined by their husbands and other family members (adding ballast to Foyster's arguments about the manipulable role of the madhouse in marital disagreements), and in three of these cases there was clear evidence of abuse, with only one woman seeming to have been insane. Witnesses stressed the employment of ruses and trickery to initiate and perpetuate these confinements, and the obstruction of contact with the outside world, in particular through being locked up and mechanically restrained night and day, having visitors refused and correspondence barred, and being "treated with Severity" by keepers.[39] The women themselves complained that they received no medicines or medical treatment whatsoever and were never even attended by a medical practitioner, or not, at least, until a habeas corpus was effected.[40]

With Miles managing to evade examination, the only madhouse proprietor personally summoned to testify by the committee was Robert Turlington, the owner of a number of madhouses in the Chelsea area and, since the 1740s, the patentee of a so-called "balsam of life."[41] Testifying that "no Physicians attend the House" and that no admissions register was kept, Turlington also "avowed that the Rule was general to admit all Persons, who were brought."[42] Indeed, Turlington openly

defined his house as performing the dual function of receiving both lunatics and "lodgers" or "boarders," a distinction that conveniently col-
lapsed in practice, although he sought to divert the blame to his agent,
King, as the person to whom he left the business. A former wool trader
who, for the previous six years, had actually run the house, King was
asked on what authority he admitted people who were merely drunk
into a madhouse. "He answered, Upon the Authority of the Persons who
brought them; and he frankly confessed that out of the whole Number
of Persons he had confined, he had never admitted one as a Lunatic during the six Years he had been entrusted with the Superintendency of the
House." Subsequently, "Upon being . . . asked, If he ever refused any
Persons who were brought upon any Pretence whatsoever provided they
could pay for their Board? He answered, No." [43] Monro and Battie both
confirmed that their experience suggested that Turlington's operations
were far from unique and that false confinements were a "frequent" oc-
currence, each citing "two particular Instances" at "different Madhouses," and the latter acknowledging "that private Madhouses require
some better Regulations . . . that the Admission of Persons brought as
Lunatics is too loose and too much at large . . . and that frequent Visitation is necessary for the Inspection of the Lodging, Diet, Cleanliness,
and Treatment." [44] Monro agreed that "Private Madhouses required Regulation," in particular with respect to their licensing, "Admission of Patients," and "Visitation." [45] However, his statement that in Mrs. Durant's
case Miles had personally "confessed" to him "that he had been imposed upon" [46] was hardly a trenchant criticism of Miles's activities and
seems to reflect the mad-doctor's personal predicament, in that he had a
vested interest in sustaining good relations with madhouse proprietors.

Two years before this inquiry, Monro had been intimately involved in
another controversial case of an allegedly insane woman, Mrs. Deborah
D'Vebre, who had been confined at Turlington's Chelsea madhouse by
her husband, a case that came before the King's Bench in January 1761.
Her supporters alleged false confinement and attempted to procure
a habeas corpus against the keeper for her release. Monro was one of
three persons (besides her nearest relation and attorney) who were ordered by the court to inspect her and to have "free access" to her "at all
proper times, and seasonable hours." [47] As a result of this inspection, during which Monro had "conversed with the woman, and [also] examined
her nurse," he delivered an affidavit that was read before the court two
days later, and that "saw no sort of reason to suspect that she was or
had been disordered in her mind: on the contrary, he found her to be

very sensible, and very cool and dispassionate [an interesting indication of the behavioral expectations for feminine conduct in this period]." Monro "personally attended in court" to back up his testimony, and the writ was duly granted, forcing Turlington to bring Mrs. D'Vebre before the judge.

Clearly, the mad-doctor's assessment of this woman's mental state was significant, although evidently not crucial, in resolving the matter. It was only once the patient herself had been presented before the court and "appeared" to them "to be absolutely free from the least insanity," and after still another inspection the following day, that the case was decided and Mrs. D'Vebre freed—both from a return to the madhouse and from the clutches of her husband. Yet, such personal inspections by the court were automatic in King's Bench habeas corpus cases, even if in criminal trials at other courts, such as the Old Bailey, just less than half of those being examined on insanity defenses during 1760–1864 testified at their own trial.[48] A negotiated separation between Mrs. D'Vebre and her husband soon followed. More broadly, the publicity the lawsuit attracted in the train of this case brought Turlington's operations in particular and false confinement in general forcibly to the attention of government.

Such cases, and Monro's and Battie's summons before the subsequent 1763 Commons inquiry into madhouses (which described them as "two very eminent Physicians distinguished by their Knowledge and their Practice in Cases of Lunacy"),[49] provide some indication of their standing as England's premier mad-doctors. Yet, the same evidence also emphasizes the limits of medical influence at this time and the reluctance that even the most prominent and respectable mad-doctors displayed—both as private gentlemen with social loyalties to their clients and as businessmen with financial interests in the sustainability of their particular branch of practice—about going overboard in agitating for intervention from the legislature. Despite Monro's and Battie's recommendations for tightening up regulations governing private madhouses, statutorily the 1763 inquiry merely resulted in a resolution from the House of Commons "that the present state of the madhouses in this kingdom requires the interposition of the Legislature [and] . . . That Leave be given to bring in a Bill for the regulation of Private Madhouses."[50] Concretely, its proceedings may well also have had the salutary, if limited, impact of damaging Turlington's reputation so effectively as to bring his business operations to a close. Certainly, we can find no evidence of him continuing in the mad-trade subsequent to this date. For more than a decade thereafter, however, nothing else was done by government, the trade in lunacy remaining as unregulated as before.

Some observers blamed this inaction on the "many objections" raised by lawyers to any legislation and the failure of the inquiry to suggest positive or explicit solutions. The Commons committee had purposefully limited the extensiveness of its inquiry, despite the fact "that a Variety of other Instances arising in other Houses offered themselves for Examination,"[51] content to establish its case on the minimum of evidence. The extreme sensitivity in elite circles to the desire for discretion in dealing with the private sphere of lunacy goes a long way toward explaining the slow pace of legislation on private madhouses in this period: "Your Committee restraining themselves out of a Regard to the Peace and Satisfaction of private Families . . ."[52] Although politicians like Charles Townshend had taken "great pains in the business," they were ultimately seen by contemporaries to have "dropped it" soon after. (Townshend himself was a notoriously fickle figure, his political allegiances tending to change like the tide during the 1760s.)[53]

During the early 1770s, momentum developed afresh for an act to regulate madhouses, as other cases of abuse came to light. Particularly notorious among these was the case of Mrs. Mary Leggatt, in which the keeper of a madhouse near Kennington Common was accused not only of falsely imprisoning her, but of assaults on her with intent to commit rape, and received the exemplary sentence of an hour in the St. Margaret's Hill pillory, six months imprisonment, and a rather nominal fine of 13s. 4d.[54] An anonymous 1772 publication addressed to the Lord Mayor and Common Council of London, which expressed wonderment and disappointment at the failure of the 1763 inquiry to result in any legislation, spoke of a long history of complaints about "the dreadful effects" of "unjust and cruel confinements, which soon break the heart, and then the brain, when dreadful despair either causes *suicide,* or continued *blasphemy.*"[55] Wedding itself firmly to an age of sensibility consciousness, the pamphlet plaintively detailed the plight of

> persons who, from a tender frame, by sudden *vexations, frights, and unkind usage,* may have their spirits hurt, and yet be very improper persons for these places; and may, by them, be rendered incurable; for, as Solomon too truly observes, *oppression makes a wise man mad* . . . this very year had we not an instance of one, who keeps such a place, standing in the pillory, and being fined, for detaining a woman no way disordered, but put in by a cruel husband? No misery on earth is equal, nor so soon destroys the brain, as quick sensibility, wounded by confinement and cruel usage; where no permission is

allowed the unhappy [word missing?] to write to any one, to see any one he wishes, or by his own behaviour to contradict reports too easily credited, too cruelly spread of him. . . .[56]

The author appealed for legislation requiring that no confinement take place without an attestation in writing from the patient's parish minister and twelve of his neighbors and a certificate of two physicians, "neither of them concerned in any such house." [57] He also recommended severe penalties for an improper confinement: a fine of £50 for any convicted madhouse master or keeper, plus imprisonment for at least three years in a county gaol. Additionally, he urged that madhouse servants and keepers be encouraged to inform on their masters by the enticement of a £10 fine payable to them for reporting such cases. (The master himself was to have the [rather minimal] protection of a right of appeal to the King's Bench, though the act that was finally passed offered no protection whatsoever.) Concluding, the author of this grand scheme urged that each house should be visited by the local parish clergyman and JP at least once a fortnight, with the inspectors guaranteed complete freedom of access.[58]

Two years later (1774), the Act for Regulating Madhouses (14 George III c. 49) *was* finally passed. Perhaps, as Porter has suggested, the prolonged delay in enacting legislation should be seen as a function of the opposition of the College of Physicians, some of whose members "had a large financial stake in metropolitan madhouses." [59] If so, it is somewhat ironic that parliament handed over the power to license and inspect madhouses in the metropolis to the College. (In the provinces, similar authority was granted to local magistrates.) There were other signs, too, that medical men had successfully lobbied behind the scenes to protect their interests: the 1772 appeal notwithstanding, commitment under the new act required only a single medical certificate, and local clergymen were firmly excluded from any officially sanctioned role in the process.[60]

The statute was, in any event, little more than a token gesture. In the first place, its provisions were exceptionally limited. Charity asylums, like Bethlem and St. Luke's, were expressly excluded from its scope, as were patients in lodgings and single care—a large proportion of the lunatic population in the late eighteenth century. Paupers were particularly likely to suffer from extremes of neglect and ill-treatment in unregulated madhouses, bearing in mind the parsimony of the parish overseers, from whose pittance the keepers had somehow to extract a profit. Yet the Act explicitly excluded them from its purview. While penalties were imposed for failing to obtain a license (a fine of £500 for unlicensed confinements of more than one lunatic, together with a £50 fine for uncertified admissions), neither the College nor the provincial magistrates had the power to reject applications. Worse still, the inspectors were both reluctant and ineffectual, since, however awful the conditions they uncovered were, they lacked any powers to sanction the offending parties. Nor was there any element of surprise in the infrequent visitations (at least one a year, between eight and five o'clock, having been the paltry, ill-conceived stipulation), so that, as a number of contemporaries complained, the legislation's "intention [was] . . . too often frustrated by their keepers knowing beforehand when they will be visited." [61] At best, therefore, the 1774 Act provided the authorities with a somewhat more complete list of the madhouses in operation, especially in the London area, and a rather more patchy and inadequate register of the numbers of private patients admitted to and confined in such establishments, together with some minimal protection against the unlawful confinement of the sane.

JOHN MONRO AND THE PRIVATE MAD-BUSINESS

John Monro's surviving case book for 1766 provides regular testimony about the close relationship of the Monros with many of the metropolitan madhouses and their proprietors. It frequently records the various madhouses where Monro visited patients and the names of the establishments to which patients were sent, often (presumably) on his recommendation. The madhouse mentioned most frequently is that run at Hoxton by John (or Jonathan) Miles (d. ca. 1773), who was at one time Warden of the Painter-Stainers Company.[62] Miles's Hoxton House was one of three madhouses operating in the area during the eighteenth century (the others being Whitmore House and Holly House). All three were to be found within a few hundred yards of each other, dotted along Hoxton Road.[63]

Miles's madhouse, located near Shoreditch Church, was established in 1695.[64] A large brick building, with quite extensive grounds for patients' exercise at its back, it was one of two madhouses especially inquired into by the 1763 Parliamentary Select Committee because of reports of false confinements there. In the event, only a solitary case was mentioned, and it was not until the 1815 Commons madhouses inquiry that Hoxton was to be subjected to a thoroughgoing investigation. The result would be damning criticisms of the way it dealt with patients, with particular attention focused upon its treatment of naval lunatics who had been sent there under contracts with the Admiralty from 1792 onward.[65]

At least sixteen patients mentioned in the 1766 case book were sent to John Miles's Hoxton House.[66] Monro's attendance on so many Hoxton cases suggests that he was one of those contemporary practitioners most frequently in medical attendance at this madhouse, as well as providing evidence of his advantageous business relations with Miles. The intimate relationship between the two men, which seems to have its origins in a still earlier connection between Miles and James Monro, is also strongly attested to by the provisions of the madhouse-keeper's will. Both John Monro and William Kinleside (Treasurer of Bridewell and Bethlem, 1768–74) were bequeathed a one-guinea gold ring by Miles, a customary contemporary symbol of friendship,[67] and the long-standing close relationship between the Monros and the Mileses, and between Bethlem and Hoxton, was continued after John Monro's and John Miles's deaths. The latter passed on the day-to-day running of his madhouse (obliquely referred to in his will—intent, as he was, on maintaining a level of secrecy and respectability—as "my Business of taking care of the persons and Maintenance of Boarders") to his widow, Margaret Preston. He also specified that Margaret could live in the two Hoxton houses and was "to carry on the said Business . . . as I have done," requiring additionally that she remain unmarried. It was to her that all profits were subsequently to be passed, his three-year-old son (Sir) Jonathan Miles (1769–?) not taking over the management of Hoxton House until he reached his majority (i.e., twenty-one years of age) in ca. 1790, as, once again, his father carefully laid down and as Jonathan himself was later to testify before the 1815 madhouses inquiry.[68] After his own father's death, Thomas Monro, as well as the Bethlem apothecary John Haslam, maintained strong ties with Jonathan Miles at Hoxton, and large numbers of patients continued to be passed from one institution to the other.[69] The institutions also seem to have shared much in common in terms of their internal arrangements, including, for example, a lack of any segregation between frantic and convalescent cases, the use of trough style beds and blanket gowns for incontinent patients, and the preference for irons over strait waistcoats. Jonathan Miles's growing success and wealth as proprietor of Hoxton House helped him rise to the positions of alderman and then sheriff (1806) of London, and to achieve a knighthood in 1807, while he further outstripped his father in also becoming Master of the Painter-Stainers in 1815.[70]

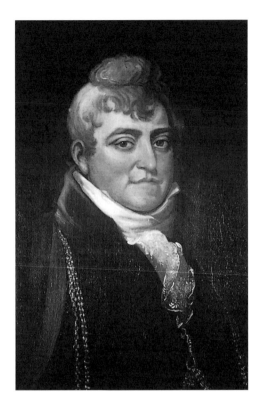

FIGURE 26. Portrait of Sir Jonathan Miles. Oil on canvas, painted by Mather Brown (1761–1831). Sir Jonathan Miles (1769–?) was the son of John Miles, proprietor of the private madhouse Hoxton House from ca. 1790 and Master of the Painter-Stainers Company. This portrait was presented by Sir Jonathan when he became Master (1815) for display in Painter-Stainers Hall, where it still hangs. Reproduced here by kind permission of the Worshipful Company of Painter-Stainers, London.

The Mileses were to amass a considerable fortune from the mad-business, in substantial measure through their Admiralty and War Office contracts.[71] It is likely that produce and livestock from John Miles's numerous farms and that of his brother-in-law were being supplied for use in the madhouse, as well as deployed strategically as gifts to influential figures in central and parochial government and in the mad-business.[72] Subsequently, the fruits of this harvest were certainly being put to such a use under Jonathan's wily hand. Testifying before the Commons

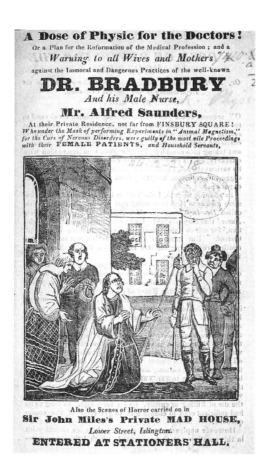

A Dose of Physic for the Doctors!

Or a Plan for the Reformation of the Medical Profession ; and a

Warning to all Wives and Mothers

against the Immoral and Dangerous Practices of the well-known

DR. BRADBURY

And his Male Nurse,

Mr. Alfred Saunders,

At their Private Residence, not far from FINSBURY SQUARE !
*Who under the Mask of performing Experiments in "Animal Magnetism,"
for the Cure of Nervous Disorders, were guilty of the most vile Proceedings
with their* FEMALE PATIENTS, *and Household Servants,*

Also the Scenes of Horror carried on in

Sir John Miles's Private MAD HOUSE,

Lower Street, Islington.

ENTERED AT STATIONERS' HALL.

FIGURE 27. Engraving depicting a scene at Sir John (i.e., Jonathan) Miles's madhouse in Lower Street, Islington (ca. 1844). Here Sir John is "standing over his victim, having a whip in one hand, while with the other he is holding a mask before his face to guard against any future recognition, in case of discovery." This madhouse was polemically described as "Hell upon Earth," a "horrid den," and "a dreary looking house at the corner of a turning, having iron bars before every window, and a garden with very tall trees at the back," where "many an unfortunate being was concealed from the light of day . . . and while chained up, whipped by their brutal keepers, until the blood gushed from the lashings inflicted." Reproduced from Anonymous, *A Dose of Physic for the Doctors* (London: E. Hancock; Lowe & Co. Printers, 1844, frontispiece and p. 12), by kind permission of The British Library. Shelfmark 1890.C 1 (10); 12403AA34(2); 7410A72(2).

inquiry into madhouses in 1815, for example, Dr. John Weir, inspector of naval hospitals, related how "Messrs. Miles," or "Sir Jonathan Miles and Company," had sent him presents of fish and game, until, that is, his conscience prompted him to put an end to the practice.[73]

Neither John Miles nor his son was medically trained. They relied instead on patients' families and friends to call in their own doctors to consult on the case and to provide the patients with whatever medical attention was felt necessary, although by 1815 there was also a medical man in more or less regular attendance.[74] The question of medical involvement in the operations of these establishments was an issue addressed critically, but to little effect, by the 1763 madhouses inquiry before which Monro testified, and it would emerge again, but considerably more forcefully, in the course of the far more searching 1815–16 madhouses inquiry.[75]

A large number of poor and pauper cases were sent to the Mileses and to other private madhouses from the mid-eighteenth century onward. Monro's case book provides a number of examples of the former of these sorts of patient. Those recorded as being in private institutions included, for example, a servant and a slave, both of whom were evidently being supported by the relatively well-off households of their masters and mistresses. There were, besides, many patients from somewhat more prosperous backgrounds—a bookseller, a tailor, and a butcher, for instance—but, unsurprisingly, no parochial patients are mentioned in the case book. Although pauper patients evidently made up the majority in most private madhouses serving the metropolis, Monro's fees were surely too steep for either pauper families or parish officials to swallow.

Poorer patients were often sent to metropolitan madhouses prior to their admission to hospitals like Bethlem or St. Luke's. Waiting lists at the charity asylums meant that admission was often delayed, though some families preferred them to their profit-oriented private competitors because their admission (and other) fees were cheaper, and there was less apparent ambivalence as to the motivations behind the retention of patients. Where families could afford the additional cost, however, private care was generally—though not universally—preferred. What determined these choices, or even the preference for confinement over domiciliary care, is difficult to assess from the surviving records. Mr. Cawthorne, for example, as the case book details, "was brought up [to London] with the intention to be put into the hospital but [for reasons not here recorded] his friends chose to leave him for some time at Mr Miles's."[76]

No doubt, to some extent it was the lesser availability of specialist medical care and private madhouses in the provinces that persuaded some families to bring their deranged members up to the city. One suspects, though, that more selfish motives were often at work: the desire to cast out a difficult or uncooperative member of the family or parish, and the need for more discretion, or even to cloak the case in anonymity—advantages that capital could most certainly provide—surely also played some role in decisions to travel to secure treatment, and in families weighing up the choice between public and private establishments. Private madhouses offered those with more capital, and those of genteel sensibilities, the promise of greater secrecy and confidentiality. Families of means, apt to take offense at the notion of private griefs and travails entering the public domain, tended to decry the mingling of anyone of superior birth in open consort with common paupers. A family's name and reputation were obviously less likely to be at risk where the patient was confined in a private place, rather than in a public institution, especially one as open to casual visitants as Bethlem. Economic fortunes could and did fluctuate, however, and accordingly the boundaries between pauper and private patients were liable to substantial flux in this period. Lunacy itself might prove such a financial drain on the resources of a middling household as to entail a descent into pauper status for certain families and their distracted members. Alternatively, both patients of means and even those of the poorest sort might be removed to private houses once the year normally allowed for them to be treated at public asylums had elapsed—for this was an anniversary of more than passing significance, since in the eyes of the hospital authorities it marked a patient's official transition from the cases defined as "curable" to the ranks of the "incurable." Private madhouses, in such cases, could serve as temporary way stations for families deciding how else to cope or waiting for a vacancy that allowed their relation to secure admission to Bethlem's incurables wing.

The fact that almost 25 percent of the cases Monro attended (or heard about) in 1766 were sent to private madhouses does seem to provide some measure of the more frequent resort to private confinement that characterized the second half of the eighteenth century, and the enlarged carceral provision available for families in the private sector. Violence was especially difficult to manage within the home, and many of the cases Monro mentions as being confined in Hoxton and other private madhouses were described as extremely mad, violent, or suicidal, reflecting the importance of the containment function of early modern institutions for the mad. Mrs. Harris, for instance, "had made attempts to hang herself before she was brought to Mr Miles's," while Miss Cutter's removal from home was probably connected with her tendency to live up to her name, Monro noting on his first visit how she had "cut her hands in several places, by striking them thro a sash window the day before in a violent hurry."[77]

A number of cases were relapses, recommitted to madhouses like Miles's for a second or third time, presumably, for the most part, because that was where they had first been treated. Mr. Buckley, for example, had been at Miles's once before "about a month" and was to be sent back for a third time on relapsing once again within a fortnight of his supposed recovery.[78] This sort of thing may have been less a matter of the private madhouse and its proprietor feeling responsible for their own cases than the family opting for a familiar and convenient recourse. Nevertheless, the rapid-fire admission and discharge of such cases reminds us once again of the fallacy in any claims (if not in terms of the discourse about madness, then in quantifiable, empirical terms at least) about a "great confinement" of the insane in the eighteenth century.

Few of those patients whose lengths of stay in private madhouses were specified in Monro's case book appear to have endured the prolonged detentions with which such establishments were often associated. More typical were cases like Miss Cutter, who "was very sensible of her complaint, & by keeping quiet, got so well as to return home in 3 weeks," or Mr. Hamilton, who "was continued under my [Monro's] care one fortnight only, & then set out for Scotland with a man to take care of him."[79] In a private case book such as this one, there can have been little motivation for Monro to attempt to manicure the record, which allows us to conclude that, much more often than not, incarceration was a temporary resort in this period, especially for private cases. Families were generally unwilling to support it for long, either financially or emotionally.

Case book entries suggest that Monro treated patients at another madhouse at Hoxton at this time. In addition to patients sent to Miles's, two other cases are mentioned who were sent to a "Mr Devic's" or "Devy's" at Hoxton. It seems unlikely that this is a reference to Miles's madhouse, and that Devic was merely the keeper there.[80] Madhouses were often found clustered in the same neighborhood, and at least one other Hoxton madhouse, Whitmore House,[81] was in business from the 1750s onward.[82]

The next most frequently mentioned madhouse in the case book was

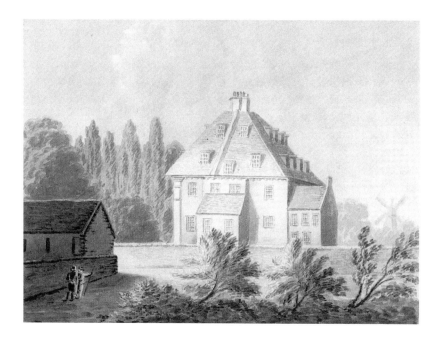

FIGURE 28. Whitmore House, Hoxton: a view from the grounds looking west, painted in the late eighteenth century. Whitmore House, one of a number of madhouses in Hoxton, was run from the late eighteenth century onward by the Warburton family, who also operated madhouses at Bethnal Green. Built by the Balm brothers for Sir George Whitmore in 1540, the house was originally moated and surrounded by formal gardens. Acquired by Richard de Beauvoir in 1680, it was leased to Dr. Meyer Schomberg (d. 1761) and transformed into an asylum by 1756, a few years before John Monro opened Brooke House. Thomas Warburton was originally employed as the gate porter at the establishment, becoming "expert at conveying liquor in to the house for keepers to dispose of among the patients." Having learned to read and write, he worked his way up to first keeper and, by the simple expedient of marrying his employer's widow, succeeded to the business when the previous physician/proprietor died. By the early nineteenth century, the inmates at Whitmore House included the son of the British prime minister, Henry Addington (d. 1823); the brother of Lord de Dunstanville; the marquess of Tullibardine, later the duke of Atholl (d. 1846); and Mrs. Priscilla Wakefield (1751–1832), the mother of the prominent early-nineteenth-century lunacy reformer Edward Wakefield. As the centerpiece of the Warburton empire, Whitmore House had an exclusively fee-paying clientele, many of whom paid very substantial sums for their confinement. According to Mitford, the duke of Atholl paid £1,000 a year for his son, and Lord de Dunstanville £1,200 for his brother. Several other patients paid well over £500, and in total, Whitmore House contained more than sixty patients, making this a lucrative enterprise indeed. Patients, however, were routinely abused and mistreated, and together with Warburton's other madhouses in Bethnal Green, the asylum became a target of the 1815–16 Select Committee on Madhouses. Thomas Warburton handed over his business to his medically qualified son John in 1829, and subsequently, Warburton's grandson, then operating the business, went mad himself, and the madhouse was closed and redeveloped in 1852. The Hackney Archives currently occupy a building that stands on the site where the madhouse once operated. Reproduced by kind permission of the Hackney Archives, London.

Michael Duffield's (d. 1798) Chelsea madhouse, where (as Cruden had been earlier) four more of Monro's cases were sent and where still another patient was recommended for admission.[83] Duffield's house was, according to Bowack, "a regular handsome house with a noble courtyard and good gardens, built by Mr Mart."[84] According to Blunt, it was located just east of Lord Shaftesbury's house (the site of which was later occupied by St. George's Workhouse), and just west of Lord Wharton's Park, now Elm Park Gardens. Duffield evidently ran several madhouses in Great Chelsea.[85] An examination of his will (dated 1798) and that of his father (who was also named Michael Duffield; d. 1761) shows that while Michael junior inherited substantial assets from Michael senior, some amount of parental disapproval (probably prompted by Michael junior's apparent marital difficulties) made Michael junior's own son (confusingly enough, also named Michael) the major beneficiary of Michael senior's inheritance. Indeed, it may have been this partial disinheritance that pushed the second Michael into the mad-business. If so, the handsome profits his will reveals suggest that trafficking in insanity enabled him to more than eclipse his comfortably-off father by the time of his own death.[86]

Michael junior failed to make any explicit mention of his madhouse business in his will. Almost certainly, however, his bequest of "the two Messuages or Tenements" plus "Appurtenances" in China Walk, Saint Luke's, Chelsea, Middlesex (where he then resided) to the surgeon-apothecary William North of Grosvenor Row, St. George Hanover Square, Chelsea, comprised the house he employed for lodging the insane. These premises and their profits were to be held in trust for his wife, Mary (who had presumably shared a hand in her husband's business), for her either to use, or else to let and receive the profits. The intimacy of Michael junior's connection with the medical profession is also attested to by the fact that he was to make North, whom he referred to as his "friend," one of his executors, leaving him £21 for his "Trouble" in executing the will. He left the remainder of his estate directly to his wife, Mary.

Other madhouses referred to in the case book include Clarke's Brooke House (about which we shall have more to say in a moment); the madhouse of Duffield's nephew, Inskip, at Little Chelsea[87] (where Cruden had also been confined—see above); Dudley's Bloomsbury madhouse; Peter Day's Paddington madhouse; and Thutton's at Bethnal Green. The slave girl Flora had been sent to Dudley's prior to her confinement at Hoxton, while Mrs. Mackenzie had already been released from Day's

Paddington house when Monro became involved in her case. However, Monro had personally attended Mrs. Walker at Inskip's, and Miss Graham and Mrs. Wilmot at Thutton's.[88]

Through the prism of the case book we can catch valuable glimpses of the close links between Monro's public and private practices. Some patients whose cases he records spent time in Bethlem as well as receiving private treatment, either in their own homes or at private madhouses. The often rapidly shifting economic fortunes of the time, and the fact that the Monros creamed off some of the richer clientele for their private businesses from among those presented for admission to Bethlem, are some of the more obvious sources of this pattern.

Metropolitan hospital practice virtually guaranteed a ready supply of private patients. Indeed, this was clearly one of the major attractions of taking up such posts. The Bethlem physicianship came with a salary of just £26 13s. 4d., plus a more or less automatic annual gratuity of £50, which would have hardly been sufficient to keep Monro in the gentrified style to which he would have wished to be accustomed.[89] It was the same salary—more, in truth, an honorary stipend—that his father and generations of Bethlem physicians had enjoyed before him,[90] and John was to receive no increment from the hospitals' governors throughout his four decades of service at Bethlem and Bridewell. Obviously, though, the fact that Monro could find time to attend one hundred private cases in a year provides a telling indication of the limited demand that his Bethlem duties were placing on his time and energies.

At least 5 percent of Monro's 1766 cases were at some point sent to Bethlem, and the case book is quite revealing about what provoked moves of this sort. Poverty, as one would expect, was unquestionably a highly significant factor in this decision. Thus, among those conveyed to Bethlem, a Mr. Tonkin, for instance, was described as a "poor man" who had "run out his substance," and Mr. Pottinger as "a bankrupt." [91] More interestingly, the substantial degree of overlap between Monro's public and private practice highlights a degree of fluidity about the criteria by which private cases were distinguished from those fit for Bedlam in this period, and it makes manifest the substantial numbers of the afflicted who were on the socioeconomic cusp. To be sure, the decision to send a patient to Bethlem rather than a private madhouse was often some sort of measure of the putative seriousness and dangerousness of patients, either to themselves or others, but even these factors were not always decisive. For example, where a patient inherited money, or was found to possess it after confinement in Bethlem, the hospital's own rules barring the moneyed as unfit patients for the charity prompted further movement between the public and private forms of provision.

FOR THE BEST AND THE WORST PURPOSES?
MONRO, MADHOUSES, AND FALSE CONFINEMENT

Although the case book testifies to Monro's wide connections with the metropolitan madhouses, it does not tell us a great deal about them, or how he regarded them. It does, nevertheless, offer a few hints. It substantiates Monro's relatively matter-of-fact attitude toward the mad-business and the types of patients for whom it catered. Monro evidently accepted that most patients he visited at these madhouses were indeed quite mad. He patently had little time for Mrs. Wilmot's request that he release her from Bethnal Green and "convey her . . . to town in my chariot," remarking that she had "been disorder'd for some years past by the account I have had of her, & by her appearance I should imagine her head to be damag'd beyond repair."[92] However, his summons by Dr. Southwell to Mrs. Walker at Chelsea[93] implies some sort of recognition among practitioners of the need for second opinions, or expert consultations, in doubtful cases.

Monro probably saw his role in visiting patients at Hoxton and other madhouses as mostly a personal matter between, on the one hand, himself and the madhouse proprietor, and on the other hand, between himself, the patient's family, and the patient. The patient was often a rather subsidiary agent in (or object of) this business arrangement and, partly as a result, often exerted only a limited influence on the decisions that were made. Personal autonomy was almost inevitably lost or sharply diminished once an individual was placed under confinement outside the domestic environment. The mad-doctor, meanwhile, operating in the limited capacity of medical consultant, appears to have left most decisions about the management of madhouse patients to the proprietor and keepers. Monro rarely seems to have felt any need to interfere with, or question, the way in which such patients were being maintained and treated, though he certainly made prescriptions for patients that required implementation by madhouse personnel, and must have occasionally left instructions about how patients were to be cared for.

In the case of Mr. Fitzgerald, for instance, Monro was unconvinced that the patient needed to be removed from home. When it proved necessary, he was prepared to state his opinion in most vigorous terms to Miles and ultimately to terminate his association with the case.[94] Yet

Monro's main quarrel here was not with Miles and the staff at Hoxton but with the patient's family, who had refused to countenance home treatment. Indeed, on this issue, Monro and Miles subsequently presented a united front. Without Monro's endorsement, Miles was evidently unwilling to continue to take responsibility for the patient (concerned no doubt about the possibility of being sued, as had occurred in a number of highly publicized contemporary cases of false confinement), and the upshot was that Fitzgerald was sent home.

Monro's case book contains some other tantalizing references to false confinement and ill-treatment in the establishments with which he was connected, and suggests why some patients might be moved from one place to another. Flora's case, for example, implies that Monro was disinclined to take accusations of abuse in the madhouses he attended at face value. Obviously, he knew where his interests lay, but he was equally aware that complaints of this sort were apt to be overblown, if not fallacious. Flora's mistress alleged that the young girl had been sent to Miles's after being "frighten'd by the ill usage of some servants at Bloomsbury," but Monro countered that it was her unmanageability, "extravagance" and morbidly suspicious refusal of medicine and food that had precipitated the transfer: "they not knowing how to manage her sent her to Mr Miles's." [95] Furthermore, he declared, she had ultimately "proved mad enough."

Mad-doctors and madhouse proprietors, who were concerned to maintain, if not augment, their "respectability" and social standing, naturally worried about the trouble and damage that might be caused to their businesses and to other patients by extremely noisy, violent, destructive, or difficult cases, and so might steer clear of placing these sorts of patients in their own houses. Indeed, this is very much the implication of Monro's account of the "very mad" Mrs. Mackenzie, the case of alleged false confinement (briefly discussed in chapter 2) reluctantly attended by Dr. Battie. Battie, in this instance, is described as "not chusing to take her into his own house," recommending instead another private madhouse or a home confinement. Yet ironically, of course, it was the very extremity of the behavior such patients exhibited that made relatives so determined to seek non-domiciliary confinement for them. Thus Mr. Mackenzie had sent his wife to Day's Paddington madhouse on Battie's advice, after complaining "that she made too much noise for him to bear her in [his own] . . . house." [96]

The surviving trial affidavits for the Mackenzie case, which have recently been admirably surveyed by Elizabeth Foyster, make it clear that this confinement was essentially about a marital conflict between Hannah and her husband, Peter.[97] Indeed, Foyster's account suggests that, through their involvement in madhouse confinements, mad-doctors like Battie and Monro may have become, at times, complacent or perhaps unwitting tools, assisting errant husbands who sought to control their "deviant," unruly wives. As she shows, Peter Mackenzie initiated the confinement after attempting to make Hannah's niece (with whom he was having an adulterous affair) mistress of the household, and he seems to have felt he "had a right to treat his wife in that way." When Hannah refused to comply with his demands, his introduction of Dr. Battie into the home understandably provoked Hannah's flight. The ensuing home confinement under the supervision of a female keeper evidently specializing in the care of the insane entailed the customary methods of restraint, such as locking her in her room, battening down the windows, and straitjacketing her when she tried to escape—a recourse that Hannah claimed caused her "violent pain" and profuse bleeding. Days later, the unfortunate woman was conveyed to Peter Day's Paddington madhouse, from which she escaped with the aid of John Sherratt ("a lawyer and well-known campaigner against private madhouses") and others[98]—only to find her husband retaliating by issuing a writ of habeas corpus against them.

Four years before this case, in 1762, John Monro had been involved with the alleged false confinement of another married woman, Mrs. Anne Hunt, in the madhouse being nominally run by William Clarke (but which Monro most likely owned), Brooke House, Clapton. Mrs. Hunt had been committed on Monro's recommendation and at the insistence of her daughter, Mrs. Threkeld, but a writ of habeas corpus had been served on Clarke for her removal on 26 November 1762. Three days later, Monro presented an affidavit via the solicitor general before the Court of King's Bench, justifying the patient's continuing detention and urging the withdrawal of the writ. He avowed not only that Mrs. Hunt had been insane from the time of her admission until "this time," but that the "lunatic . . . is now in so disordered a state of mind, that she is not fit to be brought into this Court"—an important circumstance given that, according to Eigen, medical witnesses generally participated in contemporary trials (Old Bailey trials, at least) when the prisoner was "silent" or unable to testify.[99]

Monro's affidavit seems to have been the determining factor in this case, and to have "perfectly well satisfied" the court. The main problem with the confinement appears to have been something of a technicality: Mrs. Hunt had been confined without any commission of lunacy, which left the strict legality of the process open to contest. According to Monro, though, the formalities had been deferred only because of the minority of the patient's grand-daughter and next of kin, Anne Bowen. He assured the court that, now that young Anne had come of age, the commission "will shortly be issued," and the judge agreed that the handling of the case had been "intended for [the patient's] benefit and advantage." The ultimate acceptance of Monro's affidavit of this woman's insanity, the consequent repeal of the writ of habeas corpus, and the subsequent grant of a commission of lunacy, serves less to highlight the limited means of redress available to those who had been incarcerated than to reveal the tendency for some contemporaries to exaggerate the frequency of clear-cut cases of false confinement.[100] Indeed, while Serjeant Whitaker on behalf of the crown prosecution appealed for a ruling granting "liberty to have access to and inspection of Mrs Hunt, in order to see that she was properly treated," no one else in or outside of the family appears to have had "the least pretension" to desire this course, and the court duly rejected the request.

In 1771–72, Monro was once more at the bar fending off allegations of false confinement on at least two occasions—although, as usual, he was a witness rather than a defendant. The first was the "much talked of case" of Jonathan Green of Dudley, who was the nominal "plaintiff" (actions involving the mentally suspect customarily and predictably being brought about primarily by their relatives and friends, but also involving a wide range of other actors). The action was brought against a madhouse-keeper and three other defendants and held before a special jury at the Worcester Assizes in Lent 1771. The charge (as was standard in such cases) was "assault and imprisonment," and the rather elliptical style in which this trial, by contrast with many others, was reported in the press, underlines the ambivalent constraints of discretion, even in the most "talked of" cases. As the *Annual Register* related, it was satisfactorily established during "the course of the trial that the plaintiff was unhappily afflicted with lunacy; that he was taken up and put under the care of one of the defendants, and attended by Dr Monro, for the purpose of effecting a cure, [and] a verdict was found for the defendants."[101]

Other contemporaneous actions involving Monro likewise tend to emphasize how dubious, or at least difficult to prove, many such cases were. These cases alert us as well to the significant discrepancies between various printed versions and the aptness of more popular media to distort the medico-legal record for polemical purposes. They may be contrasted, however, with one of the worst instances of abuses in private madhouses, albeit one in which Monro was only indirectly involved.

The case in question is the 1772 indictment before the King's Bench of R. Coates the Elder and his wife, Susannah the Younger, for the illegal confinement of Mrs. Ewbank for almost two months in their madhouse at Bethnal Green, at the request of an abusive husband who had taken her children from her, beaten her, and "used her very ill."[102] During the course of the trial, which lasted from 9 A.M. until 4.30 P.M., the case of Mrs. Mills was also brought forward, another woman who had allegedly been committed nefariously by her husband and had then been verbally and physically abused by Coates and his wife, and a keeper called Gunston.[103] It was the latter case that had first come to the attention of the courts, Mrs. Mills having appeared before Sir John Fielding at the assizes earlier that year, and it was Mrs. Mills herself who had brought Ewbank's case to the court's notice. Supposedly, Mills had been decoyed into Bethnal Green after being misinformed that her husband was in trouble and under arrest. Once there, it was alleged, she had been handcuffed and chained, verbally abused by the keepers as "a d[amne]d infernal b[itc]h" in a house dedicated to "mad bitches," told that "she should have her hair cut off, and her head shaved," and given "rotten beef" to eat. Still more indignities were then heaped upon her: "the stench" of her apartment "was intolerable," "as almost made her retch"; and its "appearance beyond description wretched." It was there that Mills met Ewbank, who had also been confined by her husband's artifices "for a considerable time."

Visiting his wife thereafter, Mr. Mills was apparently prompted to regret his actions, and having "declared his sorrow . . . took her home with him" within two days of her confinement. Mrs. Ewbank, on the other hand, was not released until her former co-prisoner had applied to Fielding and Justice Wilmot for a habeas corpus and a warrant against the keeper. Even then, Wilmot was obliged to attend the house in person before he could procure her liberation, finding her "apparently sane," but "in a truly piteous [sic] situation, having a hole quite through her hand" that was presumed to have been "occasioned by some violence from her inhuman keepers." Evidently, although Fielding had ordered both cases to be prosecuted, Mrs. Mills had been unwilling to bring charges against her repentant husband. This explains why it was Ewbank's case that took precedence in the proceedings when both cases were subsequently transferred to the King's Bench. Ultimately, judgment on Mr. Mills was suspended by the latter court, "till his wife thinks fit to complain of him," it being recognized "that he could not be imprisoned without ruin to both."

The straightforward narrative we have presented here tends to obscure a significant issue: contemporary accounts of both women's treatment vary considerably in their details, highlighting the problems inherent in trying to reconstruct the historical record from conflicting accounts with their own differing constructions of a case. The *Annual Register*, for example, asserts that Mrs. Ewbank was confined for a year and three quarters, while the actual law report states more reliably that she was detained for just two months. There seems little doubt that the former version—which claimed that Mrs. Ewbank was "forcibly dragged to the madhouse, by threatening to rip open her belly if she resisted"—was exaggerated for effect. Likewise, there are grounds to believe that the women's own representatives in court were prone to embroider upon reality, constructing hyperbolic images of the awfulness of their situations under confinement in order to achieve the desired impact on their audience.

More significantly for our purposes, during the course of Mrs. Ewbank's case, an explicit contrast was drawn with a previous instance of alleged false confinement in which Monro had been very much involved, namely that of Mr. Wood (discussed earlier in chapter 2). Indeed, in deliberating over the cases of 1772, the King's Bench judge made detailed and pointed reference to Monro's and others' treatment of Wood. Wood's treatment was referred to as something of a model for what had been, and should be, best practice in the confinement of the insane in private madhouses, while Monro was represented as something of an exemplar himself:

> In Doctor Monro's case, you observe, whatever would be done by the most tender husband or parent, must be the treatment; no coercion, no harshness of treatment; nothing but with the best view, subject to the assistance of the faculty. Whatever is done with any other view, all unnecessary severity, all confinement other than for the best purpose of the unhappy person's recovery; is subject to a censure proportionate to the conduct.

Proceeding to detail at greater length Monro's impeccable conduct in such cases, the judge pointed out how "in Mr Wood's case, Dr Monro was acquitted by special jury, both here and in London; it appearing there, that every thing had been done for the best." [104]

Though the 1772 case details conspicuous abuse, it simultaneously reveals the thoroughness of many of the judicial investigations that were conducted, as well as the conspicuous efforts often made to support appropriate or even "tender" treatment aimed at the patient's recovery. On the other hand, it also raises the question of potential bias in medico-legal proceedings, for not all was as it seems. The judge in both the Wood and Ewbank cases was one and the same, William Murray, earl of Mansfield (1705–93), Lord Chief Justice of the Court of King's Bench between 1756 and 1772,[105] who was thus, in part, merely reiterating the verity and wisdom of his own previous judgment. As a nationalistic Scot, furthermore, he may well have had other reasons to be favorably disposed toward his compatriot Monro.[106] Whatever the case, Mansfield provides a telling example of the decided disinclination among the judiciary to find distinguished members of the medical faculty to blame for their part in the mad-trade, lest intervention by the courts discourage doctors and madhouse-keepers from continuing to offer services generally conceived as being a social and medical necessity.

Although the Ewbank case was one in which not only false confinement but appallingly brutal treatment was fully substantiated, and which involved the adjudication of a lawsuit, significantly just two years before the 1774 Act, it was an example of how the bench was at great pains to resist the rising clamor for legislation on madhouses. Indeed, Mansfield's dicta in the case provide us with invaluable insight into the reasons for the great reluctance in elite social, legal, and governmental circles to support an act to regulate madhouses. As Mansfield expressed it: "Much has been said, and I think on a wrong foundation, of regulating these houses. The law recognizes them not; if we go to regulate them, we establish them by law." Mansfield was clearly convinced that cases arising out of alleged abuses in private madhouses were best dealt with individually, according to their "particular circumstances," whereby they might be made to "stand the strictest test." To legislate would simply provide a veil of legitimacy for bad practices, or for an unjustified confinement in a madhouse. Under existing circumstances such steps could only be regarded as acts "of authority not allowed by law," requiring "the doers [to] answer for . . . such" and to prove that they acted "with the best motives" and out of "necessity." For Mansfield, the "special jury" and the weight (and effects) of public censure upon bad conduct were the proper means of settling these issues, not the promulgation of a set of laws that would run the risk of making inveterate abuses legally justifiable—to say nothing of rendering madness in private families all too often a matter of public knowledge. Mansfield voiced a concern that was widespread in elite society when he spoke of the undesirability of requiring the moneyed insane to "always have their case made

notorious by a commission under the Great Seal," and for the "indi-
gent" to be "necessitated to that expensive remedy"—twin problems
that together explain why so few commissions of lunacy were initiated
in this period. Yet adhering to such a position required ignoring the
many previous cases of abuse in such institutions that had come to light
over previous decades. Mansfield's statement that, until Mrs. Mill's case,
he had "never heard of a madhouse, without regular medical attendance
by some of the faculty," was surely disingenuous, or at least a form of
stubborn denial, given the large body of testimony to the contrary, not
least the report made by the 1763 Commons inquiry.[107]

In reality, as we have already suggested, worries about false confinement were an extremely sensitive issue in this period, and concerns of
this sort clearly profoundly affected Monro's and other mad-doctors'
practices. They derived in part from the vigor of Enlightenment liber-
tarianism, and the vociferousness with which eighteenth-century elite
culture (in theory, at least) prized the various rights of free-born Englishmen—however inconsistently those rights may have been defined in
actual practice. The confrontation of this libertarian spirit with the unregulated and somewhat contradictory growth in the private mad-trade
(and other contemporary machinery of confinement) made the private
madhouse a particular source of concern in the popular press and magazines of the day. Meanwhile, the touchiness of the subject of false imprisonment, and the liability of mad-doctors like Monro to be sued by
patients and their friends unhappy with the withdrawal of their liberties,
prompted a range of responses from the profession. Physicians went to
increasing lengths to substantiate their authority to decide when seques-
tration was appropriate and necessary, and to persuade families of their
expertise and good intentions—but also to apprise their colleagues of
the hazards involved and the methods they should use in the diagnosis
and confinement of the insane. Thus, contemporary medical treatises
on madness regularly warned against the plausibility of the mad, and
stressed how easy it was for the mad to appear sane, at least to those in-
experienced and unlearned. Prior to any notion of monomania, or any
workable definition of partial insanity, there was a growing recognition—at the very least in medical circles—that the mad might appear
and behave like the sane in many aspects of their lives, and cunningly
strive to avoid detection of their derangement. This, in turn, placed the
onus on the mad-doctor as a diagnostic detective, and on his claims to
possess special diagnostic skills. To devise and deploy tactics to catch the
dissembling patient off guard; to find the particular nub or subject of the

patient's delusion; to discover the motions of irrationality and disease concealed beneath apparent mental calm: all these talents were trumpeted as key elements of the mad-doctor's art. The doctor was admonished to exercise vigilance and patience, and sometimes even to resort to ploys and tricks, in order to penetrate his patients' facades. The medical literature on madness was jocularly mirrored and mocked in this respect by a long tradition of Augustan satire, which pictured the world as one great Bedlam, where too many of the insane were at liberty and disguised as normal, rational citizens. Regularly, stories were relayed of madmen and dunces fooling their sober (or equally weak-headed) observers into believing that they were sane, if not great, personages.

Monro himself took measures in his practice to preclude being deceived by his patients' "seeming composure," and his case book provides some exemplary, if rather self-congratulatory, histories of the process and the means the mad-doctor typically employed to detect derangement. Monro took care not to employ techniques and ruses that might smack of quackery (such as mesmerism, or the "fixing with the eye," used by the Willises on George III and their other patients). His approach relied instead on prolonged acquaintance and careful observation, sometimes without letting patients know they were being observed. Contemporary medical texts often recommended the enhancement of the mad-doctor's investigatory power that might be gained by concealing his own identity from the guardedness of the patient. Monro's methods also involved (ideally, at least) sustained and varied inquiries and verbal discourse, and pressure on any particular points of frailty, designed to bring to light his patients' "inconsistencies." Monro's exposure of the madness of Captain Knackstone, whom he saw at Duffield's madhouse, presents us with an eloquent case in point:

> He talks very well & with coherence, & seeming composure upon the subjects of his confinement, & the ill usage he has met with on that account, & might in all probability succeed in making people unacquainted with him or his story, beleive that he was confined without reason, & they would conclude, if they enquir'd no farther, that liberty was terribly [oppressed] by the usage he rec^d. but tho he can talk with consistence & seeming moderation, let him but alone his talk is without end, even to tire himself & bring him into flurries: his actions if carefully observ'd without letting him know it, are all trifling & childish : & by those who are acquainted with him he may be brought into inconsistencies, he fancies that he has been charg'd with being register'd as a freeMason at the Devil Tavern, & on this point, if press'd, he cannot talk, so as to make himself intelligible.[108]

MONRO BECOMES PART OF THE BUSINESS

Clearly not a family to miss out on opportunities for enterprise, the Monros were quick to capitalize on the tremendous growth in the trade in lunacy that marked the eighteenth century. Not content, however, with the retainers and fees they could obtain for referring and subsequently treating inmates in madhouses run by others, at some point in the 1760s or 1770s, they entered the business more directly. Immediately following the passage of the 1774 Act for Regulating Madhouses (owing to its stipulation that, for the first time, required proprietors of these houses to obtain a license from the College of Physicians), the family involvement became a matter of public record when John Monro became the licensee of Brooke House in Hackney.[109] We can, however, trace his connections to its operations back at least a dozen years earlier, to 1762, when he was first recorded as recommending a patient be placed there, and it seems distinctly possible that he had had a close connection with Brooke House from its opening in 1758 or 1759, or shortly thereafter.[110] Granted, the establishment is not explicitly mentioned in the 1766 case book, but there seems little doubt that the two patients recorded as sent to Mr. Clarke's were actually being kept in Brooke House. Monro certainly spoke in very personal terms about these cases being "under my care," and of what "we would permit," and it seems likely that he was already receiving the profits from this institution.[111] A large number of entries meticulously record his attendance on patients held at private residencies or at other madhouses (whose names and addresses he provides us with). It seems reasonable to presume that at least a few of the remaining cases—those Monro mentions without giving any clues as to where they were treated—are patients who were seen at, or subsequently conveyed to, Hackney.

One of Monro's patients who was certainly sent to Brooke House was the print and map seller John Bennett. Bennett had been taken into partnership by Robert Sayer (1725–94) in 1777, having been Sayer's servant and apprentice from 1760, and a journeyman for him since 1773.[112] Sayer was a particularly important and well-known operator in the printing and map selling trade, employing a large number of workmen to engrave under his directions. Bennett was admitted to Brooke House in April 1783, his illness first manifesting itself around 1781 in such "violent . . . temper" and such frequent quarrels with the workmen "that they would not work any longer for the shop," while, contradictorily, he was also apt to be "very extravagant in the payment of the workmen." [113] More than likely, Bennett found the stresses of running a business too much for him, having been elevated from the rather more limited responsibilities of one of the workers, and the record of Sayer's and Bennett's output suggests that the firm was at its busiest and most pressurized during 1775–80, just before Bennett began to show symptoms of derangement. The careers of other famous contemporary engravers, including James Ward (1769–1859), John Raphael Smith (1752–1812), and William Blake (1757–1827), provide ample evidence of the demands on the health and nerves of such concentrated but monotonous work. [114]

Evidently Bennett was so insane on admission to Brooke House that "it was found necessary to confine him by a strait waistcoat" (another indication that Monro shared the Bethlem apothecary John Gozna's preference for this type of restraint over irons). He remained in confinement at the madhouse for nine months under Monro's care, finally "by Doctor Monro's consent being removed to private lodgings." While no lunacy commission was initiated in Bennett's case, soon after his release, Sayer decided to terminate their business relationship, and accordingly brought an action against his partner before Chancery in June 1784. Understandably, he was unhappy about Bennett's ability to transact business, but perhaps he was equally uncomfortable about being in partnership with a quondam lunatic whose current and continuing mental stability was far from assured. Significantly, although two apothecaries were summoned by the defense to testify at the trial, neither was able to sufficiently substantiate claims that Bennett was sound enough for business, let alone to support the assertion of one of them that he was unlikely to relapse. [115] The judge in the case, who censured all parties, including the apothecaries and Bennett's family for their poor presentations of evidence, emphasized the difficulties of determining the precise extent of Bennett's recovery. The patient might well, after all, be experiencing no more than a temporary lucid interval, which, asserted the judge, "every lunatic is supposed to have." It was common knowledge, he insisted, that "it is very frequent for persons once mad not to recover," and he could find no grounds for the apothecary's confidence as to the unlikelihood of a relapse. Called as a witness before the Old Bailey in another case during the course of the same year, the aforementioned John Gozna, Monro's colleague at Bethlem, had been emphatic that "most cases" of insanity "are subject to relapse," and—if he had been summoned—Monro might well have testified in similar terms. [116] However, neither Monro nor any other physician was summoned to the trial, while the plaintiff failed to call any medical witnesses at all.

Significantly, the judge confessed himself "astonished that neither party examined Doctor Monro," particularly given that the doctor "ought to have had frequent and recent opportunities of seeing him." In the absence of convincing medical testimony, he felt himself obliged to examine lay witnesses and the defendant himself to determine whether he was mentally competent to conduct his business partnership, and concluded that he was so "and had been so since November 1783." This was a verdict that was so much to Sayer's displeasure that he persuaded the court to direct a further legal inquiry as to the precise date when Bennett was fit to transact business, and whether he was still in such a state of mind. Whether there was ever a judicial resolution of these issues is not clear, for no record of such a hearing appears to have survived.

Retrospectively, the whole sequence of events indicates that, while expert testimony might have been gaining legitimacy with some lawyers and members of the judiciary at this time, it was far from an instinctive or automatic choice for laymen in insanity cases (whereas the court was apt to exercise considerable discrimination about the quality of such testimony). Eigen has pointed out, in his groundbreaking analysis of Old Bailey insanity trials, that as the century progressed, "medical personnel from Bethlem and St Luke's were [increasingly] well represented among the cadre of medical witnesses, as were medical practitioners from private asylums." He also noted, however, that it was (specialist) apothecaries and surgeons as much as mad-doctors who seem to have been seeking to enhance their income and status in this manner.[117]

Unlike the asylums that became such a striking and sinister feature of the English landscape during the next century, Brooke House was not a purpose-built establishment. Instead, like many another eighteenth-century madhouse, it was set up by adapting an existing set of buildings to the new task of confining the raving and the melancholic. Who provided the capital, how much was spent on the necessary modifications, and at precisely what stage John Monro became active in the enterprise are all issues that remain difficult to resolve. We *can* reconstruct, however, some aspects of the hitherto hidden history of Brooke House, drawing upon both pictorial and written evidence to give the reader some sense of what a madhouse of this sort looked like and how it accommodated its inmates.

King's House or Place, later to be known as Brooke House, was first erected on a two-hundred-acre estate in Hackney, possibly in the late fifteenth century, but certainly no later than 1532, at which time it belonged to the sixth earl of Northumberland. Subsequently, the property passed through a variety of hands, including those of Henry VIII's advisor, Thomas Cromwell, and the king himself. On the king's death, it was given to Sir William Herbert, a gentleman of his Privy Chamber, and thence sold on to a variety of aristocratic owners, ending up from 1609 onward, for a period of more than two hundred years, in the hands of the Greville family.[118]

It was William Clarke, described as "a gentleman of Hackney," who obtained a ninety-nine-year lease on the property in 1758 from one of the Grevilles, Lord Brooke.[119] It was Clarke also who appears to have set about reconstructing the existing sixteenth- and seventeenth-century buildings to accommodate a madhouse. Just over a century earlier, the well-known diarist John Evelyn had visited Brooke House and pronounced it "a despicable building,"[120] and by the early eighteenth century, the decaying structure had been roughly subdivided into a miscellaneous hodgepodge: a warren of apartments, a shop, a brewhouse, and a Presbyterian meeting house. Contemporary records leave an impression of "general squalor" and suggest that the disintegration of the building's fabric was already evident, all of which may have paved the way for its transformation into a madhouse.

Clarke, possibly with Monro as a silent partner, at once set about tearing down portions of the Jacobean structure, building a new wing to serve as the keeper's (later the superintendent's) residence and subdividing the interior to create a series of small rooms for patients, all arranged around two interior courtyards. Almost certainly, the medieval plan and conception of the house—"in which the outward aspect of a house, and the prospect from it, were regarded more as invitations to thieves and vagabonds than as amenities for the inhabitants . . . an inward facing house in which life centred around the courtyard . . ."[121]—made the conversion to its new role as a house of confinement easier. The whole project was clearly done on the cheap, with the result that "for the most part the rooms were devoid of decorative interest, many of them having been formed by the partitioning of large rooms with little care for anything beyond utilitarian considerations."[122] On the first floor, the "long gallery" of the Elizabethan house was chopped up into a series of individual cells, each equipped with its own fireplace—the successive ranks of the chimneys creating a very odd effect. Dormitories for some of the less affluent inmates, and the ladies' drawing room, occupied the south

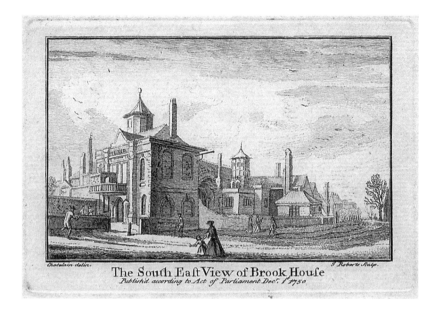

The South East View of Brook House.
Publish'd according to Act of Parliament Dec.ʳ 1 1750

FIGURE 29. View of Brooke House from the southeast in the 1750s. A drawing by J. Roberts, completed some time between 1750 and 1758, of a dilapidated Brooke House just before it was modified to serve as a madhouse. Reproduced by kind permission of the Hackney Archives, London, from *Survey of London,* plate 12b.

side, along with a more sinister pair of cells: the "strong room" and the "padded room"—clearly a nineteenth-century addition—for confinement of the particularly recalcitrant. The wing dividing the two interior courtyards was partially occupied by a "billiard room" for the use of the male patients.

Decades later Richard Paternoster, a disgruntled inmate who complained he had been corruptly confined within these walls, left us a patient's-eye view of Brooke House, which had remained essentially unaltered physically since John Monro's tenure and which was now run by John's great-grandson Henry. Henry Monro, like John, was content to leave the grubby business of running the establishment on a day-to-day basis to his resident lay assistants. As Paternoster described Brooke House in 1841:

> It is licensed for fifty patients, who are under the charge of the Misses Pettingal, Dr [Henry] Monro residing in Cavendish-square, and going only oc-

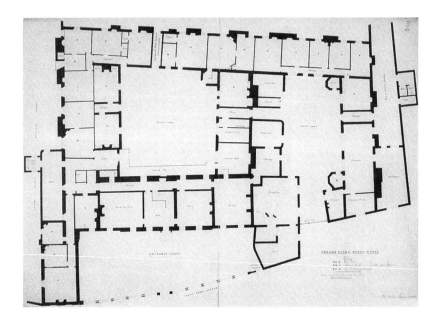

FIGURE 30. Plan of the ground floor of Brooke House, drawn by John Burlison (1842). The physical structure had remained essentially unaltered since the buildings were first adapted for use as a madhouse. Note the partitioning of space into many small rooms surrounding the two courtyards. Access to the male patients' "airing ground" was through the small passageway at the top of the courtyard on the left, while the female "airing court" is on the right side of the plan. Reproduced by kind permission of the Hackney Archives, London, from plate 4 in Ernest Mann, *Brooke House, Hackney,* 1904.

casionally to Clapton to give general orders and arrange accounts. The house is an old-fashioned and dilapidated place, to which a modern front has been attached, which fails to give any idea of what the interior is. The situation is low and damp, and devoid of any prospect. Immediately behind the house is a grass-plot, of about thirty paces square, surrounded by a high wall. This, with the exception of the gravel walk round it, was entirely under water. Beyond was an extensive kitchen-garden in which the female prisoners [*sic*] were allowed to walk. . . . Not one foot of pleasure garden, no flowers, no shady walks, no seats, nothing whatever pretty or agreeable. . . . [Set in the middle of the] green swamp [that constituted the male "airing court" was] a gloomy-looking building of about seven feet square . . . a cell for the refractory. . . . [Meanwhile, for the female patients, small rooms opened off] long galleries, some looking into a small court-yard, surrounded by buildings, and some into the green swamp where the male prisoners are allowed to walk

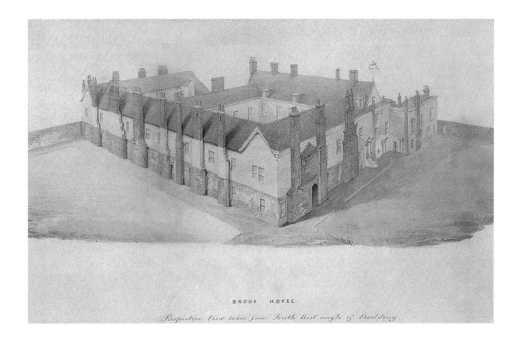

BROOK HOVSE

Perspective View taken from South West angle of Building

FIGURE 31. Perspective view of southwest side of Brooke House, painted by George Toussaint (ca. 1844). Note the serried ranks of chimneys arrayed around the courtyards, added to heat the individual rooms. Reproduced by kind permission of the Hackney Archives, London.

round and round. They were most wretchedly furnished with old-fashioned latticed windows, letting the wind in so as to defy all attempts at keeping warm . . . and with thick iron bars outside, which would effectually prevent escape.[123]

Dismal as Brooke House may well have seemed from a patient's point of view—even in a period six or seven decades previous to this description—for the Monros it was a wonderfully profitable place in which to confine many of their private patients. Small wonder, then, that although John Monro relinquished the license to Mary Hawkins in 1784 (probably in order to avoid the trouble of prosecutions that tended to be encouraged by direct ownership), he nevertheless held tightly on to his financial control over the madhouse until his death in 1791. John's son Thomas became the licensee when Mary Hawkins died in 1790. Haw-

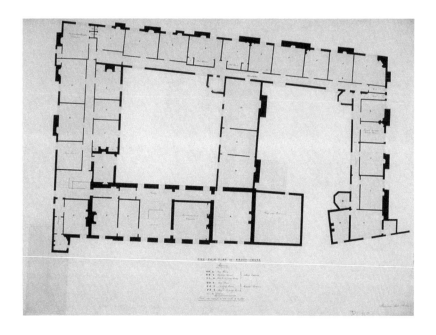

FIGURE 32. Plan of the upper floor of Brooke House (1842). Reproduced by kind permission of the Hackney Archives, London, from plate 5 in Ernest Mann, *Brooke House, Hackney,* 1904.

kins's legacy of around £11,000 in value, including a bequest of £1,000 to John and his family, evidences the prosperity of the business and its continuing intimate attachment to the Monros. John's will not surprisingly provided explicit instructions to his sons about the preservation and running in partnership of what—like the Miles's and other madhouse proprietors—he referred to and thought of as the family "business." The lion's share (50 percent) of the profits was to accrue to Thomas, as physician, in consideration that it would "in a great degree depend upon and be supported by him," and a sizable amount was held aside each year to provide for John's widow.[124]

Monro's will indicates that he owned other property in Clapton apart from Brooke House, and we know that Monro had also taken over the Clerkenwell madhouse formerly leased by his rival Battie (and left to Battie's family by his will).[125] To all intents and purposes, mad-doctors

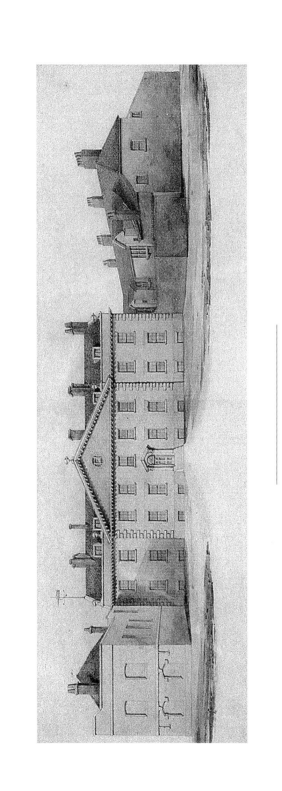

FIGURE 33. East elevation of Brooke House, painted by George Toussaint (1844). Shows the Georgian wing, built in 1758–59, in which the madhouse-keeper lived. It was this part of the house that was visible from the street. Reproduced by kind permission of the Hackney Archives, London.

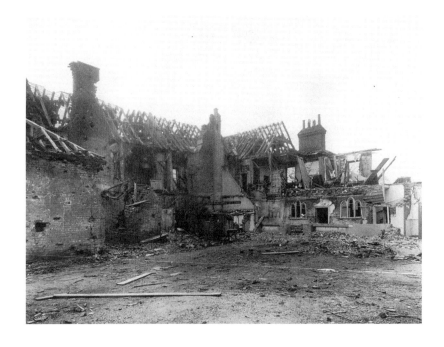

FIGURE 34. View of the wrecked northern courtyard of Brooke House after October 1940 bombing. Reproduced by kind permis- sion of the Hackney Archives, London, from *Survey of London,* plate 16b.

like Battie and Monro were running these madhouses as their own private businesses rather than merely attending patients confined in them. Still they seem to have elected to keep their madhouses as lease-hold properties, under the nominal control of keepers and other em-ployees, rather than adopting titles such as master or superintendent of such houses, in order to steer clear of the possibility of personal prosecutions.[126]

Brooke House remained the lucrative heart of the Monro family's mad-business for exactly a century more. John Monro's son Charles, a solicitor and partner in the enterprise with his brother Thomas, secured the freehold of the property from the earl of Warwick in 1820, and suc-cessive generations managed its operations until 1891. One family mem-ber, Edward Thomas Monro, the last of the dynasty to serve as Beth-lem's physician (1816–53), had the unwanted distinction of being committed as a patient to the asylum, which by then was run by his son Henry. Even after the latter's death brought an end to the family's direct involvement in the asylum's affairs, Charles Monro's descendants continued to own the estate, and to lease the madhouse to a resident superintendent.

It took Hitler's bombers to end Brooke House's nearly two centuries of operations as a private asylum. In October 1940, at the height of the Blitz, a high explosive bomb wrecked the northern courtyard and irretrievably damaged the remaining buildings. The patients were evacuated and the asylum closed, its uninhabitable ruins passing into the hands of the London County Council until their demolition in 1954–55.[127] John Monro's madhouse was no more.

CHAPTER 6

Murder Most Foul, Madness Most High

The Courtroom, the Stateroom,
and the Misty Summits
of the Mad-Doctor's Expertise

IN VAIN WOULD HIS Excusers endeavour to palliate his Enormities, by imputing them to Madness. . . . Madness only operates by inflaming and enlarging the good or evil Dispositions of the Mind: For the *Curators of Bedlam* assure us, that some Lunaticks are Persons of . . . Virtues, which appear in their highest Ravings . . . while others, on the contrary, discover in every Word and Action, the utmost *Baseness* and Depravity. . . .

> Jonathan Swift, *A Vindication of . . .*
> *the Lord C[artare]t* (1730)[1]

To say he's mad will not avail:
The Neighbours all cry, *Shoot him dead*,
Hang, Drown, or knock him on the Head.

> Jonathan Swift, *Traulus*
> (1730)[2]

The day drew nigh when our great man was to exemplify the last and noblest act of greatness by which any hero can signalise himself. This was the day of execution, or consummation, or apotheosis (for it is called by different names), which was to give our hero an opportunity of facing death and damnation, without any fear in his heart, or, at least, without betraying any symptoms of it on his countenance. A completion of GREATNESS which is heartily to be wished to every great man . . .

> Henry Fielding, *The Life/History*
> *of Jonathan Wild the Great* (1743)[3]

. . . he never in his life had seen a person more disordered . . . her Language was perfectly unintelligible and it was impossible to relate it . . . she appeared to have a consciousness of what she had done, but did not seem sensible of having committed any crime . . . in her conversation yesterday she burst out without any apparent cause into a fit of Laughter so violent as to make it necessary for her to support herself against the back of a chair. . . .

> From John Monro's testimony on the case
> of Margaret Nicholson (1786)[4]

A NOTORIOUS MURDER:
THE "FEROCIOUS" EARL FERRERS

In 1760, John Monro's visibility and reputation in aristocratic circles drew him into one of the most sensational criminal trials of the eighteenth century: the prosecution of Lawrence Shirley, Earl Ferrers, for the brutal murder of one of his servants, his steward John Johnson, a longtime family retainer. Monro's appearance on the stand marked a particularly dramatic moment in the proceedings, as the accused earl struggled vainly to save his neck.

Ferrers was an erratic, irascible man, with a family history of insanity and a record of domestic violence that had already got him into trouble with the law.[5] (Monro had, in fact, previously treated his uncle and possibly an aunt for lunacy.) On a former occasion, the earl's drinking and rages had led to him "attempting to murder his wife, Mary, a pretty, harmless woman,"[6] the "fortuneless sister of Sir William Meredith," who, he maintained, had "trepanned him into marriage [in September 1752] while he was in a [previous] state of drunkenness."[7] In fact, as King's Bench records show, Ferrers was guilty of a long history of abusive behavior toward his wife. He had threatened her life, at one point informing her that he would burn her in her bed, and on other occasions beating and attempting to strangle her.[8] Mary meanwhile appears to have made repeated and sincere efforts to cohabit peaceably with her volatile spouse. Her family was so worried about her safety that they attempted to engineer her escape, only for Ferrers to set off in hot pursuit with pistols in hand, accompanied by an armed posse of servants (including the haplessly loyal Johnson, who was later to testify in the earl's favor during separation proceedings). After flinging mortal threats against all and sundry standing in his way, Ferrers returned his wife to

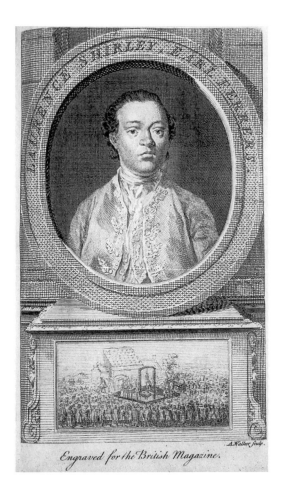

where he felt she belonged (no matter what), and kept her a virtual prisoner at his country seat at Staunton, in Leicester.

Subsequently, her anxious family pursued legal means to secure Mary's freedom from her husband's control, her brother issuing a writ of habeas corpus against the earl. Ferrers, however, refused to comply with the writ, and it had to be reissued before the case was finally heard between January and May 1757, a clear indication that he already considered himself (presumably by virtue of his elevated social status) to be above the law. In the course of the litigation, Mary had her husband bound over to keep the peace, and in order to make bail, Ferrers was obliged to provide sureties of £10,000. After the habeas corpus proceedings (held during January and 1 February), Mary initiated a separation suit in the London Consistory Court. Even then Ferrers refused to submit answers to her accusations (or "libel"), the church court then imposing its most serious sanction by excommunicating him for his contempt.[9] After a further flare-up, when (with loaded pistols) Ferrers hunted down his wife at her residence with the earl of Westmoreland and proceeded to assault her, the errant earl was taken into custody and once again compelled to enter into articles to keep the peace. It was only then, presumably at the end of her tether, that Mary determined to pursue a parliamentary action, and there followed (in January 1758) the earl's legal separation from his spouse by means of a private bill.[10] The petition brought by Countess Ferrers's brother, Sir William Meredith, initially encountered considerable parliamentary resistance, but eventually received royal assent on 20 June 1758.[11] The terms, to which Ferrers reluctantly assented, provided for her maintenance from the proceeds of his estate, and, always a man to hold a grudge, Ferrers brooded incessantly thereafter over this "theft" of what was rightfully his.

These latter proceedings reveal that Ferrers's general conduct and the extremity of his violence toward his wife not only convinced her, her family, and her servants that her life was in danger, but suggested to some that her husband was periodically insane. Ferrers himself chose to blame his behavior on the fact "that the Drinking of strong Liquor had a very unfortunate Effect upon this Deponent rendering him . . . hasty passionate and cholerick [sic] entirely altering the Natural Disposition of his Temper." One of his servants, William Hodgson, confirmed that when the earl drank "he is a madman" and would beat or strike his wife for such trifles as a chair being out of place or the supper not being ready.[12] Significantly, these were excuses the earl was to recycle but two years later, when he pled his case on the more serious charge of murder, and he himself embraced the notion that he was mad, summoning Monro as a witness in an attempt to lend the defense more credence.

In the aftermath of the separation from his wife, the management of Ferrers's estates was handed over to his steward, Johnson.[13] Inevitably, Ferrers soon quarreled with him, accusing the luckless man of plotting with his enemies to engineer his wife's settlement and of obstructing his efforts to profit from the coal that had been found on his lands. On 21 January 1760, according to Horace Walpole, "he sent away all his servants but [this] one, and, like that heroic murderess Queen Christina, carried the poor man through a gallery and several rooms, locking them after him"—the prelude to "the most barbarous and deliberate [murder]." [14] The row that then erupted was furious. Witnesses testified that when the quarrel was at its height, Ferrers shouted, "Down on your knees; your time is come; you must die," and instructed his steward to pray to God for forgiveness as these were to be his last moments on this earth.

Johnson's age, his years of faithful service, and the implacable hatred his master had displayed toward him all seem to have intensified public outrage about Ferrers's conduct. All were central elements, for example, in the *London Magazine*'s recital of the case:

> As events reached their climax, and the deadly nature of the encounter became manifest, the old gentleman expostulated with him, desiring to know in what he had offended; that he doubted not but upon examination he would find his accompts [*sic*] exact, and, as they had always been, to his satisfaction. He beseeched his Lordship to give him leave to explain them: His answer was, that he did not doubt his accounts, but he had been a tyrant, and he was determined to punish him, and insisted on his falling on his knees to make his peace with his God, for he should never rise again till he rose at the resurrection. The old gentleman then fell upon one knee, and besought him to consider his age and services; that he had been thirty years a servant in the family, and that he could never be charged with wrong to any man. [But his pleas for mercy fell on deaf ears.] His Lordship made answer . . . pulling a pistol out of his pocket, and cocking it, bid him instantly fall on his knees, and pray to God, for now was the last moment he had to live. He then obeyed and his Lordship discharged the pistol full at his body . . . [wounding him in the stomach]. [15]

After the shooting Ferrers was reported to have lifted Johnson up and asked him how he felt. The dying steward replied, "like as man who has but a few moments to live." [16] Placing him in a chair, Ferrers apparently proceeded with contradictory coolness to instruct a servant to fetch a surgeon, Mr. Thomas Kirkland. [17]

The wound, an inch wide and four inches deep, according to the coroner, was not immediately fatal, and Johnson, with some assistance, staggered upstairs to bed. Hours later his assailant once more materialized—having, over dinner with the surgeon, got drunk and into another "outragious" temper against Johnson—and demanded that the steward confess to his villainy. Ferrers being "about to drag him out of Bed upon the Floor," was only prevented by Johnson's weakly furnishing him with the confession he wanted: "I am a Villain." Ferrers was further (if temporarily) pacified by the terrified surgeon (who feared for his own life should Johnson die, and who—or so some sources said—the distempered earl had explicitly threatened if he breathed a word about the crime). Kirkland at length managed to steal out of the house and get word to a neighboring justice. A party of seven armed men was rapidly assembled and Johnson was successfully removed to the surgeon's own home. However, medical intervention proved fruitless. Before the day was out, the victim was a corpse, after which a crowd of angry tenants and colliers surrounded Ferrers's house, thwarted his attempt at an armed escape, and arrested him. Within hours, he was confined in Leicester gaol, from whence he was subsequently removed to London and imprisoned in the Tower.[18]

Three months later, in April 1760, Ferrers found himself arraigned and on trial for his life before a literal jury of his peers, 117 members of the House of Lords.[19] In Smollett's words, "The circumstances of this assassination appeared so cruel and deliberate, that the people cried aloud for vengeance,"[20] and the weeks of waiting for the trial to begin had aroused a frenzy of interest in the proceedings. To accommodate some small portion of the prospective audience, arrangements were made to transfer the trial to Westminster Hall, and the Lord Great Chamberlain was instructed to prepare a maximum of 1,070 tickets granting admission to the spectacle. The hall was specially decorated and designed for the event, fitted out with a throne under a velvet canopy for the king; a crimson velvet chair beneath that for the Lord High Steward; a tent with crimson silk curtains for the royal family and another for the great officers of the crown; and further bedecked with wool-packs covered with crimson cloth and crimson seats for the Lords Spiritual and Temporal.[21] The front benches on each side were reserved for peeresses, their daughters, and the wives of the eldest sons of peers, and eight tickets were set aside for each peer who had personally attended parliament during the current session. Demand for the remaining spaces far exceeded supply, and the Lord Chamberlain's office was besieged with requests for tickets: "The Countess Dowager of Warwick presents her compliments to the Duke of Ancaster [the Lord Chamberlain] and (if not too troublesome) will take it as a particular favour if His Grace has not disposed of all his Tickets for the Tryal of the Unfortunate Lord, if he woud [*sic*] oblige her with a couple for her daughter Lady Charlotte Rich." And again:

> My Lord,
>
> My son being come up from Oxford to hear Ld Ferrers Tryal hope you'll excuse my taking the liberty to beg yr favor [*sic*] of two places in yr Box if not all engaged and will lay under a particular obligation.
>
> Yours Grace's most obedient and humble servt Charles Sheffield.

Many more similarly phrased requests were received.[22]

The scene was thus set for Ferrers's trial to be a truly spectacular theatrical event (and one with a larger actual—if smaller virtual—audience than modern equivalents, such as the circus-like trial of O. J. Simpson). For spectacle and the carnivalesque were at the very crux of early modern notions of justice and deterrence, the *Royal Magazine* commenting that however "dreadful to him [i.e., Ferrers], the admirable magnificence of that august assembly [was], to every eye but his own, [it constituted] a scene of exquisite entertainment."[23] The earl's journey to Westminster Hall only amplified the drama and anticipation surrounding the trial, as Ferrers processed in his landau, attended by five other coaches with his own arms and livery; by nearly thirty gentlemen and twenty servants also in livery; by five hundred foot-guards out of Colonel Gore's three regiments of mounted guards; and by thirty yeomen of the guard.[24] The hall, meanwhile, was filled before 8 A.M., the press noting in particular the "great appearance of ladies elegantly dressed to hear the Trial; many of them" arriving, like Ferrers himself, "by [coach and] six [horses]."[25] Most would-be voyeurs, of course, including all those without aristocratic connections, were compelled to rely on second-hand accounts of the proceedings, with which journalists eagerly supplied them.

Eighteenth-century law was designed first and foremost for the protection of property and men of property.[26] Its formal provisions were singularly sanguinary, with as many as two hundred offenses punishable, in principle, by death. Yet, in practice, the "Bloody Code's" reliance on the terror of Tyburn was capricious rather than systematic, with many a capital criminal avoiding a death sentence—either through the intercession of judge or jury at the time of the trial[27] or through a subsequent royal pardon or commutation of sentence. Despite ideological proclamations of equality before the law, the rich and powerful were seldom caught in its coils, and rare indeed was the aristocrat (whatever his crimes) who ever faced the extreme sanction of death.[28]

Whether because he was so eminently unpleasant a character, or from the publicity that attended his heinous crime, Lord Ferrers found that he was likely to become the most conspicuous of exceptions to this rule. In desperation, and unable to refute the evidence that he had shot Johnson, he and his family sought instead to excuse his actions as the product of insanity. In his opening remarks, Ferrers sought to sway the jurors:

> My Lords . . . the grounds of this defence has been a family complaint; and I have heard that my family have of late attempted to prove me such. The defence I mean is occasional insanity of the mind; and I am convinced from recollecting within myself, that, at the time of this action, I could not know what I was about. . . .[29]

Insanity had long been recognized as a defense against criminal charges, for the question of intent was central to common law assessments of guilt and innocence.[30] However, it was assumed that such judgments could be made by any competent citizen, and required no special expertise or insight. Hence, jurors who listened to the evidence and observed the defendant were generally expected to decide his or her fate on their own, on the basis of what they heard from ordinary witnesses, with scant notion that "expert" testimony would be forthcoming on the subject.[31]

In its early stages, Ferrers's defense adhered to precedent. Various servants and family members appeared on the stand, and the earl sought, rather self-contradictorily, to use their testimony to impeach his own sanity. His first witness was John Bennefold, who had been in charge of collecting the estate's rents, and had known Ferrers for more than two decades.

FERRERS: Please to observe what you know of my Conduct, as to the State of my Mind, without having any particular Questions asked of you.

BENNEFOLD: His Lordship has always behaved in a very strange manner, very flighty, very much like a Man out of his Mind, more particularly so within these Two Years past, such as being in Liquor, and swearing and cursing, and the like, and talking to himself, very much like a Man disordered in his Senses; and then he has behaved himself as well as any other Gentleman at times.

Under cross-examination, however, Bennefold was forced into a whole series of damaging admissions. He confessed he could not say that Ferrers "was in that State of Mind as not to know Right from Wrong," and conceded that Ferrers had successfully managed his own affairs. When asked whether Ferrers's complaints about losing control of his estate were "those of a Fool, or of a Man of Understanding upon the Subject," he admitted, "I should think, of a Man of Understanding." The attorney general pushed him still harder:

ATTORNEY GENERAL: As you have known him so long, and have been ad-
                     mitted to his Familiarity, I wish you would recollect
                     One single irrational Expression that you have ever
                     heard him make use of?
BENNEFOLD: I cannot recollect any in particular.

Bennefold's testimony was only too typical of what was to follow. Another servant of ten years' standing, Thomas Godfrey, cited as an instance of Ferrers's insanity the fact that he frequently gave instructions that "were either fruitless, or opposite to his Interest, and upon those Occasions I have always found it in vain to endeavour to dissuade his Lordship from it." However, when pressed as to whether such actions proceeded "from a Tenaciousness of his Opinion, or from the Insanity of his Mind?" the witness visibly hesitated before acknowledging that to term such incidents insanity "might be going too far." Worse still, when asked why, if Ferrers were mad, he had not advised the family to proceed with a commission of lunacy, he blurted out: "I am in great doubt whether my Lord was so insane as that a Commission of Lunacy could be taken out; I should think a Commission of Lunacy could not be taken out against him." [32]

Further witnesses, including Ferrers's two brothers, the Honourable and Reverend Walter Shirley and the Honourable Robert Shirley, proved no more persuasive, each conceding that he could not provide specific instances of insane behavior on the defendant's part, nor distinguish what actions were the product of madness rather than passion.[33] That mental instability was rife in the Shirley family few could question. That Ferrers's own mental state was such as to excuse his actions remained, however, distinctly doubtful. Perhaps sensing the desperateness of his plight, Ferrers now broke with precedent and summoned John Monro to the stand to testify as an expert in his behalf.

Those charged with felonies in the eighteenth century were not entitled to plead their cases through counsel, so perforce Ferrers had to question all his witnesses himself. Horace Walpole, who observed "the pomp and awfulness" of the proceedings with a mordant eye, commented on the peculiarity of the spectacle:

> At first I thought Lord Ferrers shocked, but in general he behaved rationally and coolly; though it was a strange contradiction to see a man trying, by his own sense, to prove himself out of his senses. It was more shocking to see his two brothers brought in to prove the lunacy in their own blood, in order to save their brother's life. Both are almost as ill-looking as the Earl; one of them is a clergyman, suspended by the Bishop of London for being a Methodist; the other a wild vagabond, whom they call in the country, "ragged and dangerous." [34]

Having in extremis turned to Bethlem's doctor as his last hope, Ferrers attempted to use Monro's presumed authority to buttress his claim to be excused as mad. However, as might have been expected, the defendant's performance in his own cause proved clumsy and inept. Opening with a reference to his uncle's madness, and Monro's involvement in treating the disorder, Ferrers sought somehow to elicit testimony from Monro that would convince their lordships that he could not be held responsible for his actions, in the process providing a series of clues about his own patterns of behavior:

FERRERS: Did you know the late earl Ferrers?

MONRO: I did.

FERRERS: Did you know him in any, and what, distemper?

MONRO: I attended him as a physician when he was under the unhappy influence of lunacy.

FERRERS: You are desired to mention what are the usual symptoms of lunacy.

MONRO: Uncommon fury, not caused by liquor, but very frequently raised by it; many others there are which tend to violence against other persons or against themselves; I do not know a stronger, or a more constant or a more unerring symptom of lunacy than jealousy, or suspicion without cause or grounds: there are many others too long to enumerate.

FERRERS: Has the carrying of arms been generally a circumstance of lunacy?

MONRO: I have known it to be so, but not generally. . . .

FERRERS: . . . Please to inform their lordships whether quarrelling with friends without cause is a symptom of insanity?

MONRO: Very frequently one.

FERRERS: Whether being naturally suspicious is a symptom of insanity?

MONRO: Yes, it is, without cause, a constant one.

FERRERS: Whether going armed where there is no danger is a symptom of
           lunacy?

MONRO: That must be according to the circumstances. . . .

FERRERS: Whether spitting in the looking glass, clenching the fist, and
           making mouths is a symptom of lunacy?

MONRO: I have frequently seen such in lunatic persons.

FERRERS: Whether walking in the room, talking to himself, and making
           odd gestures, are symptoms of lunacy?

MONRO: Very common ones.

FERRERS: Is quarrelling without cause a symptom of lunacy?

MONRO: It is a very frequent attendant upon such unhappy complaints
           and they are generally malicious.

FERRERS: Whether drinking coffee hot out of the spout of the pot is a
           symptom of lunacy?

MONRO: I should think it one in the present case; it is not a general one.

FERRERS: Whether lunatics, when they are angered with or without cause,
           know what they are doing?

MONRO: Sometimes, as well as I do now.

FERRERS: Is it common to have such a disorder in families in the blood?

MONRO: Unfortunately too common.

FERRERS: Whether lunatics, in their intervals, are conscious of their being
           lunatics?

MONRO: They are conscious of it; many both in and out of their intervals;
           very few that are not.

FERRERS: Whether lunatics are apt to be seized with fits of rage on a sudden?

MONRO: Very often.

FERRERS: Without any apparent cause?

MONRO: Without any apparent cause.

FERRERS: Is there any other way of discovering whether a man is lunatic or
           not, but by the irregularity of his behaviour or his pulse?

MONRO: By the irregularity of his behaviour; I know of no other method;
           the pulse discovers nothing in general.

A LORD: Please to inform their lordships whether a person under an
           immediate visitation from God of madness, has not commonly
           a fever?

MONRO: Seldom or never, unless it may be at the first attack of the distem-
           per, or in some very violent fit.[35]

   Clearly Monro sought to use his answers to put the best possible face
on Ferrers's claim to have been insane at the time of the crime. Equally
clearly, his testimony was full of cautions and equivocations, and sensibly so. For the behaviors he was asked to evaluate might, under other

circumstances, be interpreted (both in the courtroom and more generally in society) as evidence of a bad or vicious character. Whether assessed individually or collectively, in other words, these behaviors were insufficient to compel the conclusion that everyone who exhibited them was mad, and to have attempted to assert otherwise would have invited ridicule.

Evidence of Ferrers's morbid suspiciousness, discernible in his belief that his wife, servants, and others were conspiring against him, and in such acts as carrying pistols to bed with him, was undermined by the inconclusive answers that Monro gave to Ferrers's badly framed queries. The discomfort Monro displayed in his testimony at the trial was more, perhaps, a result of the clumsy and ill-judged nature of Ferrers's examination, than of any inexperience on Monro's part. Monro, for example, not surprisingly felt unable to answer with a definitive "yes" that to carry around pistols was necessarily a sign of madness. Evidence that Ferrers's "ferocity" was heightened by drunkenness likewise did little to assist his case, and whatever Monro or any other doctor might have said would have been unlikely to nullify the strong evidence of calculating and sustained intent provided in Ferrers's conduct both prior to and at the trial.

The attorney general had presented particularly damning evidence of Ferrers's determined and remorseless motives for committing the deed. Equally damning was evidence of his planned escape, when the earl had "stood a Seige [sic] of Four or Five Hours," and armed himself with "A Blunderbus [sic], Two or Three Pistols and a Dagger," only to be foiled from slipping out through his back garden by "a bold collier." [36] According to this testimony, despite some momentary compassion in summoning the surgeon for Johnson and toward the dying man's own children, Ferrers had immediately and heartlessly informed the daughter "that he had shot her Father; and that he had done it on purpose; and deliberately." [37] If that did not suffice to appall the assembled peers, his unrepentant words to the surgeon, with whom he bizarrely ate dinner as his victim lay perishing above stairs, certainly would have managed to do so. Informing Kirkland that he had intended to shoot Johnson a second time and had only forborne due to "the Pain he complained of," he was reported to have declared "do not say . . . I repented of what I have done: I am not sorry for it . . . it was premeditated." [38]

According to Walpole, the chilling callousness, if not pleasure, the earl displayed toward his crime at the trial caused "many of the lords" to regard him with "shock" and to turn away "with detestation."[39] Furthermore, the very fact that Ferrers was capable of conducting his defense was seen by many as constituting convincing evidence in itself that his memory and understanding were intact, and that he was thus fully accountable for the crime he had committed.

Closing the case for the prosecution, the solicitor general seized upon Monro's equivocations to call into question the import of the medical evidence. Dismissing the "many . . . Symptoms" that Monro had delineated as "Marks of Lunacy"—such as "Uncommon fury, jealousy, or suspicion without cause or grounds," "causeless Quarreling," and "carrying Arms"—he emphasized that "Doctor Monro . . . did not describe any of these Things as absolute Marks of Lunacy, so as to denote every Man a Lunatick, who was subject to them. Indeed, he could not have said it, consistent with Common Sense and Experience."[40] Rather than constituting evidence of Lord Ferrers's insanity, he argued, these so-called symptoms were aspects of the malignity of the earl's character. Ferrers's "Fury" had not been "caused by Liquor, but [merely] raised by it," while "carrying Arms . . . may prove, in many Cases, a bad Heart and a vicious Mind, as well as lunacy."[41] "Do not," the solicitor general continued, "many, who are not Lunaticks, suspect or quarrel without Cause, and become dangerous to their Neighbours?"[42]

Furthermore, Ferrers's plea, if accepted, threatened to undermine the very foundations of justice, for "if the Law were to receive such excuses, it would put a Sword into the Hand of every savage and licentious Man, to disturb private Life, and public Order."[43] For the evidence had shown that Ferrers weighed and planned his dreadful act, and proceeded with deliberation, his malice "steady, cool, and premeditated." Prior to the shooting, for example, he had practiced shooting at a deal board with his pistol, and he had taken care to send others away and lock the doors before dragging the wretched Johnson off to meet his death. Citing Justice Hale's historic legal distinction between total and partial insanity, the solicitor general stressed that the second was insufficient to excuse crime, for "even felons are under a degree of this when they offend," while contrariwise even the understanding of a child of fourteen was sufficient for guilt to be ascribed. To the same purpose, he asserted a similar distinction between permanent insanity and "Lunacy, which comes by Periods or Fits." Nor was insanity proceeding from drunkenness exculpatory, as it was "voluntary [sic] contracted" (unless poison or bad medicine had been involved).[44] Acquittal because of the prisoner's mental state would depend upon a very different assessment of the case:

> If there be a total and permanent want of reason, it will acquit the prisoner. If there be a total temporary want of it, where the offence was committed, it will acquit the prisoner: but if there be only a partial degree of insanity; mixed with a partial degree of reason; not a full and complete use of reason but (as Lord Hale carefully and emphatically expresses himself) a competent use of it, sufficient to have restrained those passions, which produced the crime . . . if there be thought and design; a faculty to distinguish the nature of actions; to discern the differences between moral good and evil, then upon the fact of the offence proved, the judgment of the law must take place.[45]

Here, the prosecution alleged, Ferrers's own conduct of his defense provided decisive and compelling evidence of his capacities: "You have seen the Noble Prisoner, for Two Days at your Bar, (though labouring under the Weight of this Charge), Cross-examining the Witnesses for the King, and Examining his own, in a Manner so pertinent, as cannot be imputed merely to the Hints and Advice of those Agents and Council [*sic*] with which you have indulged him."[46] Unanimously, the assembled peers held that it was so. Having moved back to the House of Lords to consider their verdict, each rose in turn, laying his right hand on his breast, to pronounce Ferrers guilty. Brought in to hear the outcome, Ferrers was informed of their findings, rebuked for invoking insanity to excuse behavior "so black and dreadful," and reminded that "you can receive nothing but strict and equal justice."[47] In vain he now sought to retract a defense that, if anything, seemed to have further alienated those judging him, thanking them for a "Fair and Candid Tryal" and at the last insisting that

> I am extremely sorry that I have troubled your Lordships with a Defence that I was always much averse to, and has given me the greatest Uneasiness—But was prevailed on by my Family to attempt it, as it was what They themselves were persuaded of the Truth of. . . .[48]

However, neither this last-minute change of heart nor Monro's prior testimony could save him. Brushing aside his attempts at mitigation, the Lord High Steward pronounced sentence in the formulaic words usually reserved for wretches from far further down the social scale:

> Nothing remains for me, but to pronounce the dreadful Sentence of the Law; and the Judgment of the Law is, and this High Court doth award: That you, Lawrence Earl Ferrers, return to the Prison of the Tower, from whence you came; from thence you must be led to the Place of Execution . . . and when

you come there, you must be hanged by the Neck till you are dead, and your Body must be dissected and anatomised. And God Almighty be merciful to your Soul.[49]

An anonymous peer, giving the most minute attention to the reactions of the man he had just helped to usher to the gallows, commented with grim satisfaction that

> this last part of the sentence [i.e., that relating to dissection] seemed to shock the criminal extremely; He changed colour, his jaw quivered, and he appeared to be in great agitation; but [the same witness noted,] during the remaining part of his life he behaved with surprising composure, and even unconcern.[50]

At that, once Ferrers had been taken down from the bar by the Lieutenant of the Tower, to signify the close of the proceedings the Lord High Steward broke symbolically the white staff of office.[51] The sound of its snapping must have evoked, as the lords left the chamber, an eerie premonitory echo of the expected impact of the awaiting noose on Ferrers's neck.

Public interest in Ferrers's case remained at a fever pitch, and rumor and gossip about his preparations to meet his maker were rife (indeed, the insatiable interest in his fate would continue for weeks after his death). As we have indicated, England's notorious "Bloody Code" was less sanguinary in practice than in theory. Social connections were routinely employed to secure the commutation of death sentences, and Ferrers's family seems at first to have thought it could employ its social capital in this way. "His brothers and several other persons [therefore] petitioned his Majesty in his behalf. . . ." However, the authorities were bound and determined to demonstrate "that the law of England in cases of murder, makes no distinction between the first nobleman and the lowest plebeian of the realm." Who better to teach this lesson of juridical impartiality than "the chief of a noble family, even allied to the crown," guilty of what was widely considered an unusually heinous crime? So "the sovereign continued inflexible, as well knowing, that mercy shewn [sic] to some criminals, is often cruelty to the innocent."[52]

Bowing to the inevitable, Ferrers himself then wrote to his Majesty:

> to desire that he might suffer where his ancestor the Earl of Essex had suffered [within the walls of the Tower]; a favour which he had the greater hopes of obtaining, as he had the honour of quartering part of the same arms, and of being allied to his Majesty [the Earl of Essex, from whose daughter Lord Ferrers was descended, was the grandson of Lady Nellis, german cousin to

Queen Elizabeth], adding that he thought it was hard that he must die at the place appointed for the execution of common felons.[53]

However, as he failed to grasp, that was precisely what "justice" demanded if his execution was to have the desired deterrent effect, so once again the pleas fell on deaf ears.[54]

If Ferrers's trial and the journey to it had been theatrical, that was nothing when compared with the choreographed public execution that was to follow. On Monday, 5 May 1760, dressed in his wedding clothes,[55] "a light coloured Coat and sattin [sic] Waistcoat, embroidered with silver, and black Breeches," and accompanied by the serried ranks of London dignitaries, he began his last journey to Tyburn:

> He set out from the Tower at 9 A.M., amidst crowds of literally thousands. The procession was an impressive sight. First went a string of constables; then one of the sheriffs, in his chariot and six, the horses dressed with ribbons; next Lord Ferrers, in his own landau and six, his coachman crying all the way; guards at each side; the other under-sheriff's chariot followed empty, with a mourning coach and six, a hearse, and the Horse Guards.[56]

As another observer recorded,

> . . . the procession [made its way] through prodigious crowds of spectators, who all the way crowded the streets, and lined the windows. As they were passing, his Lordship asked Mr. Vaillant [the sheriff who was riding alongside him], if he had ever seen so great a concourse of people before; and upon his answering in the negative, he rejoined, "I suppose it is because they never saw a lord hanged before."[57]

The very crush of people meant that Ferrers's "passage from the Tower to Tyburn took up almost three hours," his every movement and every grimace the focus of unrelenting attention. Still, the *London Magazine* informed its eager readership, "his Lordship behaved with ease and composure during the whole time of his passage from the Tower to Tyburn."[58] Ferrers's "decent deportment" throughout this journey won him considerable respect from the assembled masses and "seemed greatly to affect the minds of all that beheld him." Indeed, "so respectful" was the crowd's behavior toward him that, according to some sources, "not the least affront or indignity was offered to him by any one . . . on the contrary, many persons saluted him with their prayers for his salvation."[59] Despite such a reception, Ferrers understandably observed "that the apparatus of death, and the passage through such crowds of people, were ten times worse than death itself."[60] At one point, "his Lordship expressed his desire of having a glass of wine and water; but on Mr. Vaillant's observing that his stopping would draw a greater crowd about him, which might possibly disturb him; he immediately replied, "'That's true, I say no more, let us by no means stop.'"

Some time later, as the tortuous procession wound toward its ineluctable end, he made one final request: "On approaching the place of execution, near which was his mistress in a coach, his Lordship observed, that he should be glad to take his last leave of a person for whom he had a sincere regard."[61] Once again, however, "the sheriff dissuaded him from [pausing on his journey], lest the sight of [his mistress] should unman him, and disarm him of the fortitude he possessed"—an objection whose weight Ferrers at once acknowledged and accepted.

The awful majesty of the public execution, designed through its powerful rituals to impress upon the meanest citizen the law's sovereign might, now ushered upon its stage a splendid symbol of its impartiality—"a peer of England, an earl of one of the best families."[62] The scene was once more meticulously rendered, in prose and in mass-produced engravings, for the many thousands of virtual witnesses unable to be physically present, journalists vying to catch every syllable the condemned aristocrat uttered, every aspect of his countenance, every detail (no matter how gruesome) attending his dispatch into the next world. On a scaffold thoughtfully supplied with black velvet cushions for the mourners, Earl Ferrers confronted his fate.

He met his end, as Horace Walpole observed (with evident satisfaction and perhaps some surprise), like the well-bred aristocrat his pedigree proclaimed him to be. "When the rope was put round his neck, he turned pale, but recovered his countenance instantly, and was but seven minutes from leaving the coach, to the signal given for striking the stage"—a marked contrast to the procession that had got him there.[63] Ferrers had "walked up the stairs with great composure and fortitude, with his hat in his hand" and had joined the chaplain on his knees, where he,

> with an audible voice, repeated the Lord's prayer, and afterward with great energy cried *O God forgive me all my errors. . . . Pardon all my sins.* Then rising, he took leave of the sheriffs and chaplain, thanked them for the civility they had shewn him, and made Mr. Vaillant a present of his watch.[64]

All had thus far gone according to the script, even the unpredictable Ferrers playing his assigned role with aristocratic aplomb. At the very last, however, things began to go wrong:

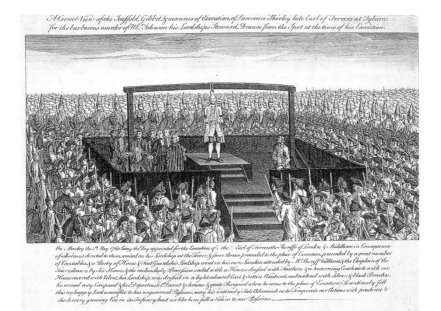

A Correct View of the Scaffold, Gibbet & manner of Execution, of Lawrence Shirley late Earl of Ferrers at Tyburn: for the barbarous murder of Mr. Johnson his Lordships Steward, Drawn from the Spot at the time of his Execution.

On Monday the 5th May 1760 being the Day appointed for the Execution of the Earl of Ferrers the Sheriffs of London & Middlesex in Consequence of their Duty directed to them, waited on his Lordship at the Tower; & from thence proceeded to the place of Execution, preceded by a great number of Constables & a Party of Horse & Foot Guards his Lordship went in his own Landau attended by Mr Sheriff Vaillant & the Chaplain of the Tower, drawn by Six Horses, & the melancholy Procession ended with a House dressed with Feathers & in mourning Coach each with six Horses covered with Velvet, his Lordship was dressed in a light coloured Coat & Sattin Waistcoat, embroidered with Silver; & black Breeches. he seemed very Composed & his Deportment Decent & Serious & quite Resigned when he came to the place of Execution: So untimely fell this unhappy lord a sacrifice to his ungoverned Passions, may his untimely Fate Admonish us to Temperate our Actions with prudence & check every growing Vice in its Infancy, least we like him fall a Victim to our Passions.

FIGURE 36. The execution of Lord Ferrers: "A Correct View of the Scaffold Gibbet & manner of Execution of Lawrence Shirley late Earl of Ferrers . . ." Shows Ferrers standing at the gallows, a hood over his head and the noose around his neck, flanked by clergy on the left and a figure who is probably the executioner on the right, and surrounded by soldiers on horses and a large crowd. This was one of a number of engravings capturing the scene of the execution for an eager audience of virtual witnesses to the hanging of the century. Taken from the *Royal Magazine* 2 (1760), p. 226. (Another, rather inferior engraving of the execution was reproduced below Ferrers's bust in the *British Magazine* 1 [1760], p. 136.) Reproduced by kind permission of the British Museum. Copyright © The British Museum.

His Lordship (by mistake) gave five guineas to the executioner's assistant. This money was immediately after demanded by the master; but the fellow refused to deliver it, and a dispute ensued, which might have greatly discomposed his Lordship had not Mr. Vaillant instantly silenced them.[65]

Worse was to follow. The authorities had planned to make Ferrers's death a swift one by using the newly invented "drop" to speed his execution. So novel was the apparatus that they decided to explain to its intended victim how the whole process would work. First, though, they . . . put on his white cap, took off his neckcloth, and put on the halter, which was a common one. He then stepped upon the little stage in the middle of the scaffold, and it was explained to him in what manner it would sink. His cap being pulled over his eyes, Mr. Sheriff Vaillant gave the signal for removing the board, by stamping with his foot.[66]

However,

As the machine was new, they were not ready [competent] at it; his toes touched it, and he suffered a little, having the time, by their bungling, to raise his cap; but the executioner pulled it down again, and they pulled his legs, so that he was soon out of pain, and quite dead in four minutes.[67]

The spectacle, already spoiled, now turned uglier still. It was customary for the body to be stripped and to remain hanging for at least an hour before being taken down and placed in a coffin, while the statute on murder required that the body be dissected and anatomized prior to any burial.[68] With this in mind, Ferrers had

desired not to be stripped and exposed, and Vaillant promised him, though his clothes must be taken off, that his shirt should not. This decency ended with him: the sheriffs fell to eating and drinking on the scaffold, and helped up one of their friends to drink with them, as he was still hanging, which he did for above an hour, and then was conveyed back with the said pomp to Surgeons' Hall, to be dissected.[69] The executioners fought for the rope, and the one who lost it cried. The mob tore off the black cloth as relics. . . .[70]

Even taken down and placed in his coffin, Ferrers—or what remained of him—was not safe from public curiosity, the *Royal Magazine* priding itself on the scoop it had obtained by including an engraving of the macabre scene of the earl's corpse on display prior to its dissection.

The morbid fascination exhibited by all segments of English society in the sordid details of his demise reached its apogee when the same magazine literature also included a vivid account of Ferrers's actual dissection, trumpeting the ironic discovery of the healthy state of his innards, which, it was stressed, would have been likely to have provided him with a remarkable longevity but for the intervention of the hangman. The enterprising reporter for the *Royal Magazine* meticulously recorded the scene:

The surgeons made a large incision from the neck to the bottom of the thorax or breast, and another across the throat; the abdomen was laid open, and the bowels taken out. Upon this occasion the surgeons declared that the entrails were remarkably sound, and that in their whole practice they never saw in any subject so great signs of long life.[71]

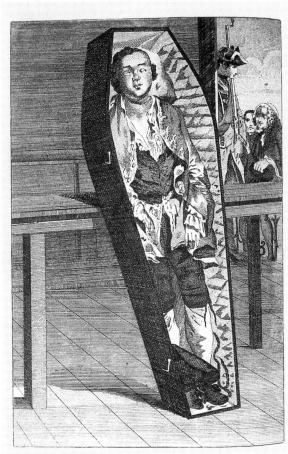

EARL FERRERS.

FIGURE 37. Ferrers in his coffin after being taken down from the scaffold, prior to his removal for dissection at Surgeon's Hall. This engraving was dated 1760 and published in the *Royal Magazine* 4 (May 1760), p. 230; the editors boasted that it "will give the reader an idea of his person, the artist having preserved a very striking likeness." The coffin was lined with white satin. Ferrers's hat and halter lay at his feet and upon the coffin lid was a plate with the inscription "Laurence Earl FERRERS, *suffered* May 5. 1760." See ibid., p. 232. (This representation of Earl Ferrers was also published in the *Memoirs* of his life [London: J. Coote, 1760].) Reproduced by kind permission of the Bodleian Library, University of Oxford. Shelfmark BOD Bookstack Vet. A5 e.286.

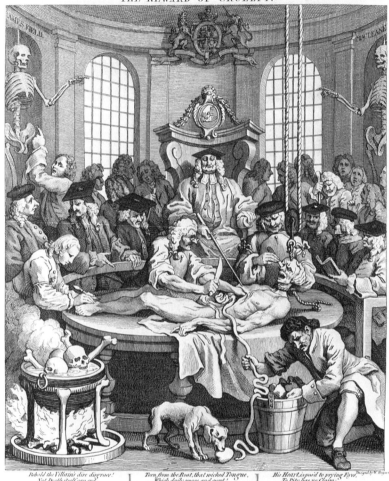

FIGURE 38. Dissection at Surgeon's Hall: the final stage in Hogarth's *Four States of Cruelty* (1751). "Foreign nations," the *British Magazine* (1760) pronounced,

will, no doubt, be surprised to learn that the law of England in cases of murder, makes no distinction between the first nobleman and the lowest plebeian of the realm. They will be amazed to hear, that the chief of a noble family, even allied to the crown, was sentenced to the ignominious death of a common felon . . . and that his body, having been delivered to the surgeons, was dissected, and exposed in public for the entertainment of the vulgar. . . .

The vulgar flocked to the scene. "Numbers of persons," the competing *London Magazine*

The bloody spectacle was intended, of course, to serve as much more than an extended source of entertainment and amusement for the masses. Against the disturbing scenes that had marked Ferrers's drawn-out death, Walpole insisted must be interposed two offsetting demonstrations of virtue: by the soi-disant madman, and by the respectable portion of the crowd that had assembled to view his demise. When all was said and done, "the universal crowd behaved with great decency and admiration, as they well might; for sure no exit was ever made with more sensible resolution and with less contention."[72]

Ferrers's courage and uncharacteristic composure at his execution, where he had seemed to many to rediscover his "gentlemanly" demeanor, had won him a degree of sympathy, not only among the masses and in the popular press, but even among some of his peers.[73] Yet over the long haul, opinion among the elite seems to have been decidedly more vitriolic. The general sentiment in their midst appears to have been not only that Ferrers deserved his fate, but that, as Walpole put it in a letter to Mann, he was "a wild beast, a mad assassin, [and] a low wretch," with a long history of violent acts, "horrid excesses," and temper tantrums, deplorably lacking in control "over his passions."[74]

Possibly seeking to offset the criticism he had received (or anticipated) for testifying in Ferrers's defense, or else at the specific request of the family, Monro had, according to Walpole, made an affidavit as to Fer-

---

(1760) noted, "were admitted to see the dissected body, at surgeons-hall, for three days; . . . [before o]n Thursday the 8th, in the evening, his lordship's remains were delivered to his friends, and carried into the country to be interred." In Hogarth's representation of such a scene, after his hanging at Tyburn, Tom Nero's corpse has his eye sockets probed by the surgeon's knife, his tongue having already been extracted, while another surgeon with rolled-up sleeves reaches into his rib cage, in what David Bindman has called "a ghastly parody of the 'Good Death'" (*Hogarth and His Times: Serious Comedy* [London: British Museum Press, 1997], p. 146). In a macabre echo of the Crucifixion, Tom's dissection takes place between the skeletons of two other criminals hanging in recesses to the left and right: on the left is that of James Maclaine, the romanticized "gentleman Highwayman" who was executed in 1750 and who was regarded as the embodiment of MacHeath. Meanwhile, the intestines spill out of Tom's abdomen onto the floor, where a mangy dog gnaws on his evil heart, and the bones and skulls of other dissected felons boil away in a cauldron. The scene is observed dispassionately by other surgeons, while a magisterial figure (possibly the president of the Company of Surgeons), seated centrally on his throne, presides austerely over the scene. Reproduced by kind permission of The Wellcome Trust.

rers's lunacy subsequent to the trial.[75] It appears that this document does not survive, but almost certainly it must have stressed factors that Monro was to emphasize throughout his career as positive indicators of madness—most especially the family history of insanity (an issue Ferrers himself had vainly attempted to bring to the fore in his own defense at the trial). Here again, however, leading contemporary public opinion flatly disagreed with Monro's verdict. Horace Walpole gave voice to the consensus when he noted that, while "the Washingtons, his grandmother's family, were certainly a very frantic race, and I have no doubt of madness in him," this was equally certainly not madness "of a pardonable sort."[76]

As we are far from the first to have noted, Ferrers's dismal demise—his death and subsequent dissection "like a common criminal"—was the subject of endless moralizing on the basic equality of all before the law of the land, his execution being cited over and over again as "an irrefutable proof of the justice of English society" and of the impartiality of its law.[77] Above and beyond the dissection of his body, Ferrers's own character was also minutely dissected to provide moralistic explanations and admonitions for the public at large about how worthy potential could end in ignominy. The earl's sad but salutary end was variously blamed on his drinking and keeping of bad company; on his overindulgent family and poor education; on his lack of religious principles and espousal of Bolingbroke's philosophy; and even on his visiting of foreign countries, which was alleged to have "obliterated" any "faint traces of virtue and religion" he had once possessed, and "rendered him impatient of controul [sic] and a slave to the inhuman passion of revenge."[78]

So mortified were some of Ferrers's friends and family by the extent of his public disparagement and disgrace, that one went so far as to publish a posthumous vindication of his character. The apologia included a letter the earl had written to explain his actions, and his own abridged edition of Bolingbroke's *Philosophical Works*.[79] Neither was calculated to win many people over, however. In the former, written while contemplating the potentially "fatal . . . consequence" of his conduct, Ferrers soberly reflected on his demonizing by society, and sought excuses for himself in drink and in mental affliction.

> In my cooler moments nobody looks on my past life with more horror than I do . . . how happy is that man, upon whose brain the cursed spirit of liquor hath no power. How granting to reflection it is to find oneself to have been a monster, in the eyes of that very society, which in sober hours it would most cordially embrace . . . [from reading] alone can [I] find relaxation and chear-

ing [*sic*] solace from the many heart aches which the wild freaks of my un-accountable brain, when crazed with drinking, but too frequently cause. . . .[80]

Quite evidently, Monro's involvement had been unable to rescue Ferrers from his emblematic fate. Ferrers and his sympathizers were predictably unlikely to have been entirely satisfied as to the thoroughness with which his mental competence had been assessed, a footnote to the condemned man's letter expressing the wish "that a complete enquiry between ideotism and lunacy, had been ordered, for the thorough satisfaction of every doubting mind . . ."[81] Yet few among the elite would have agreed with them on this score. Still, the Bethlem doctor's presence in so prominent a case had clearly established the precedent of the criminal courts turning to medical men for guidance about questions of sanity and insanity. For his successors charged with ministering to the mad, this arena would become one that was fraught with considerable symbolic significance, and all too often the site of major controversy and contestation.[82]

THE MAD-DOCTOR, MAD MEG, AND STATE COMMITTALS TO BETHLEM

The Ferrers case was only one, if the most notorious, among a number of instances in which Monro found himself drawn into highly charged legal and political arenas. He was consulted as a matter of course, for example, following the arrest of the attempted regicide Margaret Nicholson (1745?–1828), and in several other criminal and/or politically troublesome cases where insanity was strongly suspected. Once again, of course, the very prominence of the defendants in these cases further reinforced the notion of the relevance of medical expertise in matters of this sort.

Margaret Nicholson was evidently born in ca. 1745 at Stokewell, in Yorkshire, the daughter of Mr. Nicholson, a peruke maker.[83] If her social origins were humble, her education was correspondingly elementary. She learned to read only "tolerably" and to write "indifferently," and even later in life required constant recourse to a dictionary to compose her letters.[84] According to some sources, in 1786 she had been living in London for twenty-four years, her family having moved to the metropolis when she was twelve years old.[85] Her brother was a "respectable character," formerly a gentleman's servant at the Temple, and latterly a publican who kept the Three Horse Shoes Tavern in Milford Lane, in the Strand.[86] Nicholson's own respectability, however, was

more questionable. As a young woman, Meg appears to have been enticed into a relationship with an officer of the guards who took her into
his home as his mistress. Though this relationship sustained her for
some time both financially and emotionally, it tainted her reputation
and came to a sorry and premature end with his death. Her situation
grew worse when the attorney she employed to secure the annuity her
inamorato had left for her future support swindled her out of the bequest. Her indignant expostulations about this affair having fallen on
deaf ears, Nicholson decided to apply to the highest national authority
for redress. Possibly her departed lover had been one of the royal guards.
Even if not, all officers and soldiers were formally in the service of the
crown, and Meg may have felt that she had particular grounds to apply
to the king. Or, perhaps, her importunities simply reflected her conviction that the crown was supposed to be a defender of justice and rightful law. Whatever the case, it was at this juncture—or so some alleged—
that Meg's troubles began to cascade into the public domain. As one and
then another petition to the king for relief received no answer, Nicholson's frustration began steadily to mount.

If this version of events is true, the circumstances surrounding her be-
reavement alone may well have sufficed to unbalance her mind, with the
events that followed simply loading insult upon injury. In fact, though,
despite the evident appeal of this tale of a fallen woman, the entire
episode may have been a cock-and-bull story, a fiction invented by one
particular hack journalist, for most accounts failed to mention it, and,
significantly, it was omitted from the most reliable account of all, that
provided by her former landlord, Jonathan Fiske. A key witness before
the Privy Council about her assassination attempt, Fiske was a stationer
(i.e., bookseller) who penned his own account of her life in 1786 with
the firm intention of setting the record straight. As a man with whom
Nicholson had "lodged upwards of Three Years, and . . . been intimate
for many Years," he was clearly speaking about her from a much more
familiar vantage point than any other source. Fiske accused other writers of having exploited public curiosity for "mercenary" motives, dismissing their accounts as based on a tissue of "paltry fabrications, mis-
erably strung together from detached paragraphs in the news-papers,"
most of which he likewise condemned as "without the least foundations." His own narrative, although itself partly reliant on the press and
far from lacking in self-promotion and moral judgments about his former lodger, still appears substantially more sober and measured by comparison, and leaves out a good deal of the more sensational detail found

in other versions of her case. The only military connection of Nicholson's that Fiske mentioned was an artillery field officer whom Meg claimed was her "uncle" and whom she called upon when unemployed and in straitened circumstances. Indeed, Fiske and other sources placed much more emphasis on her general problems with employment and making ends meet, and on a different affair that Nicholson embarked upon in later life with a valet.

What all accounts agreed on was that, for most of her working life, Nicholson had been a housemaid, serving in "several creditable services" with "families of distinction."[87] Latterly, however, her employment history grew distinctly more checkered. Around 1780, Nicholson left one service (with a Mrs. Rice of Argyle Buildings/Mayfair) voluntarily, according to some sources, "on a pretence that she had been left a capital fortune."[88] Fiske, by contrast, claimed that it was the "delicate and chaste ideas" she "entertained" that provoked her to quit in "enraged" indignation, after hearing that "Mr R" was not married to her mistress. Indeed, according to him she threatened "to sue her master for the loss of character she must have sustained, by being seduced into so immoral a family."[89] Subsequently, she lost another of her positions with a respectable family after allegedly misbehaving with the Swiss valet de chambre, whom she had taken as her lover, although, once again, sources vary as to the circumstances. While some alleged that she was sacked by her disapproving employers, Fiske claimed that she left of her own accord and that it was her "spirit of independence" that then persuaded her to quit household service entirely. Whatever the truth of the matter, Nicholson subsequently went from one household to another, subsisting by and large through her needle, but experiencing growing difficulties in making ends meet and occasionally being forced to leave her lodgings after disputes with landlords.[90] It was around 1783, some years after being deserted by the valet, that she went to reside in the household of the Fiskes in Wigmore Street, Marylebone. Here (as Fiske himself was later to testify before the Board of Green Cloth and in his own published account of the case) she remained for about three years, continuing to make an inadequate living by taking in needlework. Latterly, however, she became increasingly fixated on the royal family, sending repeated petitions to the king and his council. Still earlier—apparently while living with the Paul[e]s and working with a Mr. Watson, a hatter in New Bond Street—she had allegedly "frequently pressed [the latter] to present Petitions in her behalf to his Majesty, saying continually, she had a large claim upon government."[91] In July 1786 she sent yet another petition to the Privy Council alleging that George III was a usurper, and that the throne was rightfully hers.

A few weeks later, on 2 August, between 9 and 11 A.M. (accounts vary), having become increasingly exasperated at the lack of response from the palace, Nicholson set out from her lodgings, determined to give the king something to remember her by. She proceeded to St. James's Park and Palace. Some sources chose to emphasize her agitation at the scene, relating how "she continued walking up and down the Park, and in the avenues to the palace, until about half past twelve," when, joining the usual crowd assembling at the garden gate for "a sight of his majesty on his arrival [or on his way to the levée], she was one of the foremost." [92] According to such accounts, displaying evident impatience and informing the other onlookers that she had a memorial to deliver to the king, she had been permitted by the crowd (or more particularly by "two gentlewomen that were known to her") to take her place at the front. On sight of the royal coach at about 1 P.M., Nicholson was then said to have pushed forward. Fiske's less melodramatic version of events, in contrast, portrays her (on the authority of one of the yeomen) more soberly awaiting the king's arrival, seated with "two other decent women on park chairs." Finding herself outflanked by the crush of people, and on the wrong side of the carriage, she was evidently allowed on request to move to the other side by the yeoman, who had noticed what seemed to be a petition in her hand.[93] What is uncontested, however, is that, as George III alighted from his carriage at the garden entrance, near Marlborough Wall, Nicholson made a show of presenting a paper folded in the form of a petition directly to him—"his majesty bending graciously forward to receive it." [94] Once within range of the royal person, however, she lunged forward with her other hand and attempted to stab him, striking out twice at the king with a knife she had concealed on her person.

Since her weapon of choice was a flimsy, worn, and old (if not blunt) ivory-handled dessert knife, the attempt (so bizarre and inept in its manner that it alone must have raised doubts as to Nicholson's mental state) was unsuccessful. At most, it merely resulted in a small tear in the king's waistcoat, although the most reliable account stressed that it "did not cut his waistcoat" at all.[95] As she commenced her second thrust, she was easily restrained and captured by the yeoman of the guard, Mr. Wright, and a royal footman, Mr. Topper, the former catching her arm and the latter disarming her.[96] Initially, having drawn back in shock, the king was reported by some to have blurted out, "What does the woman

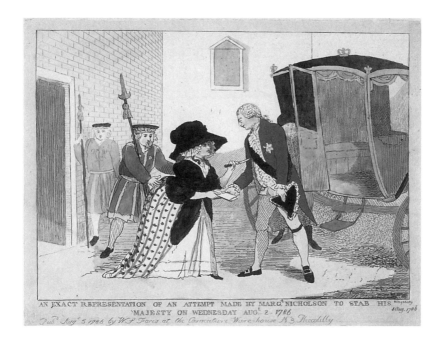

AN EXACT REPRESENTATION OF AN ATTEMPT MADE BY MARG^t NICHOLSON TO STAB HIS
'MAJESTY ON WEDNESDAY AUG^t 2 1786
Pub^d Augt 5 1786 by Wm Fores at the Caricature Ware-house N° 3 Piccadilly

FIGURE 39. Engraving of Margaret Nicholson (ca. 1745–1828) attacking George III on 2 August 1786: "An Exact Representation of an Attempt Made by Marg[are]ᵗ Nicholson to Stab His Majesty on Wednesday Aug[us]ᵗ 2 1786." George III takes a paper (a petition) from the hand of Margaret Nicholson, who simultaneously holds a knife in her left hand against his chest. A beefeater (left) steps forward to restrain her and another stands unmoved by an open door in a high brick wall. The king's coach, or "post-chariot," as some contemporaries called it, is on the right, and behind George the coachman is partially visible. This is an engraving, not a caricature, though it is drawn in the manner of one. A mezzotint of this subject is in the Carington Bowles series. The engraving is a primitively drawn and colored effort, in which the king's gracious posture, regal attire, and gentlemanly doffing of his hat to Nicholson are contrasted with Nicholson's duplicity and somewhat ridiculous out-sized garb. It was published with startling rapidity while Nicholson was still being examined by the Privy Council on 5 August 1786, by W. S. Fores, at Caricature Ware-house, No. 3, Piccadilly, as the third in a series of three satires. This engraving by Kingsbury accompanied the anonymous fifty-six-page booklet *The Plot Investigated* (see note 85), which entered a slightly different description into its title: *Ornamented with an Exact Representation of His Majesty Stepping out of his Carriage at St James's, and Margaret Nicholson in the Act of Presenting a Pretended Petition with one Hand, and Aiming a Knife at His Majesty's Breast with the Other.* Reproduced by kind permission of the British Museum, Satire No. 6973; description taken partly from Dorothy M. George and Frederic George Stephen's *Catalogue of Prints and Drawings in the British Museum,* London: Printed by order of the Trustees, 1870–1954. Copyright © The British Museum.

mean?"[97] Asked by the yeoman if he was hurt, and quickly composing himself (after "stroking his waistcoat" to verify the fact), George famously and compassionately exclaimed: "No, I am not hurt—take care of the woman—don't hurt her, for she is mad."[98] The act was sufficient, ultimately, to see Nicholson committed to Bethlem for life.[99] Yet, in the days that followed her attempt, the state of her mind and her degree of responsibility for what she had done proved to be far from straightforward matters to resolve.

The *European Magazine* reported that once George retired into the palace apartments, he calmly read Nicholson's petition, which was addressed, as was customary, "to the King's most excellent Majesty" but was otherwise completely blank. Evidently, the king's initial composure after the attack on his person did not last long, for, having "recovered himself from the surprize . . . [he] seemed greatly affected, and uttered some expressions, signifying, that he had not deserved this treatment from any of his subjects." The king had further reason to find this event particularly traumatic—for, peculiarly, according to the same source, this was the second or third time he had been attacked in this way.[100]

Outside of the palace, meantime, "a general panic" was said to have ensued among the metropolitan populace at large, as various reports circulated wildly—"and to aggravate the consternation, fictions were most plentifully added to fact."[101] Such rumors, it was reported, had "scarce got beyond the verge before several hundred persons flew to the palace and crowded the different avenues leading thereto," and—as the news filtered through that the king had survived an assassination attempt—the nobility in town allegedly "surrounded the throne with congratulations."[102] Some commentators even specified by name certain of the ladies who made public displays of their loyalty and concern, such as the duchess of Devonshire and Lady Duncannon. However, such demonstrativeness was clearly what decorum as much as affection required, and the universality and sincerity of these reactions were plainly exaggerated, more people probably being drawn to the scene by curiosity, excitement, opportunities for gossip, and the "purposes of [actually] seeing the woman," rather than by their desire to exhibit their loyalty.[103] Conflicting reports about the event seem to have been so rife, as Nicholson underwent her first examination, that the queen and the royal family were kept suspended in "great dread," until, hastening to Windsor in a vain attempt to intercept any alarm, George arrived alive and in person.[104]

Nicholson, possibly in a state of shocked withdrawal after her arrest,

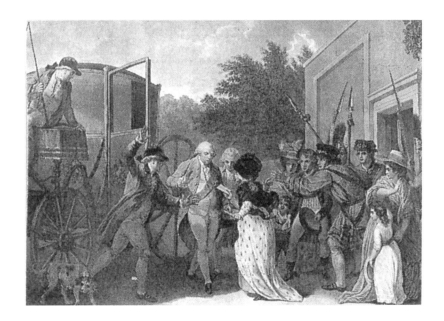

FIGURE 40. Another representation of the attempted assassination (1786), engraved by Robert Pollard (1755–1838) and etched and aquatinted by Francis Jukes (1746–1812), after an original painting (commissioned by Pollard) by the artist and literary illustrator Robert Smirke, R.A. (1752–1845), published 9 October 1786. (Smirke had also done paintings that were engraved to illustrate a whole host of literary works, including Cervantes's *Don Quixote,* the works of Shakespeare, *The Arabian Nights,* Johnson's *Rasselas,* and Montgomery's *Poems on the Abolition of the Slave Trade.* Pollard likewise did engravings for a number of literary works, including the 1785 edition of Defoe's *Robinson Crusoe* and the *Copper-Plate Magazine* [1792–1801].) Here is another example of sensational commercial opportunity providing the impetus for a remarkably rapid artistic production. In this instance, the artists skillfully recreate and accentuate the high drama of the scene. Nicholson is shown from behind with the petition in her right hand while, in her left, she wields the knife in a wide arc toward George III. The king seems caught betwixt stepping forward and backward, with his right hand raised in a gesture of appeal or self-defense. Nicholson is flanked by the yeoman on the right and footman on the left, who—while others appear transfixed and paralyzed—both reach out with rapid and vigorous movements to restrain her. To the right a woman stares at the scene, shrinking away in horror, while her child anxiously clutches at her sleeve, and to the left the king's coachman looks on with concern. A dog is the only creature apparently ignoring the drama. Reproduced by kind permission of the Witt Library, Courtauld Institute of Art, London.

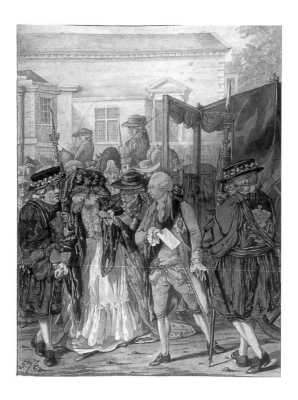

FIGURE 41. Yet another representation of the attempted regicide, drawn by the artist, printseller, and onetime actor Robert Dighton (1752–1814), in pen and black ink, watercolor, heightened with body color, possibly after Smirke, sometime between 1786 and 1791. (See Dennis Rose, *Life, Times and Recorded Works of Robert Dighton (1752–1814) Actor, Artist and Printseller and Three of his Artist Sons: Portrayers of Georgian Pageantry and Wit* [Salisbury, Wiltshire: D. Rose; distributed by Element Books, 1981].) Depicted is a nervous-looking but rather sumptuously attired Nicholson in the process of being restrained by the yeoman and footman, but still holding the knife in her left hand. Standing beside the open door of his carriage, George looks on somewhat sternly, holding the petition she has given him in his right hand. Another particularly fierce-looking beefeater stares at the scene from the right-hand side. A crowd of onlookers, royal guards on horseback, and St. James's Palace are shown in the background. In pencil: "Margaret Nicholson attempting to Assassinate His Majesty, King George III^d at the Garden Entrance of St James's Palace 2nd August 1786."

Contemporary writers and artists who depicted Nicholson paid a great deal of attention to her clothing and appearance, keen to recreate a realistic image and capture the imaginations of their potential audiences, yet they differed considerably in how they chose to portray her. She was described as "well" or "decently dressed in a black silk cloak & c." in the *European Magazine* and *Universal Magazine,* represented by some as if dressed up in her Sunday best for her unconventional audience with the king. In addition, she was said to be wearing "a flowered linnen or muslin gown, black gauze bonnet . . . [and a] morning wire cap with blue ribbons." However, Fiske

but more likely simply determined to reveal herself only to the most senior (earthly) authority, at first (and for as much as five hours) more or
less refused to speak, or at least to reply to the questions she was asked,
and appeared unmoved whenever the details of her crime were represented to her.[105] Held in the "Inner Guard Chamber," she answered in-
dignantly to questions about the attempt "that they had no right to examine her: when she was brought before the proper persons, she would
give her reasons." Subsequently, she was removed to the queen's ante-
chambers, where, addressed "by many of the Nobility," she largely
maintained her silence about her actions and motivations.[106] Finally, at
5 P.M. on the same day, after a private strip search and physical scrutiny
by members of her own sex, she was again interrogated before a special
council of the Board of Green Cloth and other important authorities, including the prime minister, William Pitt, the attorney general, the master of the rolls, the solicitor general, and a number of magistrates. Apparently, she was satisfied by this august assembly (although she needed
to be pressed to overcome some initial reticence, when she simply replied that "the King knows my motive") and, at last, she broke her silence about her cause.

Betraying "no symptoms of emotion, she answered with great firm-
ness to the various questions which were put to her."[107] Now that she
had begun to speak more freely, however, her testimony further fueled
doubts about her mental state, as she voiced in a "frantic" and "ram-
bling" manner her right to the crown:

> . . . she wanted nothing but her right . . . she had great property . . . if she had
> not her right, England would be drowned in blood for a thousand genera-

---

dismissed as fictitious depictions of Nicholson as "tall and genteel," and more reliably, if
disdainfully, described her as rather unremarkable looking, "short and clumsy . . . and
too corpulent to possess the graces," with "a
swarthy complexion, and not the most engaging features." The clothing she wore may well
have been second-hand or hand-me-down,
and for many commentators signified her
somewhat fallen-from-grace and tatty-re-
spectable servant status: "she had no more
than what were on her back, and those, ex-

cept the cloak and bonnet, were very indifferent." The fact that "a silver sixpence, & three
halfpence" (or two-pence halfpenny—accounts vary) were found in her pockets when
searched, "which was all the money she had,"
was taken as further evidence of her impoverishment (Jonathan Fiske, *The Life,* p. 39 [see
note 83]; *European Magazine* 10 [1786],
pp. 117–18; *Universal Magazine* 79 [1786],
p. 95). Reproduced by kind permission of
the Witt Library, Courtauld Institute of Art,
London.

tions. . . . On being questioned as to her right, she [indicated she] would answer none but a judge, her rights were a mystery.[108]

According to the *Universal Magazine,*

> She did not appear in the least embarrassed before the Council, answered
> some questions with consistence, and others incoherently. Her object, she
> said, was to obtain the prayer of her petition by terrifying the King, which
> she fancied the sight of the knife would have effected. . . . At intervals she
> talked of a "claim on government"—"law suit"—"just cause"—and such
> like sentences. . . .[109]

Nicholson having proceeded to mention her original petition to be
granted her "rights," it was searched for and located among various
state papers. As might be expected, however, its discovery did little to
persuade the assembled dignitaries to take her any more seriously: it was
observed to be "full of princely nonsense about tyrants, usurpers, and
pretenders to the throne"; and in most quarters, "it was found to be
such stuff and nonsense, that no notice was taken of it." [110] Yet certain
signs of "composure," including her ability to recollect her petition almost word for word, made some continue to wonder precisely how mad
she was. The *European Magazine* was not alone in thinking that there
was "method in her madness, (if she is indeed a lunatic)," citing her rational explanation when she was "asked by Lord Salisbury why she had
delivered a carte blanche" to the king. In a Tristram Shandy–like manner, which must have suggested to some that she had lucidly premeditated the act and had thus been capable of forming a sane intent, "She
answered, her ends could have been accomplished under a blank sheet
of paper, as well as by a petition in proper form." [111] There was a ready-
made doctrine available, however, to account for a situation where one
observed putatively reasonable answers and logical thought patterns
alongside evidently irrational speech and conduct: most, the *European
Magazine* included, dismissed them as merely the product of "lucid
intervals." [112]

Nicholson had evidently presented so many petitions already (she
herself put the figure at seventeen) that she was convinced that "the King
knew what she wanted." It seems unsurprising that, although they "appear to have been delivered," these petitions were found on inquiry to
have "abounded in the most glaring inconsistencies, and were disregarded at the time." More remarkably, however, Nicholson had apparently already made explicit threats to assassinate the king, one or two of
her petitions having included words that were paraphrased as follows:

"If your Majesty would wish to avoid Regicide, you will make some provision for me without delay." [113]

Given the mounting testimony—not least that from "the delinquent" herself—supporting "the strongest presumption of insanity," the fastidiousness of Nicholson's examination is striking, a point that did not escape a contemporary press always eager to tout the nationalistic virtues of English justice and liberty. As the *Lady's Magazine* put it, rather than reach an early verdict, "conformably to the legal proceedings in a free country, it was judged proper that all possible evidence should be obtained, for determining the real state of Nicholson's mind." [114] Thus, as soon as Nicholson revealed her place of residence, the key to her room was confiscated, and "in order that every possible research should be made," Lord Sydney and the Green Cloth "sent to several of the Westminster Magistrates" and ordered a search of her lodgings. [115] In addition, they summoned her landlord, Fiske, and others among her relations and acquaintances. Fiske was brought before the Board in a manner that says a good deal about the level of panic the attempt had caused, and the peremptory measures the state was prepared to sanction in crimes affecting the royal person. Removed from his stationer's shop and not even permitted time to fully dress and wash himself, Fiske was briskly transported (evidently alone and not, as some sources suggested, with his wife) under the personal escort of an undersecretary of state in a hackney coach to St. James's.

Fiske was detained for several hours in a private room, according to some sources, "without having the least knowledge, or even suspicion, of the cause." In fact, as he himself related, after being asked if he knew Nicholson, he had at least been informed (if somewhat inaccurately) that Nicholson "had been to St James's and had behaved very ill to the gentlemen of the Board of Green Cloth." [116] Such stringent but reticent precautions may imply that some harbored suspicions that her landlord had consorted in a plot with Nicholson. In the interim, within five minutes of Fiske's departure, two royal messengers were posted at the door to his lodger's room to secure its contents prior to the search, so alarming his seven month's pregnant wife—kept equally in the dark about the cause—that she "was taken ill." [117]

Eventually, Fiske was brought before the Privy Council for questioning, feeling thoroughly unprepared to appear before such an august assembly. Under examination, he seems to have presented a relatively unremarkable chronicle of Nicholson's character and conduct. Some accounts of his testimony stressed his comments on her "odd" behavior, his having observed her "frequently talking to herself" and "agitated," and his mentioning "that she said she was shortly to have a place at Court."[118] Fiske's own version, however, emphasized that she was "harmless and inoffensive . . . behaved decently and honestly," and that "I had never remarked any acts of insanity, unless talking to herself might be deemed so, and that was her frequent practice," a characteristic that he personally did not think marked her out as insane.[119] Indeed, few witnesses seem to have detected "any striking marks of insanity about her," Fiske and a number of other witnesses pointing out that she was previously "very industrious," decent and honest, "harmless [and] inoffensive," quiet and steady in manner, and literate.[120] Some persisted, even after Nicholson's confinement as a lunatic, in considering her "a keen, artful, subtle kind of woman."[121] Only her brother was quite "positive that she is insane," although she had evidently "not lived on terms of intimacy with him for a considerable time," and, in general, her relations "declared that she was the most inoffensive creature living, but that the state of her mind was very unsettled."[122] Two of Nicholson's female acquaintances were also questioned by the council, considerable attention being accorded to the issue of premeditation, and to such matters as how she had cleaned and sharpened the knife.[123]

As they grappled with these questions, the authorities, both lay and medical, appear to have concentrated on Nicholson's recent speech, behavior, and thought patterns to assess her level of responsibility for her act. More popularly oriented accounts of her case in the magazine literature, however, gave particular attention to other circumstances in her history. Some of the more censorious and judgmental represented her case less sympathetically, as that of a crazed and "audacious" assassin, an "unhappy wretch" and a "miserable woman," whose past life and "reputation" offered significant clues about her ultimately deplorable fate, and might serve as a stern warning to others. Those apt to see the attempt in more conspiratorial terms even referred to it as a "plot."[124]

Yet the reactions aroused by the Nicholson case were varied and complex. The attempt was exploited, on the one hand, for the opportunity it provided to curry favor with the king and his government, by emphasizing the monarch's virtues, the liberality of the constitution, and the mildness and civilized nature of English justice, government, and society. Even Fiske concluded his account by congratulating his "heroine . . . that her dealings were with so generous a king, and so merciful an administration."[125] On the other hand, the case also allowed for a more potentially reforming and humanitarian discourse on the duties of kingship and the deficiencies of the law. Some authors adopted both of these perspectives. In Grub Street journalistic style, for example, the author of *The Plot Investigated* hyperbolically and sycophantically lauded "his Majesty's greatness of mind . . . his command of temper—fine sensibility—humanity—and everything laudable and amiable!" Proudly and xenophobically, works like this alleged that, if the same thing had occurred "in any [other] country under heaven . . . racks and tortures would have been applied, and the jails . . . would have been filled by accusations against innocent persons."[126] While condemning the fact that lunatics like Nicholson were at large as "not only a disgrace to the laws and regulations of this country, but [also] as wanting in humanity to objects, of all others the most in need of its salutary influence . . . ," this commentator appealed explicitly for the establishment of more extensive hospitals for the insane, or else for wider legal compulsion on families and parishes to secure the insane.[127] He also took advantage of the case to appeal at length for a reform of the manner in which petitions were presented to the king—being careful, to be sure, to avoid casting aspersions on George for any inattention to the pleas of his subjects. Strategically, instead, he blamed the crown's officers for failing to read petitions, and for the way in which dangerous threats, such as those Nicholson had repeatedly made, had been ignored.[128]

These were, however, far from the only morals drawn from the Nicholson case. Quite another ideological didactic lurked ominously behind portraits that harped on how, despite being "honest, sober, [and] industrious," she was "remarkable through life for a degree of pride unusual in persons of her station"—a characteristic equally evident in her "contemptuous" replies to her eminent interrogators.[129] Although her behavior was deemed "irreproachable" in some services, including one of her first positions, with a Lady Seabright, the affectations she displayed here and elsewhere about her appearance and status were depicted by contemporaries as at the root of her ensuing mental problems, madness being commonly perceived in this period as originating in the self-delusions of those who thought themselves above their stations. Fiske certainly portrayed her endless "assiduous" attentions to her "personal attractions," to powdering her face, and the presentation of her own beauty, desirability, and gentility as vain pretensions, divorced from reality. He frequently reiterated how "her figure is not calculated to make conquests, nor is it wonderful that she has so long continued out of the matrimonial noose," and how "all the aids of dress were of little consequence in creating admirers."[130] It was to similar deflating,

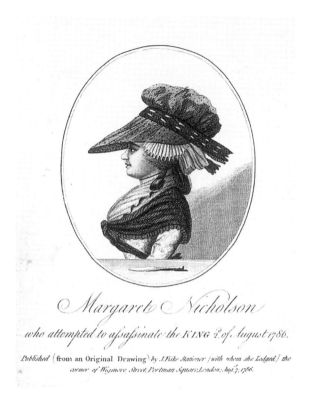

FIGURE 42. Margaret Nicholson shown in profile. Published just five days after her attempted assassination, this profile emphasizes Nicholson's rather unbecoming short, stout, swarthy appearance and somewhat eccentric style of dress; from an original drawing made by her former landlord, Jonathan Fiske, to illustrate his own published account of her adventures, *The Life and Transactions of Margaret Nicholson* (1786). The knife she used is morbidly depicted in the bottom forefront of the frame. Reproduced by kind permission of the Syndics of Cambridge University Library, from the Hunter Collection.

humbling and moralizing ends that he reproduced a drawing of her, claiming more accurately to represent her unbecoming appearance.

Likewise, her putting on of airs and graces before fellow servants and others was denigrated as "rather too assuming, and affected . . . superiority, to which she was not in the least entitled, as she had never moved in a higher sphere than that of house-maid."[131] The letters she sent up to Lady Arundel, while lodging somewhat later in the household of her husband's porter, Mr. Hopkins, and spending evenings in his lordship's house playing cards below stairs, were regarded as pure "effrontery," prefiguring her later conduct toward judges, privy councilors, and the king himself.[132] There was the implicit suggestion that the follies of vanity and pride were not only improper to this (or any other) poor woman's sex, occupation, and class, but were a route to crime and madness. More salacious authors dwelled on her dubious claims to chastity and her alleged sexual intrigues and putatively tawdry, promiscuous morals, looking askance at how she had been "enticed away" by the guardsman, "who [they alleged], after debauching her, took her into what is understood in the world of gallantry, by keeping [her as his mistress]."[133] Aspersions were even cast on her religious uprightness, for, despite her statement before the Privy Council that she had been brought up as and remained a Protestant, Fiske commented that he had never seen her go to church or chapel and designated her religion "as somewhat problematical."[134]

Yet these and other accounts could also accommodate more generous interpretations. Some recalled a series of events in her past that allowed her actions to be assimilated within a wider discourse of female fallenness, of disappointed hopes and spurned love. The same author who spoke of Nicholson's moral degradation concurrently emphasized how she had lived with her guardsman "very happily till he died," and how "cruelly" her attorney had behaved toward her.[135] Recounting at length how the prudish Nicholson (while in the employ of a lady of quality as a personal servant) had fallen from grace after becoming entangled with and then being abandoned by the valet permitted other authors to offer an even more sympathetic explanation for her mental degradation and allowed for a moral lesson to be drawn from her case to present to other (servant) women. This type of recital was coupled with a traditional admonition regarding the dangers of solitude and distress to those of a melancholy temperament.[136]

Fiske recounted with similar feeling how his former lodger had been "slighted, and then neglected" by the valet, whom she had expected to marry, castigating the fickle and proverbially venal character of the Swiss. Noting how "far affected" Nicholson had been, and that she had for some time contemplated an action against her lover to obtain "half his property," Fiske was highly disposed to attribute the origins of her insanity to "this disappointment."[137]

Accounts like these explicitly related Nicholson's case to her socioeconomic predicament, hypothesizing, for example, that the "penurious" existence she was obliged to pursue, striving to live by needlework, and the "want of nourishment attendant on it must [have] encrease[d] her mental debility."[138] By the time she elected to move to the Oxford Street house of Mr. and Mrs. Paul[e], Nicholson was evidently able to afford only "half a bed," which she shared "with their maid-servant," despite being "frequently employed" at this time by Mr. Watson, a hatter.[139] Thereafter, things only went from bad to worse. While under Fiske's roof, "want of employment, and, its consequences, want of proper necessaries" made Meg "very unsettled."[140] It was only, perhaps, on opening up her room after her ultimate confinement in Bethlem that Fiske recognized the full extent of her impoverishment, his description also serving to signify her mental degradation. "On opening the door, attended by a constable, &c. I beheld such a quantity of rags and dirt, as really quite astonished me; and all her furniture, including her miserable bed, was valued at only eighteen shillings."[141]

Generally, however, Nicholson was conceived as a victim of her own vanity and perversity of will or temperament, as much as of her environment or of an uncontrollable mental disease. Fiske was certainly convinced that her gradual descent into poverty and ill health was fueled by her pride, so that "probably she deprived herself of many a meal" to enable herself to appear "decently and genteely cloathed"—habits that only increased her propensity to talk to herself.[142] Even when she was sympathetically ordered an outfit of clothing by Lord Sydney while confined at the Coateses' (see p. 232), after it was learned that she had no more than what was on her back, Nicholson's antipathy to wearing garments that she "thought . . . infinitely too mean for her" was clearly conceived by Fiske and others as typical moral perversity and ingratitude, proceeding from her depraved and ridiculous vanity.[143]

No less judgmentally, Fiske also related her difficulties in finding decent employment to incidences of Nicholson's dishonesty, such as "cabbaging" or "over-charging" one client, and taking "unwarrantable liberties with the [dress and sewing] materials delivered to her" by another—episodes that not only lost her valuable employment, but also prevented her from ever again visiting "her old friends Mr and Mrs Paul."[144] At the culmination of his narrative, Fiske referred to recent intelligence he had received affording further proof of her "cunning and dexterity" in the art of "swindling."[145]

Equally significantly, perhaps, Nicholson had remained throughout the years preceding her crime rather isolated from her family in London and elsewhere, and somewhat estranged from her brother.[146] Her brother's reaction to the news of her assassination attempt when Fiske called on him was to observe that he rarely saw her, and that when he did they always quarreled; that she "had been insane for several years," and that it "was occasioned by her pride." Although he was at least willing to discuss with "her uncle . . . what could be done for her," and "appeared much affected when he saw her" soon after, detained at Mr. Coates's house, he was primarily concerned about how her sorry condition would affect "her aged parents." Meg herself found his visit disagreeable and spurned his assistance.[147] Apparently, Nicholson had herself applied for support to her uncle (an artillery officer at Blackheath) some time before her crime, when in dire financial straits, having anticipated and prepared for spending a week's sojourn with him. Yet this recourse too had resulted in another setback (assuming, indeed, that the visit and her uncle's so-called "respectable character" were not still other partial figments of her imagination, or psychic defenses for her endangered self-esteem). Despite her best efforts with her limited wardrobe and powder, she returned to her lodgings at Fiske's on the very evening of the day she had departed, "much chagrined and disappointed."[148] Nicholson's isolation and abandonment—her representation as spurned by past sweethearts and shunned by her family, and also "deserted" by employers "who she had . . . injured"—were thus portrayed as partly her own fault, and only partly the result of circumstances. It was at this juncture that Nicholson once again seems to have reverted to her rather delusional hopes "of a place at Court," engrossing herself in the writing of petitions to this effect and regarding herself as too busy to accept work that she had anyway begun to deem beneath her.[149] Fiske's own demands for her rent, which Nicholson strove to avoid but, ultimately, confessed she was unable to meet, no doubt increased the pressures she was under at this time.[150]

John Monro (probably alongside his son Thomas, with whom he was by then virtually sharing his practice) appears to have been summoned almost at once to examine Nicholson, after she had been brought before the Board of Green Cloth. This was a clear enough recognition that "their medical situation" made the Monros "extremely conversant with cases of insanity."[151] However, like the lay authorities, the doctors were reserved in their diagnosis, finding it "impossible to discover with certainty immediately whether she was insane or not."[152] John emphasized cautiously "that for the accomplishment of such a purpose, she must be taken under the care and inspection of one of his people for three or four days."[153] There was considerable doubt as a result about how to dispose of her. In the beginning, there had even been doubts about her sex, some thinking (or so certain sources claimed) that she was a cross-dresser who had assumed the masquerade of a female habit to expedite her design, a suspicion that had taken an examination by members of her own sex to dispel.[154] An initial suggestion that she be detained for three or four days pending a final disposal of the case was rejected as illegal, while a further recommendation that she be committed to Tothill Fields Bridewell was objected to because "she was a state-prisoner." It was agreed instead to place her in the custody of a royal messenger, Mr. Coates, so that she could be observed and examined at greater length.[155]

Evidently, Nicholson had found the hours of interrogation something of an ordeal, and after Monro had finished his questions "she appeared much convulsed, and seemed as if she was making an effort to weep, saying . . . 'tears would give her relief!'"[156] On her way to Coates's house, Meg is reported to have "declared, that she had no intention to hurt the King," but that after receiving no reply to her numerous petitions, "it was her determination . . . [rather ironically expressed] to bring matters to a point."[157] Although on arrival at the Coateses', Nicholson had "conversed for some time in a very rational manner with Mrs Coates, who was the only person suffered to be with her," she soon lapsed into "symptoms of a disordered mind."[158]

Subsequently, judging by press accounts, Monro did little more than send a keeper, or "nurse," to take charge of her (as was his usual practice), the first priority evidently being seen as securing her person, rather than offering her any medical treatment. Lord Sydney informed the king the day after her arrest that "she has been attended by one of Dr. Monro's people, and that person, as well as those who live in the house [i.e., that of Mr. Coates] looks upon her as mad."[159] Nevertheless, Fiske claimed that "Dr Monro and his son attended their patient every day" at the Coateses'.[160]

On 3 August, she was interrogated for a second time by Justice Addington, who went to see Nicholson in person at the Coateses'. On this occasion, Nicholson complained about the nature and "great number" of the previous day's questions, which she said "she did not understand," "had distracted her [and] . . . had made her deaf on one side." Otherwise, she spoke as before about her rights to the throne, which were "all a mystery," but which she kept at "the back part of her head," a site to which she regularly pointed.[161] What was different and most interesting about her testimony at this stage, however, were her statements

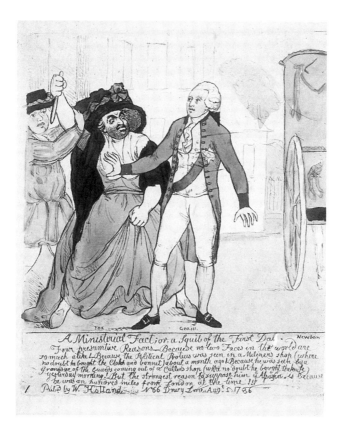

A Ministerial Fact; or, a Squib of the First Day. Newton

Four presumtive Reasons—Because no two Faces in the world are
so much alike!—Because the Political Proteus was seen in a Mileners shop (where
no doubt he bought the Cloak and bonnet) about a month ago!—Because he was seen by a
Grenadier of the Guards coming out of a Cutlers shop (where no doubt he bought the knife)
yesterday morning! But the strongest reason to suppose him y.ᵉ Assassin is Because
he was an hundred miles from London at the time!!

Pub.ᵈ by W. Holland N.° 66 Drury Lane Aug.ᵗ 2. 1786

FIGURE 43. Engraving by Richard Newton (1777–98) caricaturing Charles James Fox (1749–1806), Whig grandee and leader of the opposition to Williams Pitt's (1759–1806) Tory administration, stabbing George III, in the same fashion as Margaret Nicholson: *A Ministerial Fact; or, a Squib of the First Day.* Fox, dressed as a woman and raising his skirts with his left hand (but unshaven, thus underlining the gender incongruity of the scene and satirizing Fox as a political turncoat or cross-dresser—Nicholson herself being suspected by some to be a counterfeit woman and/or counterfeit lunatic), is shown scowling, with a knife raised aloft in his right hand to strike the king (right). George fends him off with his right hand. A beefeater (left) seizes Fox's right arm in both hands. In the background the garden front of St. James's Palace is suggested; on the right is the king's coach, seen from be-hind. Beneath the title the caption reads,

> Four presumtive Reasons—Because no two Faces in the world are so much alike!—Because the Political Proteus was seen in a Miliners [sic] shop (where no doubt he bought the Cloak and bonnet) about a month ago!—Because he was seen by a Grenadier of the Guards coming out of a Cutler's shop (where no doubt he bought the knife) yesterday morning!—But the strongest reason to suppose him yᵉ Assassin is because he was an hundred miles from London at the time!!

Published by W. Holland, No. 66 Drury Lane, 2 August 1786, as the second in a series of three satires. Reproduced by kind permission of the British Museum, Satire No. 6972; description taken in part from George and Stephen's *Catalogue of Prints and Drawings in the British Museum.* Copyright © The British Museum.

about the judges, Lord Mansfield and Lord Loughborough, to whom she had formerly written: "She said that she had brought them both into the world—they owed every thing they had to her. But she was not their mother. She never knew any man." [162]

As a childless spinster of modest and retiring, if not rather prudish, sensibilities, whose sole (recorded or alleged) sexual liaisons had supposedly culminated in the death of one lover and her abandonment by another, Nicholson's life story seems characterized by a set of circumstances that may also suggest to modern eyes—just as they did to her contemporaries—a whole variety of interpretations of her emotional and mental problems. To a significant degree, her story vividly encapsulates the social and economic difficulties of the servant classes in this period, and the particular vulnerabilities and frustrations of unmarried and far from eligible women trapped within the narrow confines of service occupations—especially those with limited personal and familial resources to call upon. Her affair with the valet had resulted in one of a series of losses of employment and a besmirched reputation that may well have tarnished her references as a servant and damaged her chances of being reemployed in that capacity. Nicholson had then been spurned and deserted by the very man who had caused her all this trouble, while her decision to quit the life of service altogether seems only to have resulted in further isolation, hardship, and disappointment. Her presumably fragile self-esteem had thus received a major series of fractures and assaults, and her biological, emotional, and social prospects of fulfillment as a wife and mother had been steadily eroded, if not shattered. Yet Margaret's own peculiarities of temperament also seem to have rendered her course an especially troublesome one to chart. Indeed, she may have found it difficult not to feel significantly responsible for her own reversals.

Just how fixated Nicholson had become on marriage as the bedrock of female potentiality is suggested by the extremity of her reaction to a fellow lodger and unemployed housekeeper at Mr. Paul[e]'s. The latter's unwillingness to consummate the marriage that she had subsequently secured so appalled Margaret that she took the leading hand in forcibly undressing her co-lodger so that nothing could prevent her from honoring her wifely duties.[163] Yet, as time went on, comparisons with other women seem only to have aggravated her own feelings of inadequacy. For example, Fiske emphasized how at a later date her friendly visits below stairs with his wife were curtailed once Mrs. Fiske gave birth to another baby. He surmised rather harshly that "antiquated virgins are not fond of that kind of vocal music, which they cannot contribute to produce." [164]

One should be careful not to take contemporary constructions of Margaret as the archetypal mad spinster too literally, or to perceive her mental state deterministically as the direct product of thwarted womanly desires. Margaret's growing poverty, the exposure of her dishonest dealings with clients, the lack of sympathy from her family, and the repeated disruption of her residences and occupations must also have placed considerable strain on her emotional and mental resources. Nonetheless, one might plausibly speculate that she may have had deep-seated psychic reasons for constructing a false but superior identity for herself and relating it to the "secret"—but frustrated—potentialities of her mind, her birthright, and her womb. In a revealing examination before the Privy Council, Nicholson was even more overtly to connect her particular demands from the king to her childlessness: "Upon being asked what she wanted of the King? her reply was, 'that he would provide for her, as she wanted to marry, and have children like other folks. . . .'" [165] Having reached the age of about forty-one by 1786, Nicholson was, at the very least, approaching (if not past) menopause, so her prospects of bearing children must long have seemed to be dwindling. Even if the hopes she still harbored on this front were not wholly illusory, her growing desperation about her womanly integrity is quite evident from her own reported testimony. Having been thrown over by her last (or only) lover when in her mid-thirties, in favor of a woman of property, must increasingly have signified to Meg the loss of her last chance for matrimonial and maternal happiness. As time went on, this disappointment may well have combined with others to provide Nicholson with additional and irresistible reasons to identify her own lack of substance with her undesirability as a spouse, and to sublimate, or translate, her inferiority and dismal circumstances into delusional hopes of succor from the highest earthly authority.

Discussing the case of the seventeenth-century prophetess Lady Eleanor Davies (or Touchet), who was sent to Bethlem in the 1640s, Roy Porter has emphasized the way in which Eleanor employed the language of bodily generation in order to articulate and legitimate her prophesying,[166] to appropriate to herself a special feminine power, and to emphasize her singular claims to insight. One wonders if Margaret Nicholson was not doing something similar with her assertions of being a virgin, a mother, and a queen, the rightful regal ruler of England, who had given birth to lords, a carrier of mystery in the vessels of her body, an important personage who held great secrets in her head. On the other hand, her mental problems seem to have antedated her abandonment by the valet, and her vulnerability had possibly been exposed after the alleged tragic end of her first great romance. Seen in another context, her delusions and somewhat hypochondriacal anxieties might be interpreted—as they probably would be by many modern psychiatrists—as rather typical features of the symptomology of functional mental illness, coupled with a repressed (or diverted) recognition that something systemic, something both mental and physical, was awry with her.

Hypothetical psychohistory and post hoc diagnosis aside, what is more significant, perhaps, is that in its own context Nicholson's testimony was dismissed by Addington and other contemporary authorities—lay and medical alike—as essentially not "worth noting," beyond the fact that it evidenced her lunacy. Yet, while Nicholson's was still another case in which the testimony of the insane was essentially seen as meaningless, it should be stressed that this was also a case in which the examination of an individual's state of mind was so searching that it took an entire week to complete satisfactorily.

The next examination had been ordered by the cabinet to be held in the Great Council Chamber at St. James's on Friday, 4 August. No doubt required to put on a reassuring public demeanor when leaving St. James's after the first examination, the king was observed to have "dispelled concerns" among the crowds by walking to his carriage with a composed and "smiling face." [167] In fact, this concealed no small unease. The royal nerves had clearly been pushed to a new edge in the intervening period between Nicholson's first and second examinations, the guard at the palace gate having been "judiciously encreased," and George, on his arrival from Windsor on the Friday at 11:50, being "for the first time in his reign . . . observed to descend from his carriage with an undrawn hanger in his hand. . . ." [168] Fear of regicide was in fact to dog George for much of his reign (see figure 48 on p. 251).

Once again, "the concourse of people" drawn on 4 August "to see the King . . . was considerable," "every avenue of the court" being "filled with people," and the levée room being mobbed by a whole range of nobility and gentry, "most of the foreign Ministers, and an infinity of commoners." The occasion had even dragged out of courtly retirement "many old Peers who had not been at St James's for . . . years." [169] While

such a reaction was hailed by the press as testimony to the profound affection and relief "universally" felt among the populace, court etiquette,
existing patronage, and hopes of future preferment no doubt also recommended this continued show of concern.

Soon after the king's arrival, and his receipt of further congratulations on his "happy escape" by this crowd of ministers and others,
Nicholson—readied for the occasion by the Coateses as ordered—was
duly brought before the Privy Council for yet another session of questioning. At this examination she claimed to have been thinking about the
regicide for about a week before attempting it, raising once again the
possibility of rational premeditation. Behaving in "a very wild and extravagant manner," she was observed to lose all signs of her previous
"collectedness" and to say nothing "in the smallest degree intelligible."
Reasserting her right to the throne, she maintained that it was sanctioned by Lords Mansfield and Loughborough and that "it was a cause
in which she would live and die." She had been "provoked to . . . attempt his Majesty's life by revenge" because he had failed to answer her
petitions.[170]

Monro and his son, attending the Council of State, were now prepared to opine more confidently "that having paid every proper attention to the culprit, and particularly having visited her that morning . . .
she was insane." In consequence of this evidence, Nicholson was re-
manded again into Coates's custody and it was felt unnecessary to summon Nicholson herself to appear at "any further examination."[171]
Doubts evidently remained, however, as to the precise timing and extent
of Nicholson's intellectual derangement. One observer theorized that
the crime itself and "the defect and recollection of its infamy" would
have been "enough, on reflection, to render the most callous mind disordered."[172] Subsequently, reaching new heights of meticulousness,
the authorities dispatched messengers far and wide, "to every part of
the kingdom where . . . she at any time resided," so that a thorough inquiry could be made as to the origins of "her present appearance of
insanity."[173]

On her return to the Coateses' home, Nicholson was observed to
have been

in a very placid humour, owing to the excellent treatment which she received
from Mr Coates, who made it his study to render the miserable woman as
comfortable as the remorse of her own mind, and her own unfortunate situation would allow. During the evening she requested to play a game of whist,

which Mr Coates complied with, and part of the time she was perfectly collected.[174]

The final examination by the council was suspended for a further four days, until 8 August. It was a delay that was mostly welcomed by the various commentators, who emphasized the wisdom of waiting "till some certain opinion could be collected by medical men."[175] In the intervening period, John Monro, accompanied by his son Thomas, seems to have been afforded ample opportunity to assess her mental state in the thorough way he had desired, Nicholson evidently being "daily visited by the two physicians."[176] Both Monros were summoned to the 8 August meeting, along with several other witnesses,[177] but it seems to have been their expert opinion that carried most weight.

Despite the Monros' initial hesitancy in pronouncing her insane, now that they had enjoyed the advantage of examining her regularly over the course of several days, both were convinced that she was indeed quite mad, John declaring her the worst case he had ever seen. Earlier questions about whether Nicholson was counterfeiting madness were now authoritatively dismissed by the Monros. While, for example, one witness (probably one of the Coateses) reported Nicholson's earlier enjoyment of a whist party, any uncertainties as to how usual it was "for Persons insane to be capable of Playing Cards" were met by the Monros averring tersely that this was "frequently" the case.[178] Setting to one side his earlier equivocations, John insisted

> that he never in his life had seen a person more disordered; that her Language was perfectly unintelligible and it was impossible to relate it; that she appeared to have a consciousness of what she had done, but did not seem sensible of having committed any crime; that in her conversation yesterday she burst out without any apparent cause into a fit of Laughter so violent as to make it necessary for her to support herself against the back of a chair; that he thinks from her account she must have been in this situation about ten years; that she always got upon the subject of her right to the Crown and the mystery; that he had not the least suspicion that her Madness was Counterfeited; that he hardly ever saw a clearer case of Insanity.[179]

Interestingly, the Monros' prolonged examination of Nicholson—although partially reliant on the patient's own account—seems to have convinced them that hers was a chronic case, so that the relevance of her more recent history as a servant and as an abandoned sweetheart was dismissed in their diagnosis. The introduction of the letters found at her lodgings addressed to Lord Mansfield, Lord Loughborough, and General Bramham, proclaiming her right to the throne, lent further weight to their verdict. Thus, at last, a week after her arrest, following this final prolonged interrogation before Justice Addington and the Privy Council, Nicholson was committed to Bethlem, never having been brought to trial for the crime. As Fiske pointed out sardonically, she had "now, as she has often devoutly wished, obtained a place under government, and probably she will continue in it for life."[180] She was indeed ordered "confined for life, supported in case of sickness; but while in health to be employed, and made useful," as her lunacy was regarded as "of that kind as not to affect her manual operations."[181]

At 11 A.M. on 9 August 1786, Nicholson was transported to Bethlem in a hackney coach with all due care. She was accompanied by a substantial, but relatively sympathetic, escort—namely, Mr. and Mrs. Coates, "another lady, and the nurse" (evidently the same nurse supplied by the Monros on 2 August). The Coateses even took the precaution of pretending that they were taking her "on a party of pleasure," a standard ruse in the confinement of the insane to avoid any trouble or resistance on the way to the madhouse (see chapter 5). The oblivious Margaret was observed to be "in very good spirits, and talked very rationally the whole of the way," her mood only altering slightly when she came within sight of Bedlam's walls, which she recognized immediately.[182] On her arrival at the hospital, according to Fiske, "she was admitted [as was customary] at the back door," where she was awaited by Monro in person, the doctor engaging her in "conversation . . . for some time" [a rather less than standard display of attention].[183] Fiske and the press reports also related how the Bethlem steward, Henry Weston, "received her with great tenderness and politeness" and "behaved with much kindness to her."[184] She and her party were accorded the special privilege of being invited to dine with him (Weston probably being curious for a closer inspection of such an unusual new inmate). Over a long supper, Meg "appeared perfectly collected, except," that is, "when the name of the King was mentioned," which provoked her to declare that she was expecting the king to visit her in her new quarters.[185] In a manner that must have presented Meg with a post-prandial foretaste of her life to come and the kind of conformity that indeed seems to have been expected of patients at Bethlem, Coates was to firmly admonish her to "patiently and quietly submit to the regulations of that place," a request to which Meg was said to have "composedly replied" her own simple but firm assent: "Certainly."[186] More leniently, she was informed that she was to be "indulged with pen, ink, and paper" to write to her friends, and at 4 P.M. "was conducted to her cell, which had been

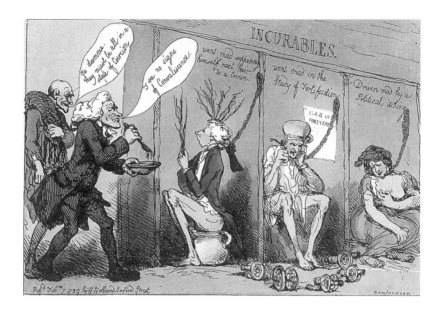

FIGURE 44. *The Hospital for Lunaticks,* by Thomas Rowlandson. This hand-colored etching by Rowlandson (1756–1827) was published on 7 February 1789. It depicts the prime minister, William Pitt the younger (1759–1806), sitting on a chamberpot in a hospital cell (probably supposed to be Bedlam). An inscription above him reads, "went mad supposing himself next heir to the Crown" (recalling Nicholson's delusive claims), and he is shown with his straw-fashioned symbols of office: a straw scepter and a straw coronet. In the next cell, Charles Lennox, fourth duke of Richmond and Lennox (1735–1806), is represented with his chamber pot on his head and encircled by a protective battery of cannons, having been driven mad "in the Study of Fortification." (See Charles Lennox, *An Answer to 'A Short Essay on the Modes of Defense Best Adapted to the Situation and Circumstances of this Island'* [by James Glenvel (1750–1817); London: Printed and sold by J. Alman, 1785].) Adjoining that cell in its turn is a woman, commonly assumed to be Jane, duchess of Gordon (1746–1812), who has become insane

through "Political itching"—a reference, perhaps, to the duchess's notorious political and sexual intriguing, and carrying the implicit suggestion that her strumpetry led to her contraction of "the itch," or venereal disease. Her London house in the Mall was not only the social center of the Tory party, but the site of regular drawing room parties, over which the famously beautiful duchess presided with equally famous wit and coarseness of speech (see http://www.robertburns.org/encyclopedia/GordonJaneDuchessofGordon17461511812.400.html). All three of the lunatics are represented as "INCURABLES," evidently being lodged in the hospital's incurables wings and chained by their necks to the walls of their cells. On the left, a bald and vicious-looking attendant declares, "They must all be in a state of coercion." This is an opinion concurred in by a bewigged physician or apothecary stirring and examining a recent stool, who sees "no signs of convalescence." Reproduced by courtesy of the British Museum (BM 7504). Copyright © The British Museum.

previously furnished with new bedding & c. for her reception" (an attention to a welcoming cleanliness and comfort that, Bethlem's records confirm, distinguished Weston's period of stewardship at the hospital). Immediately thereafter, "a chain was put round her leg, and fastened to the floor," a procedure that—if Nicholson had not already anticipated it—does not seem to have altered her outward "composure." Indeed, she may well have appreciated the steward's concern in this matter, as reported by the *European Magazine:* when he asked "if the chain hurt her leg, as it should be altered if it did? She replied, 'No, not at all.'" The consideration with which Nicholson was treated is also testified to by the fact that Coates was reported to have "waited near an hour" at the hospital for her to write some letters "which she wished to send by him," despite the fact that (once again) she was unable to translate intent very fully into action: in point of fact, "she did not attempt to write anything."

While the press and the public repeatedly and far and wide thanked "the blessing of Providence" for the king's escape,[187] Nicholson began to settle in to her new abode. The secretary of state, Lord Sydney, had insisted that "the most strict and proper Care be taken of her," and there was clearly intense concern in the government and at the hospital about her potential dangerousness. Consequently, almost immediately after her admission, all visitors to her were excluded unless accompanied by a governor and, for the next half year, monthly examinations were made of her by the Bethlem committee.[188] Commenting in 1787, the Kent specialist on insanity William Perfect used her case to emphasize the dangerous unpredictability of the insane, and the need to be careful not to be premature in arresting treatment and confinement:

> The late happy and providential escape of his majesty from the horrid attempt of assassination, from the hand of an infatuated maniac, appears in itself sufficient to determine all those persons under whose care and protection such unfortunate persons are, not to let them venture at large.[189]

It was evidently in partial response to such fears that Nicholson was initially confined to her apartment and kept in chains. A year later, however, all mechanical restraint was removed on the queen's order.[190] Soon afterward, Nicholson was transferred to the incurables wards, following a further verbal message from George III and still another examination by the Monros, this one undertaken in the presence of the Bethlem committee and the undersecretary of state, Evan Nepean. The king's message, which was conveyed as before by his undersecretary, expressed his

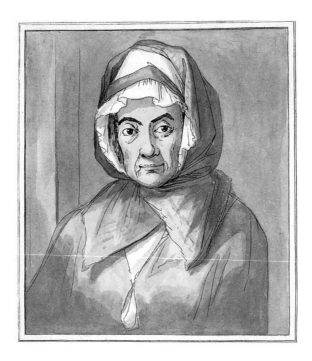

FIGURE 45. Portrait of Margaret Nicholson toward the end of her life (ca. 1828) and long confinement in Bethlem. Nicholson is shown here in a white linen bonnet, blue head scarf/ hood, and brown top. The etching was engraved by the draftsman and antiquary John Thomas Smith (1766–1833) after his own painting (ca. early nineteenth century). Nich- olson's rather drab dress and tired, worn facial features seem to be intended to reflect the ravages of time and confinement on what had formerly been portrayed (by some artists) as her good looks. Reproduced by kind permission of the British Museum, engraved portrait series. Copyright © The British Museum.

appreciation for the governors' "great Care and Attention in their Treatment of Margaret Nicholson" and requested her continuing detention.[191] As an incurable, the would-be assassin was once again placed in chains, a restraint that was only lifted in 1791 on the motion of two governors. Nicholson seems to have lingered on Bethlem's galleries quite peacefully for decades.[192] At length, she died in the hospital on 14 May 1828, aged about seventy-seven, more than forty-one years after being admitted, having outlasted her similarly long-lived intended victim.

As a case in whom royalty and the government, as well as the Bethlem governors and staff, took a special interest, Nicholson seems to have been treated carefully and relatively sympathetically, continuing, for example, to be provided with writing and reading materials when she requested them. On a broader stage, her crime and her delusions of grandeur, not to mention the irony of her connection to a king who himself was adjudged mad within just three years of her admission, ensured that she would continue to inflame the public imagination. As with the Ferrers case, contemporary pamphlets and magazines went to some lengths to satisfy and further "excite the public curiosity," few more so than the *Lady's Magazine,* which, accepting the inevitability of the interest the case created, promised to do its best "to gratify our fair Patronesses."[193] Within days of the attempt, one enterprising author managed to produce a 56-page shilling booklet, comprehensively detailing her case even before it had been resolved and gathering together a host of disparate accounts from the diurnals and from street gossip, determined to satisfy the public with all the "minutiae" of the case.[194] He even managed a major exclusive, puffing his narrative up in its title as being the first to include details of the genuine motivation behind Nicholson's attempt (i.e., the alleged affair with the guardsman).[195]

Virtually overnight, as a result, Meg Nicholson became one of Bethlem's star attractions: characterized by writers and etched and painted by artists more than any of her fellow inmates, she was sought out by all the hospital's most distinguished visitors (as well as by a variety of lesser figures). This artwork and the numerous anecdotes supplied by Nicholson's visitors, and by her biographers and obituarists, reveal how she continued, throughout her long confinement, to remain a figure of fascination and of somewhat mawkish curiosity in the eyes of both medical men and the public at large.

Despite (or perhaps because of) their competing claims to be the most "exact" representation of her case, textual or narrative portrayals of Nicholson veered markedly between the relatively sympathetic and the sharply critical. While certain depictions (especially those written in later Victorian and Edwardian times) morbidly romanticized her history, others offered condemnatory readings of her as vain, degraded, and vicious. Pictographic representations of her case betray a similarly contrary, even contradictory, set of social constructions. Some displayed a rather beautiful, refined lady, in sumptuous attire, glamorizing Nicholson in accordance with popular contemporary images of disappointed, spurned women, or alluring heroines—a stereotype popular long before

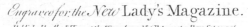

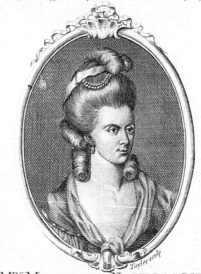

M.^{RS} MARGARET NICHOLSON,

who attempted to Stab *the* King *of* Great Britain *.*
Aug.t 2 1786, and being judged Insane *was sent to* Bedlam
Aug.t 9 1786, where it is supposed she will remain for life.

283

FIGURE 46. Line engraving of Margaret Nicholson from the *New Ladies Magazine* (1786). One of many contemporary depictions showing her looking rather stunning, with her hair fashionably, if not luxuriously, dressed and beaded (and recalling the fascination in modern times with figures such as Myra Hindley). (She was also described somewhat less glamorously in the magazine literature as "rather short, of a very swarthy complexion, which gives her the appearance of a foreigner"— *European Magazine* 10 [1786], p. 118; *Universal Magazine* 79 [1786], p. 95; *Lady's Magazine* 17 [1786], p. 386.) Evidently her life sentence to Bethlem was already thoroughly expected. "Mrs MARGARET NICHOLSON, *who attempted to* Stab *the* King *of Great Britain Aug.t* 2 *1786, and being judged* Insane *was sent to* Bedlam *Aug.t* 9 *1786, where it is supposed she will remain for life.*" Published by Alexander Hogg at the Kings Arms, No. 16 Paternoster Row, London, 30 September 1786; apparently engraved by Isaac Taylor (1730–1807) of Stanford Rivers, the mapmaker and engraver, who had also done capital plate engravings for *The Curiosities, Natural and Artificial, of the Island of Great Britain* (1775), William Pain's *The Builder's Pocket-treasure* (1776), and Batty-Langley's *The Builder's Director* (ca. 1790).

As for Myra Hindley, since her conviction and indefinite detention in a special hospital in the 1960s along with Ian Brady for the appalling (tape-recorded) torture and murder of young children (the notorious "Moors murders"), she has became the incarnation in

the mid-Victorian invention of femmes fatales. (Nicholson's case, it should be remembered, came to public attention just seven years before the onset of the Gothic romantic literary and artistic cult of the "fair maid," Crazy Jane, the melancholy madwoman whose ceaseless lamenting for her departed lover was made famous by Matthew Gregory Lewis's [1775–1818] 1793 ballad.)[196] Most educated eighteenth-century writers, however, were disposed to condemn the glamorization of madness, crime, and (female) criminals, and, correspondingly, narrative and artistic portraits of Nicholson tended more often to present her as ugly and bizarre, outfitted in ridiculous garb, a thwarted spinster who might be pitied but was far more to be blamed for delusively and perversely refusing to accept her lot.

Underlying this ugly/beautiful polarity[197] in pictorial and literary depictions of Nicholson are important class and gender constructions of the poorer or servant classes, and more especially of femininity and the female body. It is noteworthy that the compassionate and/or glamorizing view of Nicholson was less prominent in contemporary representations than more didactic, censorious perspectives. Without question, Nicholson's age and the particularly grave, if not heinous, circumstances of her crime counted against her. More than that, however, at least until after the turn of the century, prevailing trends in contemporary culture made romanticizing her case distinctly difficult. A major theme in prevailing class/gender attitudes, embodied in a whole series of decidedly derogatory narratives, criticized women who tried, or appeared, to

---

British culture of female psychopathology. There have been endless books and articles about her, while her photograph has been reproduced again and again in contemporary press and other publications, and she has recently and notoriously become the subject of artistic representation, in Marcus Harvey's gargantuan portrait *Myra,* prominently featured and vandalized in the "Sensation" exhibition during 1997 at London's Royal Academy. Both despite and because of the persisting and often morbid fascination with her case, she has also become something of a cause célèbre for liberals who continue to campaign for her release, much to the chagrin and dismay of the families of her victims. See Pamela Hansford Johnson, *On Iniquity, Some Personal Reflections Arising out of the Moors Murder Trial* (London, Melbourne [etc.]: Macmillan, 1967); Jonathan Goodman, *The Moors Murders: The Trial of Myra Hindley and Ian Brady* (Newton Abbot: David and Charles, 1986); Jean Ritchie, *Myra Hindley: Inside the Mind of a Murderess* (London: Angus and Robertson, 1988); and Janie Jones and Carol Clerk, *The Devil and Miss Jones: The Twisted Mind of Myra Hindley* (London: Smith Gryphon, 1993). Reproduced by kind permission of the British Museum. Copyright © The British Museum.

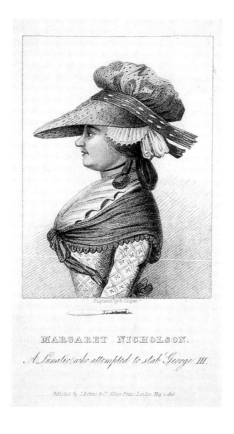

FIGURE 47. Line engraving of Margaret Nicholson: "A Lunatic who attempted to stab George III," by R. Cooper (probably Richard Cooper, ca. 1730–1820); shows Nicholson in a bonnet, within a square frame, and is clearly modeled on Fiske's drawing (see figure 42). Outside the frame, exemplifying the morbid fascination with the macabre that lay behind many of these sorts of representations, the knife she used is also represented. It is displayed (in order to add a touch of chilling realism) as if actually tacked on to the wall beneath the portrait. Published by J. Robins & C. Alburn Press, London, 1 May 1816. Reproduced by kind permission of the British Museum. Copyright © The British Museum.

present themselves above their stations. Eighteenth-century elites were strikingly hostile to those women whose backgrounds and conduct, once thrust into the public eye, seemed to identify them as proud, vain, deceitful, and self-indulgent. Of course, many, if not most, of these productions on the theme of Nicholson emanated not from literary haute couture, but from the popular press. Yet Grub Street was just as disposed to cheap exposure of tawdry female morality and to inverse class snobbery as to sensational romanticization. The dominant discourse was especially critical of those who were deemed licentious enough to make irrational sacrifices to fashion. Efforts were made to expose such women and to show them up for what they truly were—incongruous, fake, ugly, loose, tatty-genteel (or plain crazy). In a society generally averse to the imposition of sumptuary laws on dress or other novel "continental" constraints on traditional liberties—despite some English agitation in their favor—the discursive domain was the main or even the exclusive arena where such limits might be asserted.[198]

Yet, however paradoxical it may seem, even in the mid-eighteenth century there was concurrently a tendency—one associated with the cults of sensibility, nascent romanticism, and the picturesque—to romanticize women with emotional/socioeconomic afflictions.[199] Literary representations like Samuel Richardson's Pamela (a young woman from the same servant classes as Nicholson who ends up marrying her master) reflect the positive potential being recognized in this era of tremendous social mobility (even) for women, for the virtuous and talented to overcome persistently forbidding and formidable social barriers. Richardson was a leading figure in the new "age of sensibility" literature. His hypersensitive portrayal of Pamela's woes, and his championing of her entitlements as a person and particularly as a *female* of virtue, were replicated in numerous other contemporaneous portrayals of women (though, to be sure, they were simultaneously savagely burlesqued in Henry Fielding's *Shamela*). Richardson's novel may be seen as just one sign of the broadening feminization of polite culture that was also, to a lesser extent, mediating contemporaries' readings of Nicholson's case. While higher ranking professional and occupational roles remained essentially beyond women's reach, marriage (according to writers like Richardson) offered a perfectly legitimate arena within which women might employ their innate and authentic qualities (in particular character, virtue, and beauty) with a view to the enhancement of their own social circumstances. Unfortunately for Nicholson, of course, respectable marriage was not only an elusive, but ultimately a rather self-delusional goal—which was precisely, in the eyes of some commentators, the circumstance that had so plainly impelled her toward acts of immodesty, self-abasement, and degradation.

Another subtext of particular pertinence when one seeks to sift the various meanings discernible in representations of the Nicholson case is the contemporary preoccupation with crime, vice, illicit activity, and social advancement prosecuted or achieved under false or counterfeit guises. Depictions of Nicholson that dwelled on the fantastical, fraudulent, or counterfeit elements in her identity and self-presentation (contrasting these defects with the noble dress and deportment of the regal object of her fixation) seem to link her own allegedly disreputable origins and intentions with other contemporary figures who were seen to prey on their betters. The prostitute and the highwayman[200] are perhaps the most obvious examples of this discourse about dissembling. In order to ply their trades, these exemplars of the morally disreputable classes customarily dressed above their social stations, an apparently trivial social infraction in the context of their other challenges to conventional morality and the social order, but one that was nonetheless a common preoccupation in contemporary commentaries. The peculiar obsessions one observes here derive in substantial measure, we suggest, from aggravated anxieties about declining distinctions between the classes—especially the lower/middle ranking classes and the gentry/nobility—as money, and more widely purchasable fashions, seemed to be eroding the stable divisions of rank in a steadily commercializing, consumerist society.[201]

Yet, there was no simple polarity in contemporary representations of Nicholson. For, as historians of eighteenth-century fashion and the masquerade have argued, rather than any dichromatic set of cultural and social distinctions, sartorial forms presented highly unstable messages in this period.[202] In part, this was because of the very absence of "exact," let alone photographic/scientific, forms of recording and presenting appearances. Hack writers, engravers, and artists, competing in a free and eager market for the consumption of spicy yarns and portrayals, were at liberty to attribute to Nicholson more or less whatever physical attributes they chose to adopt in presenting her case. When Fiske attempted to discredit all competing accounts by asserting the superiority of his own eyewitness view of Nicholson, he was also—and as much for moral as for documentary reasons—at pains to repudiate the glamorized images of her that had been peddled within, or alongside, these other "authentic" accounts. His inclusion of his own drawing of her on the first page of his *Life*, then, was in one sense a rhetorical device to claim narrative superiority. Yet, while he was at once signifying the partiality of contemporary constructions, he was inevitably, perhaps, doomed to fail to constrain the continuing accretions and fashioning of her identity in the years that followed, and to be just as prone in his own time to fictionalize and construct as to "truly" document her history.

As early as 1786, Fiske's and two other published accounts vied with each other to provide the most authentic memoirs of her life.[203] That same year, the provincial mad-doctor William Perfect even included her in his book of "select cases" delineating the various "species of insanity."[204] Marie Sophie von la Roche offered a particularly detailed description of Nicholson, whom she visited less than two years after her admission and found (as usual) "tidily attired, her hat upon her head, with gloves and book in hand." Margaret was in the midst of writing a letter to "the prince"—a missive that, despite her "good hand," she worried was too untidy for his majesty to see.[205]

As with a number of other rather voyeuristic accounts of Nicholson at Bethlem, Sophie's narrative must be taken with several grains of salt, for it was suffused with the affected emotionalism and sentimentally tinted curiosity that were so characteristic of the "age of sensibility." Hence Sophie's ostentatiously drawn contrast between her own "tearful glances" at other "pathetic" young women patients and her unease when faced with Nicholson: "I shuddered at seeing a person with murderous instincts," who "fixed her horrible grey eyes wildly on us."[206] Flavored with saccharine overtones, Sophie's Candide-like narrative was constructed to reflect well on the medical régime at Bethlem under Monro. It concluded with a portrait of how "kindly" Nicholson was addressed by the Bethlem apothecary, who, evidently concerned to ensure that she had enough pens and books, called "a nurse" to provide her with "fresh ones" and promised to send her another volume of reading matter.

The French traveler Jacques de Cambry (1749–1807) provided a more politically pointed depiction of Nicholson two years later. The occasion of his visit to see her in 1788 constitutes one of the not so rare exceptions made to the hospital rule that denied male visitors access to female patients. Like Sophie, de Cambry found Margaret very properly attired in a black hat,[207] sitting reading Shakespeare's *The Merry Wives of Windsor*.[208] (It may be no accident that Shakespeare was apparently one of Monro's "favourite authors.")[209] Subsequently, he sought to use her case to make more general analogies between the much vaunted liberties of the English and the prevalence of arbitrary imprisonment in pre-Revolutionary France. The treatment of cases of attempted regicide in France (and elsewhere in Europe) were notably harsher in the second half of the eighteenth century. In particular, the horrific drawing and quartering of Francis (R. F.) Damiens in 1757, after he, like Nicholson, had made an incompetent, if not mentally suspect, attempt on a king (Louis XV) with an unlikely knife, had sent shock waves through Europe.[210]

The relevance of the comparison was not lost on contemporary commentators. The *European Magazine* itemized not merely the Damiens case, but the whole history of regicides and attempted regicides in Europe since the seventeenth century. More pointedly, it noted how "most of the miscreants . . . were insane" and that, in France, not only Damiens's, but "all these diabolical attempts were made while the kings were in or coming out of their carriages surrounded by their guards."[211] The poems, or *Posthumous Fragments of Margaret Nicholson*, published in 1810 (see below), portray Nicholson herself gruesomely, if not enviously, celebrating the Damiens affair:

> Yes Francis! thine was the dear knife that tore
> A tyrant's heart-strings from his guilty breast.[212]

The last attempt on the king's life in England before Nicholson's had been directed at George's grandfather, George I, and this too had culminated in the execution of the (allegedly insane) offender,[213] but numerous minor trespasses and assaults on royal property and personages had been dealt with more mildly by the Green Cloth in the intervening period—the offenders in a number of such cases ending up in Bethlem. There had been two assaults by mentally deranged individuals on George III himself in the years preceding Nicholson's more serious attempt. The fear of regicide reached almost fever pitch in the years that followed, with the execution of the French king, Louis XVI, and the assassination of Gustavus III of Sweden, in 1792, not to mention the murderous assaults and plots of notorious Bedlamites like James Hadfield (ca. 1772–1841) and Bannister Truelock in George's later years.[214]

Contemporaries seem to have experienced a palpable morbid frisson from reading accounts of such a notorious case being shown to visitors, and for nearly four decades a variety of scribblers exploited their readers' apparently endless appetite for gossip about Nicholson. As the anticipatory excitement conveyed in Sophie's narrative makes clear, Margaret was treated as a moving and macabre object of display for Bethlem's visitors, and few seem to have seriously scrupled playing their assigned roles in the performance: "'And now,' said the supervisor, door key in hand, 'I will show you Mistress Nicholson.'"[215] Years later, the failed assassin still captured the public imagination (again, not unlike Myra Hindley). She was the "Noted Female" who formed the subject of the small volume of burlesque verses, or *Posthumous Fragments* (men-

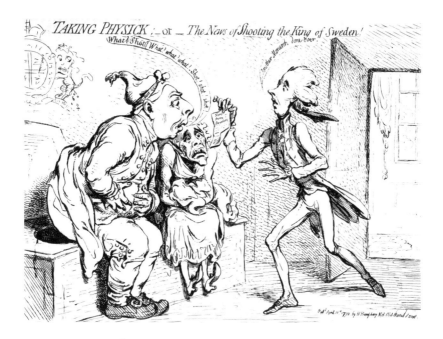

FIGURE 48. Etching of George III (1738–1820) and his queen, Charlotte Sophia (1744–1818), in a latrine (1792): "Taking physick—or—The news of Shooting the King of Sweden!" This etching by James Gillray (1757–1815) satirizes the royal reaction to news of the assassination of the king of Sweden, Gustavus III. The grossly agitated king and queen receive a message from the emaciated William Pitt, who rushes in bearing "news from Sweden," exclaiming: "Another Monarch done over!" The horrified king, clutching his bloated stomach, stammers: "What? Shot? What? What? What? Shot! Shot! Shot!"—a reference to George's well-known repetitive style of speech. The band of the king's nightcap reads: "Honi Soit qui M . . ." Behind him the lion of the royal arms is excreting, mirroring the king's terrified state. Published in London by H. Humphrey, 11 April 1792. For a description, see the Wellcome Institute Library Iconographic Collection (Videodisc Frame No. 11561) and British Museum, Catalogue of Political and Personal Satires, vol. 6, London, 1938, No. 8080. Reproduced by kind permission of The Wellcome Trust, London.

tioned above), written by Shelley and Hogg in 1810 during their student days at Oxford, and edited by Nicholson's nephew, John Fitzvictor.[216] Purporting to comprise an indication, if not an exemplary parable, of how "energy and native genius" might be perverted to "phrenzy and despair," these poems also reeked of rather exploitative voyeurism.[217] On the one hand, they were an excuse for a loosely veiled, radical republicanist critique of the tyrannies and oppressions of monarchical government. On the other hand, they represented the far from dead Nicholson ("my unfortunate Aunt") "posthumously," her current existence as a fate worse than death, yet one that offered superb material for morbid romanticizing and eroticizing. Thus, Nicholson was depicted drowning in "tides of maddening passion," castigating George as heartless and reminding him and Charlotte of their transience on this earth, while lamenting the death of her own heart and spirit. Lost in despair, tortured by agony and enthusiastic torments about horrors and hellfire, tormented by visions of storms, nightmares, and banshees, and racked by waves of anguish, her madness and confinement in Bedlam were identified as a living death:

> YES! all is past—swift time has fled away,
> Yet its swell pauses on my sickening mind;
> How long will horror nerve this frame of clay?
> I'm dead, and lingers yet my soul behind.[218]

As late as 1823, by which time Margaret was deaf and a compulsive snuff-taker, a hospital insider (probably a former keeper) presented a long account of her among the 140 patients he depicted in his even more unapologetically voyeuristic *Sketches in Bedlam*.[219] Self-evidently, the aura of spectacle had not ended at Bethlem with the end of promiscuous visiting!

Though she was certainly the most famous of Bethlem's politically charged inmates, Nicholson was far from unique. Indeed, when apparently insane individuals were sent to Bethlem by royalty or some other notable political authority, Monro could expect to be asked to make a special diagnosis. The year after Nicholson's admission, for example, Thomas Stone was sent to Bethlem from Tuthill Fields Bridewell, along with "a Verbal Message" from the king requesting his admission, and Monro and his son Thomas examined him. Stone, "a heavy looking man, about 33 years of age" and "a native of Shaftesbury,"[220] was the son of a floor-cloth painter and had trained as an attorney. He came to the attention of the authorities after writing "a very extraordinary letter" to the queen, "mentioning a very warm passion which he had conceived of her eldest daughter; and hoping, if their majesties approved of the idea of his marrying her, he and the princess royal would be a very happy couple."[221]

Not content to rest his suit there, Stone appeared in person at St. James's Palace "and begged of leave to be introduced in form, as from not having received an answer, he conceived his proposal was acceded to." Finally, on the presumptuous suitor taking his amorous quest to Kew, "he was seized and confined till he could be taken to the public office in Bow-street to be examined."[222] Paralleling Nicholson's case, "a great many papers on the subject of love were found upon him, addressed to her Serene Highness the Princess Royal." Among these were the following lines, which were submitted to Monro for examination:

> To her Highness the PRINCESS ROYAL
> Thrice glad were I to be your willing slave,
> But not the captive of the tool or knave;
> With woe on woe you melt my sighing breast,
> Whilst you reject your humble would-be guest.[223]

Stone was examined before the Monros, as well as "several [other] of the faculty and some justices of the peace," who had little trouble making up their minds, "evident marks of insanity having appeared in many parts of his conduct." According to the *Annual Register,* his "conversation" alone made it clear that he was "a lunatic," and to clinch matters—in the fashion of a crazy Swiftian projector—he had previously written to a Mr. Deleval proposing a plan to pay off the national debt. The decisive factor that determined the outcome of his case was plainly the bizarre (and potentially dangerous) attachment this unlikely Prince Charming had formed to one of the royal family. Stone had apparently become fixated on the princess at least five months previously, when he saw her at the theater, although his illness seems to have manifested itself much further back: ". . . his heart was stolen from him three years ago, and till last March he did not know who was the robber, till being at a play, he saw the princess royal . . . up at the two shilling gallery."[224]

Stone continued to write letters to the king during his first year's stay at Bethlem, and there is evidence that George III personally perused them. Their contents clearly encouraged the monarch to request Stone's continuing detention, and this time it was Thomas Monro who examined the patient and declared him "incurable and fit."[225] Transferred to the incurables wards in 1788, Stone was, like Nicholson and a number of other state committals, to spend the rest of his life in Bethlem, and died there in 1805.[226]

John Monro must have been relatively well accustomed to dealing with such political committals. Twenty years before this, it was Monro who let the Bethlem committee know about a patient who was to be conveyed by royal authority to Bethlem, another Board of Green Cloth case who had been troublesome within the Verge (roughly a fifteen-mile radius) of the court. This particular individual was one of a host of such cases who were sent to the hospital from the late seventeenth century onward.[227]

Monro also gave expert testimony as to the insanity of Richard Hyde, who was accused of riotous assembly and destruction of property in 1780 and acquitted as insane. Shortly after his arrest, as well as prior and subsequent to his trial, Hyde was confined at Bethlem.[228] Here, he was kept specially isolated from visitors, being only "permitted to Walk in the Gallery" on days when visitors were not present "and then not till after one o'Clock," with notice for him to be brought before the Old Bailey Sessions immediately when summoned for trial.[229] Monro testified that he had attended Hyde's father, William, when insane in 1771, and that, although the son was not insane on that occasion, he was very much so when Monro saw him the following year and his malady "increased extremely" within the next few weeks.[230] Monro's testimony appears to have been far from conclusive in this case, however. The majority of substantive evidence regarding Hyde's (and his family's) mental state was provided by lay witnesses, by a Dr. Coombes who had seen Hyde and found him insane just a month previous to the trial, and by the accused himself, who regularly (and rather simple-mindedly) interjected himself into the proceedings.

Such cases suggest that, as physician to Bethlem and mad-doctor extraordinaire, John Monro gradually, if only partially, carved out a place for himself as one of the first expert witnesses on insanity. However, his appearances at the law courts in this capacity seem few and far between, and the status of such expertise remained distinctly open to question in this period. As Walker has observed, in Hyde's case, Monro was kept waiting "for several days with great inconvenience" at the Old Bailey before his affidavit was permitted to be read in absentia. The frustrating bureaucracies of the courtroom must have actively discouraged busy physicians from seeking regular involvement in legal matters. Certainly, medical witnesses remained a limited, although increasing, presence, in insanity trials before 1800, and were rarely called by the accused.[231]

THE MAD-DOCTOR AND THE MAD KING: THE ROYAL MALADY AND THE END OF MONRO'S CAREER

The continuing ambivalence of the mad-doctor's status is reflected less in John Monro's rare courtroom and stateroom appearances than in the plethora of mocking references to him, and the factual and apocryphal stories about him, that circulated in contemporary literature. Numerous contemporaries from Fielding to Walpole satirically portrayed Monro, even more prominently than his father, being granted the somewhat unenviable honor of presiding over the madnesses of the nation. For example, ridiculing a host of his political adversaries and others whose conduct he disapproved of (including the "mad Lord" George Gordon, "Lord Bolingbroke [who] is in a mad house," Lord Pomfret, and his own nephew, Lord Orford, who "ought to be there"), Horace Walpole joked that "were I on the throne I would make Dr Monro a groom of my Bedchamber."[232]

Such jests were normally less to the discredit and discomfort of Monro than to those of his putatively mad charges. While some gossips spread the probably apocryphal story of how some of Monro's patients had wanted to boil him in the Bethlem kitchen kettle, or copper boiling pot, "in hope of making their broth better," others alleged that this story had in fact been told about Battie and St. Luke's.[233] More generous assessments were made by fellow professionals, such as the medical statistician Dr. William Black (1749–1829), who received Monro's aid in his compilation of statistics on mortality around 1788 and described him as "learned and venerable" with an "accustomed liberality and affability."[234]

Sophie von la Roche was extremely complimentary about Monro on her visit to Bethlem in the 1780s.[235] Portraying him as an enlightened physician of his time, Sophie reported approvingly "the cleanliness, order and gentleness with which these wretched folk are tended" and "the affectionate care taken not to hurt them." She also lauded the physical conditions at Bethlem, describing the fresh air and recreation patients could enjoy in the hospital's "fine gardens," the "comfortable beds," "spacious and bright . . . living-rooms . . . with windows up above," and the material comforts made available to the patients, "many" of whom "are provided with tables, books, and writing materials." The "inspector" who conducted her (evidently John Gozna, the apothecary) attributed this system to "Dr Monro's institute," claiming that "he had forbidden them to ill-treat or frighten any one of the unfortunates either by word or threat or mien."

As the resident medical officer, however, it is Gozna to whom Sophie accords primary credit for what she observed. In her portrayal, he comes across as a particularly "humane" man, if not an anticipator of "moral management." His introduction of strait waistcoats at Bethlem and tactful avoidance of words like "fool" and "madman," for which he allegedly substituted the word "ill," were marked out for particular praise, and Sophie enthusiastically quoted his therapeutic precepts. Insanity, he told her, "is a fever of the mind, tender, gentle handling is the only cure and persistent tenderness and kindness must inevitably have a salutary effect"; whereas, if "the fever has proved infectious to the body," he tried "to relieve it by diet and medicines."

It has to be stressed once again, however, that Sophie, who "wept for joy, and blessed Monro and the inspector," and on leaving Bethlem solicited "blessings for the wise, humane doctor and noble committee," viewed the institution through spectacles that were strongly rose-tinted by naiveté and affected sensibility. Whatever Monro's or Gozna's ideals and claims about the régime at Bethlem, the reality was considerably harsher. The reports of other visitors spoke of high levels of restraint, of semi-naked patients, of primitive conditions, and of exploitation and rough handling of patients by keepers.[236]

Just three years after testifying in the case of George III's attempted assassin, Margaret Nicholson, Monro received his one and only consultation from the royal court when the king himself succumbed to what was widely conceived to be a mental malady. This summons came during the first bout of George III's supposed madness, in 1788–89. Assailed by questions and cross-examinations about the king's case from both sides of the house, the royal physicians had been repeatedly asked to offer a prognosis. In particular, both Whig and Tory politicians demanded to know whether the doctors thought the king's condition was permanent. Although some sources (especially those in opposition, who favored a regency) declared "that the best-informed persons believed the King's insanity to be incurable,"[237] the royal physicians were unable to agree on the matter, and the government (whose political fate depended upon the king's recovery) was naturally at some pains to persuade the public that the opposite conclusion was warranted. It was on this particularly fraught issue that Monro's opinion was sought.

At the insistence of the House of Commons, the royal physicians had already obtained access to the records of Bethlem, to permit comparisons with the fate of other patients of the king's age. In the event, the rather incomplete nature of Bethlem's admission books made them of little use for such a purpose. According to the mad-doctor and medical polymath William Rowley (1742–1806), on examining these books to see whether the majority of those with the royal malady recovered, Sir Richard Warren had evidently succeeded in calculating that the chances were three to one against recovery, but had provided the information too late to be of use.[238] Francis Willis, on the other hand, asked by the Commons in January 1789 whether he had consulted the registers of any public or private receptacle for the insane, dismissed statistics derived from such sources as completely unhelpful, for "they do not give you any Account of the particular Symptoms of the Malady when taken in to the Hospital."[239]

While, in previous times, Walpole would have been happy to make Monro groom of the royal bedchamber, those in George III's court during the 1780s seem to have been far from keen to summon the physician of Bedlam to the palace. Some prominent political figures expressed wonderment, as Anthony Storer put it, that obscure private physicians like Dr. Anthony Addington (1713–90, proprietor of a Reading madhouse, whose only publications had been on scurvy) were summoned to attend King George, while Monro's assistance was "never called in." Surely, they suggested, "his opinion may have been very important."[240] During the same month, those who leaned toward a regency, such as Sir Gilbert Elliot (1751–1814), the first earl of Minto, were confidently declaring "that the best-informed persons believed the King's insanity to be incurable."[241]

Other politicians, like Edmund Burke (1729–97), appealed explicitly for the direct intervention of the Bethlem physician, hoping by this means to resolve the vexed question of curability. Yet while Burke clearly regarded Monro's experience of hundreds of cases as making him more authoritative than any royal physicians, Monro was never brought in to attend the king in person. He was merely asked informally by the royal physicians about the seriousness of the royal malady and the likelihood of recovery. Sir Lucas Pepys (1742–1830), who also emphasized (when it suited him) that Monro "has seen more Patients than any Practitioner ever did see," was apparently assured by the mad-doctor that most cases "did recover."[242] However, he and some of the other physicians were probably keen to interpret Monro's comments in the most positive possible light in order to retain their own authority over the royal malady.

Fox and his allies, however, their fortunes tied closely to the possible regency, clearly had the ear of still another of the king's physicians, Sir Richard Warren (1731–97), who made it evident that he was far from happy with the regular and misleadingly optimistic press statements he was asked to sign as to the king's health. Seeking to bolster the skeptics' case, Warren (who had become a governor of Bethlem in 1776 through Monro's recommendation) wrote directly to Monro in January of 1789 soliciting his opinion as to the "symptoms of incurability."[243] The Bethlem physician's relatively explicit answer, given by return of post, is recorded in the records of the College of Physicians. Being sick, Monro was obliged to dictate his opinion to his wife. In politically expedient terms, and being careful not to take sides, the Tory mad-doctor declared,

> I should look upon that Insanity as likely to prove Incurable which comes on towards the middle stage of life without any known cause to which it is to be attributed unless it may be a family complaint. The symptoms are great deprivation of sense: tending to fatuity: every tendency to that disposition is to be dreaded when the disorder is not checked by Medicine or management: where there is a want of natural sleep.[244]

Although Warren's special consultation with Monro seems to suggest some recognition of his expert knowledge, what is perhaps more striking still is how little reference was made to John as the crisis continued. He was asked neither to attend in person nor for any advice on treatment or management. By contrast, his son Thomas was to be paid a handsome sum for his attendance on George III in a subsequent bout of the royal malady during 1811–12.[245]

The royal physicians were plainly determined to maintain authority over the king's case (although preferably not at the expense of their reputations). Furthermore, when it was finally decided (significantly, by William Pitt the younger[246] and his government, rather than by the royal physicians themselves) that major outside intervention was called for, the preference was not for a consultation with a Bethlem physician, but rather for bringing in a country physician-clergyman, the Reverend Dr. Francis Willis—the proprietor of a private madhouse at Greatford, Lincolnshire.[247] Perhaps this reluctance to involve Monro reflected the continuing ambivalence of some in the highest medical and governmental circles toward those occupying office at Bethlem. However, another scenario (advanced at the time by Sir Gilbert Elliot and other sources close to the Prince of Wales and hostile to the prime minister) seems more likely: that Willis's intervention was sought by Pitt in the hope of locating a more cooperative medical man and a diagnosis more to his liking. As "the other physicians" were not "sufficiently subservient," the opposition alleged that summoning a provincial mountebank was Pitt's only way of maintaining the illusion of an expected recovery.[248]

In discussing Willis's credentials to treat the king, historians have stressed the remarkable nature of his summons "from the depths of the Lincolnshire countryside."[249] It should be remembered, however, that

Willis was famous in the city, as well as the country, and held an appointment as visiting physician to Thomas Warburton's Whitmore House asylum in Hoxton, on a salary of £200 per annum.[250] It was from this madhouse that keepers were sent to assist in attending George III, and the self-made and rough-hewn Warburton himself had also initially ministered to the king (much to the latter's distaste, George finding Warburton's long nose and other presentational incongruities fearsome and repellent).[251]

If Monro was a significant absence from the king's side during the 1788–89 breakdown, this was partly explained by the simple fact that he was old and in failing health. His shadow, nonetheless, still flitted across the palace walls. Once in the driving seat, Willis was quick to claim legitimacy and endorsement for his harsh and controlling methods toward the king by reference to Monro's own practice. Clearly he saw this as one way to stave off questions and criticisms he was facing from the royal physicians, and from people in the Commons and the royal household like Elliot and Greville, who felt that "Willis has done all sorts of mountebank things."[252] Emphasizing the influence professional men might exert over the mad, Willis related the ease with which he had managed some patients he had received "from Doctor Monro," who "fell into his proceedings immediately, having been already 'broke in, as Horses in a menage,' as his expression was."[253]

Monro had professed himself averse to the use of fear and intimidation toward the insane in his *Remarks,* and Greville, who plainly disapproved of the low-bred Willis, may have exaggerated what he felt to be rather barbarous methods to use on a sovereign of the realm. Yet this animal-taming approach was legitimated to a considerable extent by a long tradition of mad-doctoring and by recommendations in contemporary medical treatises as to the importance of breaking the will of the stubborn maniac.[254] On still another front, Willis also claimed the backing of Monro when it came to the isolation of George III from the queen and other visitors. According to Greville, after complaining about the disturbing effect that "new faces" had on the king, Willis flatly refused to admit any more visitors, rhetorically appealing to Monro as follows: "'Ask Doctor Monro, or any one,' said the Doctor, 'if they would allow any to go to a Patient, but those under whose immediate care they were.' 'No,' continued he, 'they would not admit another soul.'"[255]

Unwilling to provide a firm endorsement of the methods of the mad-doctor who was supplanting them, when the royal physicians were questioned about the king's illness earlier in the same month (January 1789),

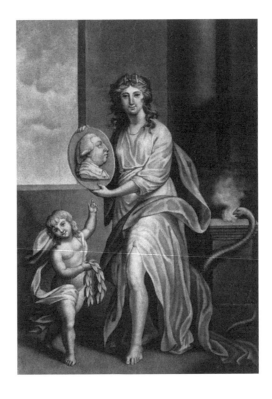

FIGURE 49. "The triumph of Hygiea. From a transparency of the happy recovery of the KING, March the 10th 1789, exhibited at Lord Howard de Walden's," a mezzotint published in London in 1789, probably by James Parker (1750–1805). The goddess of health, Hygiea, holds a relief of King George III, in celebration of his recovery from madness. George suffered bilious attacks in 1788, to which were added growing mental problems. On 19 February 1789, the chancellor announced his convalescence, but only on 10 March (the date cited on this print as the date of his recovery) did he resume his authority. This description is derived from the *Dictionary of National Biography* and the Wellcome Institute for the History of Medicine Library Iconographic Collection (Videodisc Frame No. 7928). Reproduced by kind permission of The Wellcome Trust, London.

they had similarly cited Monro. Asked, for example, whether it was "usual" for a specialist "to be consulted" as to who and when a patient was to be visited and attended by, Sir Lucas Pepys described the typical attendance with Dr. Monro as follows: ". . . he and I consult and settle the Time of Attendance—the Apothecary goes in without his Leave—and there is a certain Attendant or Two always with the Patient." [256]

By the time the king had recovered sufficiently to resume his office, Monro's health had deteriorated. It had actually begun to fail early in the 1780s. Somewhat ironically, like a number of his own patients, Monro had been struck down with a paralytic stroke in January 1783. A year later he was still, as he wrote to the Bethlem treasurer Richard Clarke, "much out of Order and . . . not yet quite well recovered," and on his request his son Thomas was allowed to substitute in his stead, "till my health shall be more perfectly reestablished": a "kindness" for which Monro expressed his deep gratitude to the Bethlem committee.[257]

Subsequently, John recovered sufficiently to continue to practice. However, the improvement was only temporary. Becoming increasingly frail and ill in ensuing years, he gradually delegated his Bethlem duties to Thomas, who was officially appointed as his assistant in 1787 "by the unanimous consent of a full general court."[258] Thus, just as *his* father had before him, John secured the succession of the Bethlem physicianship to his own heir—though the formal transfer of full authority did not occur until John's death four years later.

Having gradually retired from city life and from the active pursuit of his profession after 1787, Monro died at Hadley, Barnet, on 27 December 1791,[259] at the age of 77. He was buried in Aldenham Churchyard, Hertfordshire.

During his lifetime, Monro was the source of occasional benefactions to Bethlem and Bridewell through his friends and associates, as in 1778 when he received £50 from Isaac Hawkins Brown of Bloomsbury "for the use of Bethlehem Hospital."[260] Somewhat surprisingly, however, although he had given the standard donation on becoming a governor, Monro left nothing himself in his will to the hospitals.[261] Instead, his not inconsiderable wealth was dispersed among his three surviving sons, Charles, Thomas, and James, and his widow, Elizabeth.[262]

Monro had originally planned to pass on the family business and practice to his oldest son, John (1754–79), but the latter's premature death frustrated this scheme. Trying to secure his children's future some years earlier, in 1785, he had obtained the nomination and appointment of his two middle sons, Charles (who had studied law at Oriel College, Oxford) and Thomas (who had also initially embarked on a legal career), as governors at Bethlem and Bridewell. Replacing his oldest brother, Thomas then switched to medicine and gained his M.B.[263] By default, it would seem, as the only medically qualified child, it was Thomas who became John's choice as his successor.

Although all his private madhouse business and his considerable

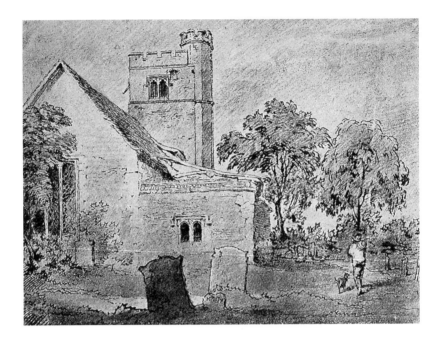

property were bequeathed to his three surviving sons, the profits of the business were split unevenly, 50 percent going to Thomas in recognition of his labors and the remaining 50 percent split between Charles and James. Out of the profits, they were also to provide the not inconsiderable annual allowance of £500 for the support of their mother, with the bulk of this money reverting to Thomas on his mother's death. When we add to this large and thriving business and its associated properties the large cash legacies that Monro also provided—£2,500 to his wife (who continued to live with her son James until her death in 1808), £3,000 to Charles on his marriage, another £3,000 for Thomas on his marriage, and £2,000 for James on top of the £2,000 his father had already given him "for his advancement"—we can begin to see just how extraordinarily lucrative the eighteenth-century mad-business proved to be for the man who was perhaps its preeminent practitioner.

Notes

PREFACE

1. "Mad-doctor" was the term commonly employed by eighteenth-century contemporaries to designate those medical practitioners who specialized in treating the mad. Embedded within the term, of course, is the sly parodying suggestion that their profession was a "mad" one.

2. See Jonathan Andrews and Andrew Scull, *Customers and Patrons of the Mad-Trade: The Management of Lunacy in Eighteenth-Century London* (Berkeley: University of California Press, 2002).

3. For a more extended discussion of this point, see Andrew Scull, Charlotte MacKenzie, and Nicholas Hervey, *Masters of Bedlam: The Transformation of the Mad-Doctoring Trade* (Princeton: Princeton University Press, 1996), chap. 1.

4. Just as we have drawn upon a wide range of visual material to enrich our discussion, so too we begin each chapter with a series of epigraphs drawn from a variety of contemporary sources. These should be read with care, for in kaleidoscopic fashion they reveal and refract the multiple meanings of madness in eighteenth-century English culture. (We are grateful to Laura Harger and Sue Carter for suggesting that we make this aspect of our analysis explicit.)

5. William Ll. Parry-Jones, *The Trade in Lunacy: A Study of Private Madhouses in England in the Eighteenth and Nineteenth Centuries* (London: Routledge and Kegan Paul, 1972).

6. William Belcher, *Address to Humanity* . . . (London: Sold by Allen and West and by the author, 1796); *Voices of Madness: Four Pamphlets, 1683–1796,* ed. Allan Ingram (Thrupp and Stroud, Gloucestershire: Sutton, 1997), title page and pp. 130, 132, 134, 135.

7. James Boswell, *Life of Johnson* (1791), ed. R. W. Chapman (Oxford and New York: Oxford University Press, 1985), pp. 1225–56.

8. See Sir Thomas Browne, *Religio Medici, Hydriotaphia, and the Letter to a Friend [Upon Occasion of the Death of his Intimate Friend],* ed. J. W. Willis (1643; Bund and New York: Scribner, Welford, and Co., 1869), pp. 178–89:

> In this deliberate and creeping progress unto the grave, he was somewhat too young and of too noble a mind, to fall upon that stupid symptom observable in divers persons near their journey's end, and which may be reckoned among the mortal symptoms of their last disease; that is, to become more narrow-minded, miserable, and tenacious,

unready to part with anything, when they are ready to part with all, and afraid to want when they have no time to spend; meanwhile physicians, who know that many are mad but in a single depraved imagination, and one prevalent decipiency [i.e., deficiency]; and that beside and out of such single deliriums a man may meet with sober actions and good sense in bedlam; cannot but smile to see the heirs and concerned relations gratulating [*sic*] themselves on the sober departure of their friends; and though they behold such mad covetous passages, content to think they die in good understanding, and in their sober senses.

9. See Thomas Greenhill's (1681–1740?) *Nekpokydeia: Or, the Art of Embalming; Wherein is Shewn the Right of Burial, the Funeral Ceremonies, and the Several Ways of Preserving Dead Bodies in most Nations of the World* . . . (London: The author, 1705).

10. Norbert Elias, *The Civilizing Process.* Trans. Edmund Jephcott from *Über den Prozess der Zivilisation* (Oxford: Blackwell, 1994).

CHAPTER 1

1. Alexander Cruden, *The Adventures of Alexander the Corrector, with an Account of the Chelsea Academies, or the Private Places for the Confinement of Such as Are Supposed to Be Deprived of the Exercise of their Reason* (London: For the author, 1754), part 2, pp. 29–30.

2. Quoted in Thomas Monro's essay "Vicious and Foolish People Considered Insane," *Essays on Various Subjects* (London: Printed by J. Nichols & Sold by G. G. J. J. Robinson, 1790), p. 69. This is Thomas Monro (1764–1815) of Magdalen College, Oxford, who also published an edition of the Sophist Alciphron's *Epistles,* and not John Monro's son Thomas (1759–1833), who attended Oriel College, Oxford.

3. This document is currently in possession of the Jefferiss family, distant relatives of the Monros.

4. Although seeming destined at one point to become the Bishop of Argyll, Alexander refused to take the oath of allegiance to William and Mary. For basic biographical information on the Monros, see *Dictionary of National Biography (DNB);* William Munk, *Roll of the Royal College of Physicians of London,* vol. 2 (London: Royal College of Physicians, 1878), pp. 113–15, 183–85, 414–15; Evelyn Dorothea Monro, "Five Physicians of the Fyrish Family," *Clan Munro Magazine* 3 (1951), pp. 27–31; Denis Leigh, *The Historical Development of British Psychiatry* (Oxford: Pergamon, 1961), pp. 51–56; Cecil S. Emden, *Oriel Papers* (Oxford: Clarendon Press, 1948), pp. 158–60; *Gentleman's Magazine* (henceforth *GM*); Joseph Foster, *Alumni Oxonienses: The Members of the University of Oxford, 1715–1886,* 4 vols. (Oxford and London: Parker, 1887–78; Nendeln, Lichtenstein: Kraus Reprint, 1968).

5. Alexander Cruden, *Mr Cruden Greatly Injured* (London: Printed for A. Injured [i.e., the author], 1739), p. 24; Cruden, *Adventures,* part 1, p. 25.

6. W. S. Lewis, *Horace Walpole's Correspondence* (New Haven: Yale University Press and London: Oxford University Press, 1937–83), vol. 19, Horace Mann to HW, 4 Jan. 1746, p. 191, and notes 3–7. Monro's companions were his fellow Oxonians Rowland Holt (ca. 1723–86), M. A. Oxon., 1745, who became MP for Suffolk 1759–68 and 1771–80, and Richard Phelps (ca. 1720–

71), B. A. Oxon., 1744, whose political career reached its summit with the appointment as undersecretary of state (northern department), 1763–71.

7. Ibid., Mann to HW, 16 Jan. 1746, p. 196.

8. Ibid., Mann to HW, 16 May 1747, p. 400.

9. For this appointment, see, e.g., ibid., p. 191, note 6; *GM* 11 (1741), p. 278; *Daily Advertiser* (8 July 1741); Munk, *Roll,* vol. 2, p. 183.

10. See Linda Colley, *In Defiance of Oligarchy: The Tory Party, 1714–60* (Cambridge: Cambridge University Press, 1982); Colley, *Britons: Forging the Nation, 1707–1837* (Pimlico, 1994; London: Vintage, 1996).

11. C. Webster, "The Medical Faculty and the Physic Garden," *The History of the University of Oxford,* vol. 5, *The Eighteenth Century,* ed. L. S. Sutherland and L. G. Mitchell (Oxford: Clarendon, 1986), 683–723, quote on p. 701. For more background on these traveling fellowships, see also Ivor Forbes Guest, *Dr. John Radcliffe and His Trust* (London: The Radcliffe Trust, 1991).

12. Lewis, *Correspondence,* vol. 19, HW to Mann, 7 Feb. 1746, p. 210.

13. Ibid., vol. 30, HW to Lincoln, 13 Oct. 1741, p. 30 and notes 15–18. Sir Edward Hulse (1682–1759), M.D. 1717, was physician to George II.

14. Lewis, *Correspondence,* vol. 33, HW to Lady Ossory, 17 Dec. 1780, p. 254.

15. C. H. Iyan Chown, "The Lethieullier Family of Aldersbrook House," *Essex Review* 26 (1927), p. 10.

16. Lewis, *Correspondence,* vol. 37, Conway to HW, 14 July 1751, p. 309 and note 16.

17. Munk, *Roll,* vol. 2, p. 184.

18. John Monro's nominations as governors, once he himself became Bethlem physician and governor, included Sergeant Leigh, a solicitor in Lincoln's Inn Fields, and Dr. Richard Warren (who was later to treat George III's madness; see chapter 6 of this volume). William Battie, meanwhile, successfully nominated Dr. John Lewis Petit (who had served as censor with Monro in 1768–69), among others. See Bethlem Court of Governors Minutes (henceforth BCGM), 27 April 1769, 21 Nov. and 12 Dec. 1776, pp. 254–55, 533, 539.

19. John Monro, *Harveian Oration* (1757), or "The Annual Lecture from Harvey's Foundation," translated version held in Royal College of Physicians Library, pp. 1–2.

20. Ibid., pp. 4–5. John Radcliffe (1650–1714) was a famous English physician, Oxford benefactor, and founder of Oxford's infirmary.

21. Ibid., pp. 5–6.

22. BCGM, 21 June 1751, p. 15.

23. *London Evening Post* (henceforth *LEP*), no. 3708 (23–25 July 1751).

24. *Read's Weekly Journal or British-Gazetteer,* no. 1428 (11 Jan. 1752); A. Z., *An Address to the College of Physicians, and to the Universities of Oxford and Cambridge; Occasion'd by the late Swarms of Scotch and Leyden Physicians, &c. . . . to which is Added, a Compleat List of all the Regular Physicians. By an Impartial Hand* (London: Printed for M. Cooper, 1747); Derek A. Dow, *The Influence of Scottish Medicine: An Historical Assessment of Its International Impact* (Carnforth, Lancashire, England: Parthenon, 1988).

25. *Annals/Registers of the College of Physicians,* in the Royal College of Physicians Library, London, 3 April and 25 June 1752, vol. 11, fols. 139, 141, 143, 145, and 25 June 1753, vol. 12, fol. 6; John Monro, *Oratio anniversaria ex Harveii instituto, habita 1757* (London: 1758).

26. Munk's *Roll,* vol. 2, p. 183, wrongly claims that Monro was also censor in 1785, but in fact this was Donald Monro; see *Annals/Registers of the College of Physicians,* 16 Sept. 1785, vol. 15, fol. 82. Monro was regularly chosen censor under the presidencies of Drs. Thomas Reeve and Thomas Lawrence, and became the senior censor in 1772. Monro's stablemates as censors were Drs. James Hawley, Charles Feake, and Thomas Wilbraham (1754); Drs. Thomas Lawrence, William Pitcairn, and William Cadogan (1759); Drs. Richard Brocklesby, Richard Tyson (great nephew to Edward Tyson, a former Bethlem Physician), and Edward Barry (1763); Thomas Gisborne, Richard Tyson, and John Lewis Petit (1768); Thomas Brooke, Richard Jebb (with whom he attended Lord Orford; see chapter 4), and Donald Monro (1772); and, finally, Isaac Schomberg, Henry Revell Reynolds, and John Rawlinson (1778). See *Annals/Registers of the College of Physicians,* vol. 12, fols. 22, 83; vol. 8, fol. 100; vol. 14, fols. 11, 21, 103. John Monro never, however, served as censor in company with Battie, nor was he ever chosen as censor during Battie's presidency, although the rival maddoctors certainly attended many ordinary committees of the College together.

27. Battie was president in 1764–65, Harveian Orator in 1746, and Lumleian (or Surgery) Lecturer in 1749–54; he was also censor during 1747–48, 1749–50, 1758–59, and 1760–61, and *Consilarii* in 1760–61. Munk claimed that he was also elected censor in 1763 (when Monro was also serving in this capacity), but this appears to have been another error. Monro took over from Battie as elect on the latter's resignation in December 1771. Battie was celebrated in the College for his "powerful influence upon their debates and councils" and as "a most admirable speaker, close, pointed, and impressive." See *Annals/Registers of the College of Physicians,* vol. 11, fols. 20, 32, 61–63; vol. 12, fols. 97, 148; Munk, *Roll,* vol. 2, p. 141; John Nichols, *Literary Anecdotes of the Eighteenth Century,* vol. 8 (London: Nichols, Son, and Bentley, 1812–15), pp. 552–53.

28. Among the previous residents in this house was the Reverend John Cowper, father of the poet William Cowper (1731–1800), who famously suffered a mental breakdown and spent eighteen months, during 1763–65, in Nathaniel Cotton's private madhouse in St. Albans. Cowper seems to have inherited the house (No. 7) from his father, who was an occupant from 1750–56, owning it jointly along with his brother, and renting it out subsequently. See *The Letters and Prose Writings of William Cowper,* ed. James King and Charles Ryskamp, vol. 1 (Oxford: Clarendon Press, 1979), p. 86, notes 1 and 2.

29. See poor rate book for 1769 in Holborn Public Library, High Holborn. The poor rate was a contemporary tax upon those with property worth 40s. or more, the proceeds of which went toward parochial relief of the poor.

30. In 1780, when there was a fire in the Barnet district, Monro and his family were caught in a friend's house between two others that were on fire, and forced to flee to a Mrs. Smith's at Hadley. See *The Autobiography and Correspondence of Mary Granville, Mrs Delaney: With Interesting Reminiscences of*

King George the Third and Queen Charlotte, ed. Lady Llanover (London: Richard Bentley, 1862), vol. 2, letter from Mrs. Boscawen, 10 June 1780, p. 535.

31. Monro harbored the dispensary at his home for seventeen months, from 24 April 1769 to the end of September 1770, hosting the meetings of its committee of physicians there, until the dispensary was transferred to East Street. See William Joseph Marie Alois Maloney, *George and John Armstrong of Castleton: Two Eighteenth-Century Medical Pioneers* (Edinburgh and London: V. E. & S. Livingstone, 1954).

32. See, e.g., George and John Armstrong, *Proposals for Administering Advice and Medicines to the Children of the Poor* (London: s.n., 1769); T. E. C., Jr, *On Why a Hospital for Sick Children Would be Impracticable, According to Dr George Armstrong, Founder of the First Dispensary for the Infant Poor in England 1772* (London: s.n., 1785); John Armstrong, *The Poetical Works of J. Armstrong, M.D. With the Life of the Author* (London: Printed for C. Cooke, 1796); George Armstrong, *An Essay on the Diseases Most Fatal to Infants. To Which are Added Rules to be Observed in the Nursing of Children: with a Particular View to those who are Brought up by Hand . . .* (London: T. Cadell, 1767); H. Bloch, "George Armstrong (1719–1787), Founder of the First Dispensary for Children," *American Journal of Diseases of the Child* 143 (1989), pp. 239–41.

33. See Maloney, *George and John Armstrong of Castleton;* Maloney, *John and George Armstrong at Edinburgh* (Edinburgh: Printed by Oliver and Boyd, 1950); William B. Ober, "John Armstrong, M.D. (1709–1779): A Scot in London," reprinted from *New York State Journal of Medicine* 65.21 (1 Nov. 1965), pp. 2711–17; F. N. L. Poynter, *A Unique Copy of George Armstrong's Printed Proposals for Establishing the Dispensary for Sick Children* (London: 1769; Norwich: Jarrold, 1957), reprinted from *Medical History* 1.1 (1957), pp. 65–66.

34. Bronwyn Croxson, "The Public and Private Faces of Eighteenth-Century London Dispensary Charity," *Medical History* 41 (1997), pp. 127–49; Irvine S. L. Loudon, "The Origins and Growth of the Dispensary Movement in England," *Bulletin of the History of Medicine* 55 (1981), pp. 322–42.

35. Some of these dispensaries were set up through the auspices of practitioners and others with nonconformist and antiestablishment leanings. For example, John Coakley Lettsom, a Quaker and a critic of the metropolitan medical establishment, was a founder of the Aldersgate Street Dispensary in 1770. See Lindsay Granshaw, "'Fame and Fortune by Means of Bricks and Mortar': The Medical Profession and Specialist Hospitals in Britain, 1800–1948," *The Hospital in History*, ed. Lindsay Granshaw and Roy Porter (London and New York: Routledge, 1990), p. 201.

36. See *St James' Gazette* (20–21 April 1769), p. 3, col. 3, (25–27 April 1769), p. 2, col. 2, (9–12 Sept. 1769), p. 2, col. 13; *The Public Advertiser* (11–13 Oct. 1769), p. 1, col. 3.

37. John Armstrong himself was a poet of some note and his much reprinted *The Art of Preserving Health* (1744) was republished again in 1795, together with Akenside's work, while in the same year it was critically assessed by Aikin. See Mark Akenside and John Armstrong, *The Pleasures of Imagination; A Poem, in Three Books. To Which is Added, The Art of Preserving Health; A Poem, in*

Three Books (New York: Printed by Wayland & Davis, for L. Wayland, 1795); John Armstrong, *The Art of Preserving Health; A Poem, in Three Books . . . To Which is Prefixed a Critical Essay on the Poem by J. Aikin. M.D.* (London: T. Cadell, Jr. and W. Davies, 1795); Lewis M. Knapp, ed., *The Letters of Tobias Smollett* (Oxford: Clarendon Press, 1970); Knapp, *Dr. John Armstrong, Litterateur, and Associate of Smollett, Thomson, Wilkes, and Other Celebrities* (Colorado: s.n., 1944), pp. 1019–58, reprinted article.

38. Bethlem Grand Committee Minutes, 9 Oct. 1728. His opponents included four well-connected and well-established physicians: Richard Tyson (1680–1750); Charles Bale (d. 1730), F.R.C.P., F.R.S.; William Ruty, F.R.S. (1687–1730); and Sir Richard Manningham (1690–1759), F.R.S.

39. On the establishment of a general pattern of endogamy in the recruitment to eighteenth-century professions, see Geoffrey Holmes, *Augustan England: Professions, State, and Society* (London: Allen and Unwin, 1982).

40. E.g., Brislington House and the Fox family, and Ticehurst House and the Newington family.

41. Alexander Pope, *The Dunciad, Variorum: With the Prolegomena of Scriblerus* (London: Printed for A. Dob, 1729).

42. Alexander Pope, *Imitations of Horace, Second Epistle of the Second Book of Horace,* in *The Works of Alexander Pope,* ed. Whitwell Elwin and William John Courthope (London: John Murray, 1871–89), vol. 2, pp. 70–71, p. 169; vol. 3, p. 382. See also Lewis, *Correspondence,* vol. 18, HW to Mann, 4 May 1743, pp. 224–25 and note 8.

43. John Monro's address was given as St. Paul's Churchyard at this time. He was elected as a governor just a year after his father had been given the same honor, and made the standard benefaction of £100; BCGM, 15 and 27 May and 15 July 1747, pp. 323, 325, 330. Rawlinson's antiquarian and topographical interests may well have influenced John's own developing preoccupations.

44. John's official appointment as sole physician, although mentioned in the press, is not recorded in the Bridewell and Bethlem Court of Governors Minutes. Thus we cannot be sure whether there was a contested election, although it seems that, apart from the motions to elect another joint physician (discussed in the next paragraph), John succeeded his father without challenge. The question of his salary was settled on 19 Jan. 1753 (BCGM, p. 97). James's assets were bequeathed in two equal shares at his death, one to his wife, and the other divided equally between his two sons and unmarried daughter. He had already provided for his married daughters and their family members, but apologized in his terse will for the guinea he bequeathed to each of them, "because I do not Expect to dye in Circumstances able to do more." See will of James Monro, PRO Prob 11/798, q.n. 302, fols. 250–51.

45. The proposer—whose name was unrecorded—presumably had John in mind.

46. BCGM, 21 June 1751 and 24 Nov. 1752, pp. 9, 91.

47. *LEP,* nos. 3694, 3706, and 3708, 20–22 June, 18–20 and 23–25 July 1753.

48. The motion of 1752 for a joint physician was resoundingly defeated, by seventy votes to twenty-seven, the first in 1751 having succeeded by sixty-nine

votes to thirty-eight. No poll was considered necessary in the even more re-sounding defeat of the second motion of 1751 for a third joint physician.

49. Previously, as the *London Evening Post* commented, the apothecary's duties "to prepare the Medicines . . . [and] to attend the Patients in both [hos-pitals had] . . . for many years past . . . been much neglected." (See *LEP,* nos. 3596, 3614, 3633, 3639, 3643, 3650, 3658, 3660, 3682, which cover af-fairs at Bethlem and Bridewell concerning the apothecary and his shop over the entire period 6 Nov. 1750 to 23 May 1751.) The proposal to make the apothe-cary resident, first considered by the grand committee of twenty governors on which both Monros sat, was initially rejected, but this decision seems ultimately to have been rescinded, the apothecary being required "to reside" in the shop. Nevertheless, those apothecaries who sued for the post evidently preferred ways of avoiding residence, offering "Constant Attendance," or attendance through a journeyman/servant instead. While the governors were prepared to allow the apothecary to attend on occasion via "his servant," ultimately they permitted the man they did elect, Thomas Winder, to keep a "labourer," rather than a full-fledged "Representative or Assistant," as they were advised to do by the *Lon-don Evening Post.* See Bethlem Grand Committee Minutes (henceforth BGCM), 5 Dec. 1750, in Bethlem Sub-committee Minutes (henceforth BSCM), p. 211; BGCM, 14 Dec. 1750, in BCGM, 19 Dec. 1750, p. 476; Jonathan Andrews, "Bedlam Revisited. A History of Bethlem Hospital c1633–c1770," Ph.D. diss., University of London, 1991, p. 272, note 112.

50. BCGM, 16 May 1750, p. 446.

51. Although the apothecary was the only medical officer with an apartment at Bethlem, he had evidently gone out of the hospital to eat and was only now granted "the provision of the House" (as enjoyed by the other resident members of the inferior staff); BCGM, 22 Dec. 1768 and 9 March 1769, pp. 236, 251.

52. BGCM, 17 Jan. 1751, in BSCM, p. 219; BCGM, 25 June 1772, p. 349.

53. The committee was comprised of ten governors, who (besides Monro and the other medical officers) included William Battie. The apothecary's post was for the first time restricted to an unmarried man who was to be permitted a single female servant. Apart from his Bridewell duties, he was to attend Beth-lem every morning at the very least and "Report to the Physician any Neglect he may observe in the Management of the Patients." He was to attend and see to the proper administration of all vomits and purges, and order medicines for the shop every week through the committee. Finally, he was to "have the manage-ment of the Patients during the Absence of the Physician." This last order seems especially significant given the criticisms that were subsequently to be leveled upon the Bethlem physician's head in 1815. See BCGM, 17 Jan. 1751 (in BSCM, p. 219); BCGM, 22 Dec. 1768 and 9 March 1769, pp. 236, 251; BCGM, 25 June 1772, p. 349; BCGM, 27 Jan. 1786, p. 225.

54. This situation was further reflected in the apothecary's salary, which was raised from £80 to £100 in 1786 on the recommendation of a Bethlem Committee on which Monro (along with his son Thomas) also sat. See BCGM, 27 Jan. 1786, p. 225.

55. BCGM, 16 May, 1 Nov., 19 Dec. 1750, 1 Feb., 4 April, 22 May 1751, pp. 446, 467, 476, 480–81, 493, 6; BGCM, 5 and 14 Dec. 1750, 17 Jan.,

7 June 1751, in BSCM, pp. 211, 213, 219, 243. For more on the apothecary at Bethlem, see Andrews, "Bedlam Revisited," pp. 271–73.

56. The surgeon's own role was partially altered at this time, the Court of Governors moving further away from the contractual model by which medical attendance had been formerly provided and, in the process, relieving the expenses of patients' families for surgery. Thus, in 1761, the surgeon was forbidden to claim individually from patients and their friends for each wound he treated on patients' admissions, and in compensation his salary was increased by £10 per annum. Monro was not present at the court that decided this. See BCGM, 28 Oct. 1761, p. 387.

57. Cruden, *Mr Cruden Greatly Injured*, p. 27.

58. BCGM, 27 Jan. 1763, p. 46.

59. Ibid., 11 May 1763, p. 52. In this instance, Dr. Smith seems to have been unable or unwilling to come up with the certificate of settlement and sureties required for her admission, and she was ordered discharged back to her place of abode; BSCM, 4 June 1763.

60. On average, for example, there were six governors present at subcommittee meetings during 1733–35 in James Monro's time, and five at subcommittee meetings during 1753–55 in John Monro's time. See Bethlem Committee and Sub-Committee Minutes for these years.

61. On the general significance of hospital appointments for the development of medical careers in this era, see William F. Bynum, "Physicians, Hospitals, and Career Structures in Eighteenth Century London," *William Hunter and the Eighteenth Century Medical World,* ed. William F. Bynum and Roy Porter (Cambridge: Cambridge University Press, 1985), pp. 105–28. See also Jonathan Andrews, "A Respectable Mad-Doctor: Richard Hale, F.R.S. (1670–1728)," *Notes and Records of the Royal Society of London* 44 (1990), pp. 169–203.

62. For the details, see the publication by an anonymous Doctors' Commons lawyer, *Trials for Adultery: Or, the History of Divorces. Being Select Trials at Doctors Commons, for Adultery, Fornication, Cruelty, Impotence, &c. From the Year 1760, to the Present Time. The Whole Forming a Complete History of the PRIVATE LIFE, INTRIGUES, and AMOURS of many Characters in the Most Elevated Sphere. TAKEN IN SHORT-HAND, by a CIVILIAN,* vol. 2 (London: Printed for S. Bladon, 1779), pp. 2–3, case 3, *Thomas Brookes M.D. v Harriot* [sic] *Brooke,* libel given 23 May 1767.

63. See Malcolm Nicolson, "The Art of Diagnosis: Medicine and the Five Senses," *Companion Encyclopedia of the History of Medicine,* ed. William F. Bynum and Roy Porter, vol. 2 (London: Routledge, 1993), pp. 806–810; Roy Porter, "The Rise of Physical Examination," *Medicine and the Five Senses,* ed. William F. Bynum and Roy Porter (Cambridge and New York: Cambridge University Press, 1993), pp. 179–97.

64. Anthony Trollope's (or rather Sir Lionel Bertram's) definition of a profession: see *The Bertrams,* vol. 1 (London: Chapman and Hall, 1859), p. 154.

65. For the persisting importance of "gentlemanly" attributes among elite practitioners, see Christopher Lawrence, "Incommunicable Knowledge: Science, Technology, and the Clinical Art in Britain, 1850–1914," *Journal of Contemporary History* 20 (1985), pp. 502–20. On the general significance of gen-

tlemanly personal identity in the solution of problems of credibility and authority in early modern Britain, see Steven Shapin, *A Social History of Truth: Civility and Science in Seventeenth-Century England* (Chicago: University of Chicago Press, 1994).

66. Such carping extended even into the nineteenth century. See Malcolm Nicolson, "The Introduction of Percussion and Stethoscopy to Early Nineteenth Century Edinburgh," *Medicine and the Five Senses,* ed. William F. Bynum and Roy Porter (Cambridge: Cambridge University Press, 1993).

67. *The World* 23 (1753), p. 138.

68. On Bethlem's patients as "curiosities," see *GM* 18 (May 1748), p. 199. From Pepys to Boswell, diarists record visits to Bethlem, often with family, friends from out of town, and children in tow, in search of "extraordinary" or "remarkable" spectacles.

69. For a famous example of these floods of crocodile tears, see the visit of Henry Mackenzie's "man of feeling" to Bedlam (*Man of Feeling*, ed. Brian Vickers [London: Cadell, 1771; London and New York: Oxford University Press, 1967], pp. 73–74):

> . . . their conductor led them first to the dismal mansions of those who are in the most horrid state of incurable madness. The clanking of chains, the wildness of their cries, and the imprecations which some of them uttered, formed a scene inexpressibly shocking. Harley and his companions, especially the female part of them, begged their guide to return: he seemed surprised at their uneasiness and was with difficulty prevailed on to leave that part of the house without showing them some others, who as he expressed it in the phrase of those who keep wild beasts for show, were much better worth seeing than any they had passed, being ten times more fierce and unmanageable.

70. Samuel Richardson, *Familiar Letters on Important Occasions*, ed. Brian W. Downs (London: 1741; London: Routledge, 1928), letter 153, pp. 200–02, and letter 160, pp. 217–20.

71. Mackenzie, *The Man of Feeling*, chap. 20, p. 30.

72. Michel Foucault, *Madness and Civilisation: A History of Insanity in the Age of Reason* (London: Tavistock, 1971), trans. and abr. from *Histoire de la Folie à l'âge classique* (Paris: Librairie Plon, 1961), p. 70.

73. BCGM, 21 Nov. 1770, pp. 316–17.

74. See John Monro, *Remarks on Dr Battie's Treatise on Madness* (London: Clarke, 1758), p. 39, and chapter 2 of this volume.

75. Making a sharp distinction between public/hospital and private attendance was but one of many of his father's practices that Thomas Monro was to adopt when he succeeded to the Bethlem physicianship and control of the family's private mad-business, with ultimately disastrous consequences for his reputation and career. Testifying before the 1815 Select Committee on Madhouses, for example, Thomas Monro acknowledged that the routine evacuations he ordered for Bethlem's inmates were of little use in their cure, and offered in his defense that this "has been the practice invariably for years, long before my time; it was handed down to me by my father, and I do not know any better practice." Asked "Would you treat a private individual patient in your own house in the same way as has been described in respect of Bethlem?" he responded truculently, "No, certainly not. In Bethlem, the restraint is by chains, there is no such

thing as chains in my house. They are fit only for pauper lunatics; if a gentleman was put in irons, he would not like it." Testimony of this sort infuriated the lunacy reformers in Parliament, and within a year their pressure on the governors forced Monro from office. See House of Commons, *Report, together with the Minutes of Evidence . . . from the Committee Appointed to Consider of Provision Being Made for Better Regulation of Madhouses in England* (1815), first report, p. 95.

76. BCGM, 20 June 1765, pp. 132–37.

77. Ibid., pp. 135–36.

78. BCGM, 19 March 1766, 22 Dec. 1768, pp. 152, 236; BGCM, 12 Jan. and 22 March 1769, in BCGM, pp. 449–50; BGCM, 22 March 1766, in BSCM, p. 186; *Bethlem Committee Book* and BSCM, 21 April and 8 Dec. 1764, 6 April 1765, 30 Sept. 1769, 9 Dec. 1775, 16 Oct. 1779, 28 Oct. 1780, 17 Nov. 1781, 1 April 1786. It is worth noting, however, that records of attendance at such meetings were not always comprehensive guides to who was actually present.

79. BCGM, 22 Dec. 1768, 27 April 1769, pp. 236, 249–51.

80. BGCM, 27 Oct. 1769, in BCGM, 21 Nov. 1770, pp. 316–17. Interestingly, although John Monro was an absentee from the latter court meeting, which authorized the ticket system, William Battie was present, along with the surgeon, Richard Crowther, and the well-known London doctor William Pitcairn.

81. Thomas Bowen, *An Historical Account of the Origin, Progress and Present State of Bethlehem Hospital* (London: s.n., 1783), p. 11.

82. BSCM, 4 Feb. 1792, p. 54.

83. BCGM, 21 Oct. 1762, 20 June 1765, pp. 62, 133.

84. BCGM, 20 June 1765, p. 135.

85. Norris was an American seaman confined in Bethlem on 1 Feb. 1800. In 1812, an inspecting party led by the Quaker land agent Edward Wakefield came across him encased in a remarkable restraining apparatus:

> . . . a stout iron ring was riveted about his neck, from which a short chain passed to a ring made to slide upwards and downwards on an upright massive iron bar, more than six feet high, inserted into the wall. Round his body a strong iron bar about two inches wide was riveted; on each side of the bar was a circular projection, which being fashioned to and enclosing each of his arms, pinioned them close to his sides. This waist bar was secured by two similar iron bars which, passing over his shoulders, were riveted to the waist both before and behind. The iron ring about his neck was connected to the bars on his shoulders by a double link. From each of these bars another short chain passed to the ring on the upright bar. . . . He had remained thus encaged and chained more than twelve years.

See Edward Wakefield, "Plan for an Asylum for Lunatics," *The Philanthropist* 3 (1812), pp. 226–29. James Tilly Matthews was admitted to Bethlem three years earlier, on 28 January 1797, after he had made threats against the government. At various times, he exhibited a remarkable array of delusions and hallucinations. He nonetheless appears to have been a harmless and cooperative patient, and both he and his family vainly petitioned for his release during almost two decades of confinement. Matthews openly kept detailed notes of the scenes he observed and the events he was told about—records the Bethlem medical officers dismissed as the scribblings of a madman. However, when the Norris case spawned a scandal that led to the first major parliamentary investigation of the lunacy question in the nineteenth century, the 1815–16 Select Committee on Madhouses, Matthews's writings contributed to a detailed indictment of the Bethlem régime. For discussion of these cases, see Scull, Hervey, and MacKenzie, *Masters of Bedlam*, chap. 2; Roy Porter, introduction, *Illustrations of Madness*, by John Haslam, ed. Roy Porter (London: Rivington, 1810; London: Routledge, 1989).

86. Monro, *Remarks*, pp. 47, 52; William Battie, *Treatise on Madness*, ed. Richard Hunter and Ida Macalpine (London: Whiston and White, 1758; London: Dawsons, 1962), p. 94. The Scottish specialist on nervous disorders George Cheyne also denied the efficacy of blisters in nervous disorders; George Cheyne, *The English Malady . . .* (London: Printed for G. Strahan and J. Leake, 1733), p. 207.

87. Nehemiah Curnock, ed., *The Journal of the Reverend John Wesley* (London: Epworth Press, 1938), vol. 2, entry dated 17 Sept. 1740, pp. 385–86; Richard Hunter and Ida Macalpine, *Three Hundred Years of Psychiatry, 1535–1860: A History Presented in Selected English Texts* (Oxford and New York: Oxford University Press, 1963), pp. 422–23.

88. For an instance of this discrimination over treatment under Monro, see, e.g., the case of Jane Little; BCGM, 29 Nov. 1787, p. 287.

89. E.g., the women's basketman was instructed to "Assist the Gallery Maids in Bathing Bleeding Shaving and giving the Patients their Medicines." BCGM, 20 June 1765, 9 July 1772, pp. 137, 359. For references to cold baths and bathing at Bethlem, see, e.g., BSCM 18 Oct. 1777, 24 April 1790.

90. Monro, *Remarks*, p. 52.

91. Both Cheyne and Battie, however, expressed much deeper reservations about bleeding; Battie, *Treatise*, pp. 94, 96; Monro, *Remarks*, pp. 50, 52, 55, 57; Cheyne, *English Malady*, p. 207. For more on the Battie-Monro debate about therapies, see chapter 2.

92. Bryan Crowther, *Practical Remarks on Insanity; to Which is Added a Commentary on the Dissection of the Brains of Maniacs; with some Account of Diseases Incident to the Insane* (London, Edinburgh, and Dublin: Printed for Thomas Underwood, Adam Black, and Gilbert and Hodges, by G. Hayden, 1811), pp. 43–44. Setons were threads drawn through folds of skin to maintain an issue or opening for discharges.

93. Lord Wharncliffe, ed., *The Letters and Works of Lady Mary Wortley Montagu* (London: Standard Edition, 1893), Lady MWM to Countess of Bute, 20 Oct. 1755, pp. 289–90.

94. George Man Burrows, *An Inquiry into Certain Errors Relative to Insanity; and their Consequences; Physical, Moral, and Civil* (London: Printed for Thomas and George Underwood, 1820), p. 151.

95. See Bethlem Auditor's Accounts, e.g., for 1760–73.

96. See chapter 2.

97. BSCM, 15 Nov. 1766 (Monro's attendance on this committee is not recorded). The dark cell was probably employed earlier at Bethlem with the idea of correcting patients' false ideas by depriving them of visual sensations, and Wesley alleged that James Monro had employed confinement "to a dark room" in the case of Peter Shaw around 1736. Curnock, *The Journal of the Reverend*

John Wesley, vol. 2, entry dated 17 Sept. 1740, pp. 385–86; Hunter and Macalpine, *Three Hundred Years of Psychiatry,* pp. 422–23. Influenced by pervasive Enlightenment symbolism and penetrating scientific insights on optics, contemporary medical and lay writers seem to have been increasingly critical of the damaging effects of light deprivation on the mental faculties in this period. See, e.g., *LEP,* no. 6014 (15–17 May 1766), pp. 3–4, where commentary on the proposed alterations in window tax are met with the following attack on

> those who turn day into night, and choose darkness rather than light—surely it can never be the policy for a Protestant Free State to confine the bodies of their most useful members in darkness, which, in length of time, will have an effect upon their minds, and reconcile them to a religion as destructive to the interests of the Community, as the deprivation of light is to that of Individuals.

98. For John Haslam's conservatism on this front, see *Observations on Insanity* (London: Rivington, 1798), pp. 126–27:

> In the most violent state of the disease, the patient should be kept alone in a dark and quiet room, so that he may not be affected by the stimuli of light or sound, such abstraction more readily disposing to sleep. As in this violent state there is a strong propensity to associate ideas, it is particularly important to prevent the accession of such as might be transmitted through the medium of the senses.

99. BSCM, 17 July 1779.

100. See, e.g., BSCM, 5 Nov. 1757, 4 April 1761.

101. E.g., forty-two men and forty-seven women were granted leaves of absence during 1783–85; see Bethlem Auditor's Accounts, 1782–1810.

102. E.g., BSCM, 18 Jan. 1772.

103. The new rules established, for example, that patients should not be furnished with anything without the physician's wish, unless a "Special Necessity" existed, although previous and subsequent orders concerning abuses with provisions hint at the inveteracy of the corruption, peculation, and other abuses of inferior staff. BCGM, 20 June 1765, pp. 133, 135, 136; BGCM, 4 Sept. 1778, in BSCM.

104. BCGM, 20 June 1765, pp. 133, 137.

105. Ibid., pp. 135–36.

106. Ibid., p. 135.

107. BSCM, 13 March 1779.

108. Bethlem Steward's Accounts, 16–23 June 1764, 24–31 May 1766.

109. For further mention of strait waistcoats and their suppliers in Bethlem's records, see, e.g., BSCM, 25 Feb. 1786; BGCM, 18 Dec. 1793 and 29 Jan. 1794, pp. 20, 22; for mention of chains, see, e.g., BSCM, 13 March 1779, 15 Sept. 1785; Bethlem Steward's Accounts, 5–12 June 1773. See also Andrews, "Bedlam Revisited," pp. 204–18.

110. For references to Gozna's introduction of strait waistcoats, which he seems to have regarded as less likely to cause sores and wounds to patients, while permitting them greater freedom to walk about the hospital, see, e.g., Bethlem Steward's Accounts, 30 Jan.–6 Feb. and 27 March–3 April 1773; Marie Sophie von la Roche, *Sophie in London, 1786. Being the Diary of Sophie v. la Roche,* trans. and ed. Claire Williams (London: Jonathan Cape, 1933), pp. 167–68.

Bethlem seems to have gone back to chains under Haslam, who contended that chains were less restricting and more humane.

111. BCGM, 8 Aug. 1753, p. 120; BGCM 24 Aug. 1753, in BSCM, p. 366; BSCM, 11 Oct. 1753, p. 375.

112. BCGM, 20 June 1765, p. 135.

113. Ibid., pp. 133, 135; BSCM, 23 Jan. 1779.

114. BSCM, 30 May 1778, 5 June 1779, and 28 Oct. 1780.

115. BSCM, 19 Sept. 1778.

116. BSCM, 21 Dec. 1771.

117. E.g., BCGM, 20 June 1765, pp. 133–34, 136, 137; BSCM, 24 April 1790.

118. On the other hand, a few physicians in this period were gradually recognizing the value of hands-on dissection for the investigation of what the mad-doctor divine William Pargeter referred to as "the *Pathology of Mania.*" Samuel Foart Simmons (1750–1813), physician to St. Luke's 1781–1811 and later physician to George III, appears to have conducted numerous post mortems on his insane hospital patients, while even private physicians were finding a few rare opportunities to dabble in dissection. Pargeter himself had investigated the state of the brain in three of his own maniacal cases by 1792. Significantly, however, neither doctor published his findings on the subject in any detail, and Pargeter emphasized the "uncertainty" as to whether the post mortem appearances were causes or effects. William Pargeter, *Observations on Maniacal Disorders,* ed. Stanley W. Jackson (Reading: Printed for the author, 1792; London and New York: Routledge, 1988), pp. 13–14.

119. Haslam, *Observations on Insanity;* Crowther, *Practical Remarks on Insanity.* See also Crowther's *The Rabies Piratica, its History, Symptoms, and Cure; and the Furor Hippocraticus or Graeco-mania, with its Treatment* (London: G. Hayden, 1810).

120. Marshall was born in Fifeshire, and after an early education in Glasgow and Edinburgh, he studied medicine from 1777 in London, gaining qualifications as a surgeon and physician. He gave private lectures in anatomy to medical students and set up his own anatomical school and dissection room at Thavies Inn, London. See Samuel Sawrey, ed., *The Morbid Anatomy of the Brain, in Mania and Hydrophobia; with the Pathology of these two Diseases, as Collected from the Papers of the Late Andrew Marshal[l], M.D. Many Years Teacher of Anatomy in London* . . . (London: Printed for Longman, Hurst, Rees, Orme, and Brown, 1815).

121. BSCM, 28 Oct. 1780, 25 May and 17 Aug. 1782. More often than not, measures at Bethlem were taken by lay committee members in a somewhat piecemeal, after-the-fact manner, which seems to reflect the rather removed nature of oversight, medical or otherwise. For example, it was not until 1767 that, with a mind to preventing escapes, violence, and suicides, servants were ordered to search patients for and confiscate any boxes with locks and keys, as well as "Razors Penknives or other Offensive Instruments." In 1779, a committee on which a younger Monro sat took the rather belated additional precaution of engraving the order that patients were not to be given "Knives or Instruments of any kind" on visitors' tickets. BSCM, 20 June 1767, 22 May 1779.

122. Theodore M. Brown, "The Changing Self-Concept of the Eighteenth-Century London Physician," *Eighteenth-Century Life* 7.2 (Jan. 1982), pp. 31–40; Donald Monro, *Observations on the Means of Preserving the Health of Soldiers . . .* , 2nd ed., 2 vols. (London: Printed for J. Murray and G. Robinson, 1780). For earlier discussions of such issues, see Sir John Pringle, *Observations on the Nature and Cure of Hospital or Jayl Fevers* (London: London: A. Millar and D. Wilson, 1750); Pringle, *Observations on the Diseases of the Army* (London: 1752; Philadelphia: Edward Earle; Boston: D. Mallory & Co.; printed by Fry and Kammerer, 1810). Monro's library included both of these works by Pringle (although his copy of *Diseases of the Army* was the 1765 edition). He also had a copy of Donald Monro's *An Essay on the Dropsy and its Different Species* (London: D. Wilson and T. Durham, 1755). See John Monro, *Bibliotheca Elegantissima Monroiana. A Catalogue of the Elegant and Valuable Library of John Monro, M.D. Physician to Bethlehem Hospital, Lately Deceased; which will be Sold by Auction by Leigh & Sotheby . . . April 23d, 1792, and the Fourteen Following Days, (Sundays Excepted) . . .* (London: For Leigh and Sotheby, 1792), nos. 1073, 1199, 1639. It should be noted that this catalogue only includes those books sold on or after Monro's death, not those he bequeathed to his son Thomas.

123. Monro, *Remarks*, p. 39.

124. BSCM, 20 June 1765, pp. 133, 135.

125. BGCM, 15 Sept. 1785, in BSCM; BSCM, 24 Sept. 1785.

126. BCGM, 20 June 1765, p. 133; BSCM, 29 Aug. 1778.

127. A "watch-house" was a place where the parish watch-keepers would lodge between their patrols of the streets, and where those they apprehended were temporarily detained.

128. BCGM, 27 Jan. 1763, pp. 46–47.

129. Monro, *Remarks*, p. 38. John Monro's 1766 case book is reprinted in full in Jonathan Andrews and Andrew Scull, *Customers and Patrons*. For references to patients keeping quiet, see, e.g., case book, pp. 34, 48, 67.

130. BCGM, 27 Jan. 1763, p. 47. Although the committee's words appear to manifest the limits to such concerns for patients and the relatively rudimentary provision being offered the poor insane at this time, it should be remembered that the free circulation of air into lunatics' cells had long been deemed a restorative influence. Furthermore, only parts of Bethlem were unglazed, and its records make it difficult to say precisely what proportion of patients' cells were open to the elements.

131. [Joseph Pote], *The Foreigner's Guide: Or, a Necessary and Instructive Companion both for the Foreigner and Native: In their Tour Through the Cities of London and Westminster*, 4th ed. (London: Printed and sold by H. Kent, T. Hope, J. Joliffe, and T. Pote, 1763), as serialized and reproduced in the *Royal Magazine* 5 (1761), p. 60. This guide was originally published in 1729 (London: J. Pote), but was popular enough to be regularly reissued and revised, with new editions in English and French *(Le guide des étrangers)* in 1730, 1740, 1752, and 1763, and even a Dutch edition published in Amsterdam in 1759.

132. Ibid.

133. BCGM, 20 June 1765, pp. 136, 137.

134. BSCM, 19 and 27 March 1757, pp. 6, 8; BCGM, 20 June 1765, pp. 133, 135.

135. BSCM, 29 Jan. 1780, 19 July 1783.

136. BCGM, e.g., 15 Nov. 1781, 21 Nov. 1782, pp. 19–20, 70.

137. Ibid., 20 June 1765, pp. 135, 136, 137.

138. BSCM, 17 Jan. 1778. See also 25 Feb. 1778, where this is made part of the "Cutter's" early morning duties, he being the servant responsible for serving patients' meals.

139. BCGM, 20 June 1765, p. 135.

140. BGCM, 30 Oct. 1778, in BSCM; BSCM, 13 Dec. 1783.

141. BSCM, 26 June 1768, 17 July 1779.

142. As in 1774, when he was one of six committee members who suspended the porter; BSCM, 28 May 1774.

143. See, e.g., BSCM, 14 Sept. 1771; BCGM, 20 June 1765, pp. 132, 135.

144. E.g., BSCM, 1 Feb. 1783.

145. BSCM, e.g., 8 Sept. and 13 Oct. 1764, 4 March 1769, 4 and 18 Sept. 1784, pp. 106, 113, 346, cases of Elizabeth Gibbs, Mary Green, Elizabeth Chilton, and Miles Slater. Not all such cases were barred, however, and it is not always clear why some were and some were not.

146. See, e.g., BSCM, 24 Sept. 1774.

147. BCGM, 20 June 1765, pp. 137–38.

148. Ibid., p. 138. For the deferral of such admissions, see BSCM, e.g., 1 Nov. 1760, p. 302.

149. See, e.g., BSCM, 13 Nov. 1773, 20 Oct. 1774, 29 Nov. 1783, 28 Aug. 1784, 1 Sept. 1787, 24 Nov. 1791; BCGM, 29 Nov. 1787, pp. 287–88.

150. E.g., see *LEP*, no. 5992, 29 Mar–1 Apr 1766, p. 3, col. 4, p. 4, re. Spital sermon at St. Brides: Bethlem Hospital, patients admitted 211, cured 150, buried 40, and remaining 271. For the increase of cells at Bethlem and Monro's presence at the court and committee meetings that effected this, see, e.g., BCGM, 5 Aug. 1784, 29 Nov. 1787, pp. 155–56, 283–85.

151. See, e.g., various published Spital reports for the London hospitals; BGCM, 3 July 1759, p. 220, where a tabulation of admissions reveals an average of ca. 183 during 1752–58; Bowen, *An Historical Account*, p. 7.

152. BSCM, 16 Oct. 1784.

153. BGCM, 27 Sept. 1783, in BSCM.

154. BGCM, 25 April, 11 July 1789.

CHAPTER 2

1. Monro, *Remarks*, p. 36.

2. Moses Mendez et al., *The Battiad*, first canto (London: G. Smith, 1750). *The Battiad* was a satire directed against William Battie when he, as president of the College of Physicians—along with the censors and fellows of the college—opposed the admission of Isaac Schomberg to become a licentiate. The case is discussed in more detail in note 17 of this chapter.

3. *Considerations upon the Usefulness and Necessity of Establishing An Hospital as a Further Provision for Poor Lunaticks,* manuscript dated 1750.

Thirty thousand copies of this text were ordered to be printed in October 1750. See St. Luke's General Committee Minutes, 23 Oct. 1750, p. 16, at archives of St. Luke's Hospital, Woodside.

4. John Noorthouck, *A New History of London, including Westminster and Southwark. To Which is Added, a General Survey of the Whole, Describing the Public Buildings, late Improvements* (London: Printed for R. Baldwin, 1773), cited (inaccurately) in C. N. French, *The Story of St. Luke's Hospital* (London: William Heinemann, 1951), p. 10.

5. *European Magazine* 6 (1784), p. 424.

6. *Royal Magazine* 8 (1762), pp. 59–60.

7. Battie remained true to this standpoint on display even in his funeral and burial arrangements, being buried according to his explicit instructions at Kingston, Surrey, "as near as possible to his wife . . . without any monument or memorial whatever"; Munk, *Roll,* vol. 2, p. 142.

8. Endorsing the Bridewell and Bethlem governors' decision to continue the lavish and expensive Easter and St. Matthew's Day entertainments, despite the disdainful eschewal of such spectacles by other charities, the *London Evening Post* (no. 3820 [11–14 April 1752]) emphasized their utility in terms of "the Encouragement of the Social Virtues" and the embodiment of "the Grandeur and Dignity of the City." This was starkly contrasted "to the mean Methods made Use of by the Rival Charities lately set up by generous and disinterested Persons," although the disparity can be overdone, for St. Luke's governors did enjoy an annual dinner graced by persons of "distinction" held at Grocer's Hall and other similar institutions. As the *LEP* mentioned, the Bethlem governors' decision came at the same time as Hogarth was appointed a governor, but the irony is that Hogarth's *The Industrious and the Idle Apprentice* (1746) had explicitly attacked the excessive gluttony and greed of mayoral and civic feasts. As a magistrate, Henry Fielding was savagely critical of St. Luke's on still other grounds, discovering that his efforts to move insane persons from the gaol to the madhouse were frustrated by the hospital's Byzantine rules and regulations. *The Covent Garden Journal* 41 (23 May 1752), p. 437 and 43 (30 May 1752), pp. 439–40, reprinted in Henry Fielding, *The Covent Garden Journal and A Plan of the Universal Register Office,* ed. Bernard A. Goldgar (Oxford: Clarendon Press, 1988). Weeks later he satirized the baroque admissions requirements imposed at St. Luke's, reprinting the hospital's rules in their entirety and then spoofing them in a parallel set of rules for a notional "Hospital for the Reception of the Widows of poor Clergymen." See *The Covent Garden Journal* 45 (6 June 1752), in Fielding, pp. 254–55, emphases in the original. (We are most grateful to Akihito Suzuki for this reference.)

9. Significantly, the proposal of the Bethlem board to extend the hospital by a further fifty-two cells was made by the Bethlem grand committee just three weeks after *Considerations Upon the Usefulness and Necessity of Establishing St Luke's* (which refers to the want of space at Bethlem) had been ordered to be printed by its governors, on 10 Oct. 1750. The intimate connection of these initiatives is also indicated by the involvement of George Dance the Elder, surveyor of London, who was contracted to design the 1750–51 St. Luke's buildings. George had been present (as a governor of Bethlem) at the Bethlem grand com-

mittee meeting of 31 Oct. 1750, which supervised the expansion. Ultimately, the committee agreed to add just twenty-four new cells, as the *LEP* put it, "to obviate an unreasonable Objection of Delays in taking in Patients." See *LEP*, no. 3650, 12–14 March 1751; BCGM, 1 Nov. 1750, p. 467; St. Luke's General Committee Minutes, 10 and 23 Oct. 1750, and the copy of the *Considerations* at St. Luke's Hospital, Woodside archives.

10. See *LEP*, nos. 3621, 3625, and 3650, 3–5 and 12–15 Jan., and 12–15 March 1751.

11. James Monro died on 7 Nov. 1752 at Sunning-Hill, Berkshire.

12. For Battie's election as a governor and his receipt of his charge, see BCGM, 18 June and 1 Oct. 1742, pp. 148, 163.

13. Battie's father was the Rev. Edward Battie. For biographical accounts of Battie and his family, see, e.g., Nichols, *Literary Anecdotes*, vol. 4, part 3, pp. 599–606; Richard Hunter and Ida Macalpine, "William Battie, M.D., F.R.S., Pioneer Psychiatrist," *The Practitioner* 174 (1955), pp. 208–15; Hunter and Macalpine, Introduction to the facsimile edition of William Battie, *A Treatise on Madness*, and John Monro, *Remarks on Dr. Battie's Treatise on Madness* (London: Dawson's, 1962), pp. 7–21.

14. His notoriously anti-Papist grandfather, after whom he was named, had risen from being rector of Alderton and Baudsey and vicar of Hitcham, Suffolk, to become the king's chaplain and prebendary of St. Paul's, so his family was hardly bereft of social connections.

15. Nichols, *Literary Anecdotes*, vol. 4, part 3, pp. 599–600, 603. According to Nichols, Battie obtained the Craven scholarship through the influence and favoritism of Andrew Snape (1675–1742) D.D., the Eton headmaster and provost of King's College, beating Dr. Thomas Morrell to the prize. Hunter and Macalpine indicate that Battie was a favorite pupil of Snape's at both Eton and King's, while Snape had a considerable influence on Battie's and other contemporary physicians' views of insanity, as a result of his Spital Sermon, published in 1718 and reissued in 1731. See *Three Hundred Years of Psychiatry*, pp. 302–05. Battie's gratitude for this assistance later led him to establish a scholarship worth £20 per annum at King's College, Cambridge, modeled on the Craven scholarship. Nichols, *Literary Anecdotes*, vol. 1, part 4, p. 689; Munk, *Roll*, vol. 2, p. 142.

16. See Munk, *Roll*, vol. 2, p. 142, and also Nichols, *Literary Anecdotes*, vol. 8, part 4, pp. 552–23; John H. Jesse, *Memoirs of Celebrated Etonians*, vol. 1 (London: Bentley, 1875), p. 18 et seq.

17. During the 1750s, Battie as a censor and then president took the College of Physicians into prolonged and costly, although successful, litigation against Dr. Isaac Schomberg (1714–80), twin brother of Dr. Ralph Schomberg (1714–92). Schomberg, a German-born, baptized Jew, was brought up in England, but obtained his M.D. from Leyden (1745). He was banned from practicing medicine in London (as his father had done) after writing an uppity letter to the College in 1746 declaring his right to do so. Attempting to bypass the College regulations and to strengthen his claim by gaining a Cambridge M.D. (1749) and by becoming naturalized as British (1750), he subsequently renewed his application to the College. However, his demands for a licentiateship and admission

as a candidate of the College without examination were dismissed as equally presumptuous, and when he ultimately agreed to be examined by the censors as a licentiate he was failed. He promptly took the College to court, but this action also failed. It was not until 1765 (once again, under Battie's presidency) that Isaac finally gained a licentiate and was admitted as a candidate. However, he was not made a fellow until 1771. The affair prompted the issuance of a satirical poem spoofing Pope's *Dunciad*. *The Battiad* (1750), penned by the Bethlem governor Moses Mendez (with the assistance of Paul Whitehead and Schomberg himself), depicted Battie as "worldly," and a "low buffoon . . . madly emulous of vulgar praise," and drew a comic contrast between such traits and his otherwise sober and "grave" aspect, his learned and literate accomplishments, and his rather ponderous bedside manner. See Moses Mendez et al., *The Battiad*, first canto; also cited in Munk, *Roll*, vol. 2, pp. 141–43; Nichols, *Literary Anecdotes*, vol. 4, part 3, p. 606. See also the contemporaneous satire on the members of the College attributed to Ralph Schomberg, *Ietro-Rhapsodia: Or, a Physical Rhapsody* (London : J. Robinson, 1751); and Alex Sakula, "The Doctors Schomberg and the Royal College of Physicians: An Eighteenth Century Shemozzle," *Journal of Medical Biography* 2 (1994), pp. 113–19.

Monro did not gain his own candidacy and fellowship at the College until 1752–53, and his attitude to the Schomberg affair is difficult to chart, although he was certainly present at numerous committees that dealt with the case and is unlikely to have sided with Schomberg against Battie and the College. After Battie's death, once the controversy had subsided, Monro was to serve jointly as a censor with Schomberg in 1778. See *Annals/Registers of the College of Physicians*, esp. vol. 11, fols. 22–24, 26–27, 33–34, 62–64, 68–69, 80–83, 85, 89, 123–24, 126, 152, 155; vol. 12, fols. 7–8, 10–11, 14, 16; vol. 14, fol. 103.

18. Henry Godolphin served as Eton's provost between 1695 and 1732. Nichols (see note 19, below) claimed that he was ninety-four years old when he sent Battie his coach, but this is impossible as he was only eighty-five when he died.

19. Nichols, *Literary Anecdotes*, vol. 4, part 3, p. 601. Like his father, Thomas Monro was appreciative of the importance of presentational style for physicians, disdainfully referring to the "shabby kind of carriage" used by the Prussian Dr. Kallerselto, doctor to the "potentates of Europe." Thomas Monro, *Olla Podrida, a Periodical Paper, Published at Oxford* (Dublin: Printed by P. Byrne, 1787), no. 8 (5 May 1787), p. 54.

20. Nichols, *Literary Anecdotes*, vol. 8, part 4, pp. 552–33, 599; vol. 4, part 3, p. 727.

21. Ibid., vol. 8, part 4, p. 553; Denis Leigh, *The Historical Development of British Psychiatry* (Oxford: Pergamon, 1961), p. 56; *Gentleman's Magazine* 46 (1776), p. 287.

22. For Battie's burial, see Nichols, *Literary Anecdotes*, vol. 4, part 3, p. 601; for Monro's gravestone, see "Letters relating to the illnesses of George III," Royal College of Physicians, MS 3011/48. Monro's inscription reads: "Here also lieth the body of John Monro MD Father of the above Charlotte Monro who departed this life the 27th day of December 1791 in the 77th

year of his age." In death there was, however, one important difference: whereas Monro left behind three sons, one of whom carried on his practice and the family mad-business (his daughter Charlotte and son James having predeceased him), Battie had three daughters with his wife (herself the daughter of an Eton underschoolmaster), and had no immediate male heir to whom he could bequeath his business. In an odd twist, it was Monro who would take over the operation of Battie's Clerkenwell madhouse.

23. Battie, *Treatise*.

24. Ibid., p. 1.

25. Ibid., p. 2.

26. *Reasons for the Establishing and Further Encouragement of St. Luke's Hospital for Lunaticks; Together with the Rules and Orders for the Government Thereof, and a List of the Governors and Benefactors* (London: H. Teape and Son, 1751; reprinted in 1763, 1786, 1817, 1819, and 1836). A copy of the pamphlet in its draft manuscript form is in St. Luke's Hospital, Woodside archives. For its drawing up, see St. Luke's General Court Minutes, 26 June 1751; St. Luke's General Committee Minutes, 17 July and 23 Oct. 1751. The publication is quoted in Richard Hunter and Ida Macalpine's introduction to the facsimile edition of Battie's *Treatise* and Monro's *Remarks,* p. 15. Hunter and Macalpine provide here a very valuable survey of the Battie-Monro debate, which has, however, been largely superseded by the excellent analysis in Akihito Suzuki, "Mind and Its Disease in Enlightenment British Medicine," diss., University of London, 1992, pp. 221–68.

27. Battie, *Treatise,* pp. v, vi. It seems plausible that Battie's own early career difficulties helped to foster his commitment to opening up the avenues of medical knowledge (as he was to attempt to do in another way by endowing the aforementioned [see note 15] scholarship at King's College, Cambridge, thus providing the sort of sponsorship that had helped him to launch his own career).

28. Ibid., pp. 93–94.

29. Ibid., p. 68.

30. Ibid., pp. 68–69.

31. William Battie, *The Annual Lecture delivered in the Theatre of the Royal College of Physicians of London from Harvey's Foundation, 18th October 1746, Royal College of Physicians,* London, MS 1024/409, a translation of his *Oratio Anniversaria in Theatro Collegii Regalis Medicorum Londinensium ex Harvaei Instituto Habita die xviii Octobris, 1746* (London: J. Whiston, 1746).

32. Ibid., pp. 1–2.

33. Ibid., p. 6.

34. Ibid., p. 5.

35. Ibid., p. 3.

36. Ibid., p. 9.

37. Ibid., pp. 5–6.

38. John Monro, *Harveian Oration* (1757), or "The Annual Lecture from Harvey's Foundation," translated version held in Royal College of Physicians Library, p. 4: "Radcliffe . . . was . . . a true disciple of nature. He observed her with attentive eyes and unmoved countenance. . . . He made use of simple medica-

ments, showing plainly that nature is helped by a few but oppressed by a great number of them."

39. Monro, "Advertisement," *Remarks*.

40. I.e., Richard Mead (1673–1754), physician to St. Thomas's Hospital and himself a physician who wrote on insanity.

41. Monro, *Harveian Oration*, pp. 5–6.

42. Monro, "Advertisement." Given these views, it comes as no surprise that Monro published nothing on medical matters besides his response to Battie and his *Harveian Oration*. Battie, by contrast, apart from his editions of Aristotle's *Rhetoric* (*De Rhetorica Seu Arte Dicendi . . .* [Cambridge: G. Thurlbourn, 1728]) and Isocrates' *Orations* (*Isokratous Hapanta. Isocratis Opera Quae Quidem Nunc Extant Omnia. Varias Lectiones . . .* [London: C. Davis, J. Whiston, and B. Dod, 1749; Cambridge: 1749]), was additionally to produce two medical works in Latin: a version (*De Principiis Animalibus Exercitationes Viginti Quatuor . . .* [London: 1751; London: John Whiston & Benj. White, 1757]) of his Lumleian lectures (which displayed his thorough grounding in eighteenth-century physiological and pathological theory); and a book (*Aphorismi de Cognoscendis & Curandis Morbis Nonnullis ad Principia Animalia Accommodati* [London: John Whiston & Benj. White, 1760]) of medical aphorisms, covering a wide range of diseases.

While Monro was a reluctant publicist on insanity, somewhat contradictorily he was a great collector of books on the subject, his library containing most of the major sixteenth- to eighteenth-century works, including Timothy Bright's *A Treatise of Melancholie* (London: Vautrollier, 1586); Richard Baxter's *The Signs and Causes of Melancholy . . .* (London: Cruttenden & Cox, 1716); Jacques Ferrand's *Erotomania, or A Treatise Discoursing of the Essence, Causes, Symptoms, Prognosticks, and Cure of Love, or Erotique Melancholy* (Oxford: Printed by L. Lichfield and sold by Edward Forrest, 1640); John Donne's *Biathanatos: A Declaration of that Paradoxe, or Thesis, that Self-homicide is not so Naturally Sin that it may Never be Otherwise . . .* (London: Printed for Humphrey Moseley, 1648); William Rowley's *A Treatise on Female, Nervous, Hysterical, Hypochondriacal, Bilious, Convulsive Diseases . . .* (London: C. Nourse, 1788); P. Fring's *A Treatise on Phrensy . . .* (London: Printed by T. Gardner, 1746) (which was dedicated to John's father, James); William Perfect's *Methods of Cure in Some Particular Cases of Insanity, the Epilepsy, Hypochondrical Affections, Hysteric Passion, and Nervous Disorders . . .* (Rochester: Fisher, 1778); Harper's *Real Cause and Cure of Insanity* (1789); Thomas Fallowes's *The Best Method for the Cure of Lunaticks . . .* (London: For the author, 1705), and, also, not surprisingly, Battie's *Treatise on Madness* (1758). See John Monro, *Bibliotheca Elegantissima Monroiana. A Catalogue of the Elegant and Valuable Library of John Monro, M.D. Physician to Bethlehem Hospital, Lately Deceased; which will be Sold by Auction by Leigh & Sotheby . . . April 23d, 1792, and the Fourteen Following Days, (Sundays Excepted) . . .*, nos. 424, 595, 661, 732, 1155, 1362, 1644, 1652, 1666 (London: For Leigh & Sotheby, 1792).

43. Monro, *Remarks*, pp. 2–3.

44. Ibid., emphases in the original.

45. See his other publications: *Oratio Anniversaria; De Principiis Animalibus; Aphorismi de Cognoscendis et Curandis Morbis.* This latter work was based on physiological principles informed by Boerhaave.

46. On the general significance of trust in the construction and maintenance of the social order, see Steven Shapin, *A Social History of Truth: Civility and Science in Seventeenth-Century England* (Chicago and London: University of Chicago Press, 1994), passim, esp. pp. 8–15, 34–36, 193.

47. Compare, too, one of the central elements in his defense of his father James: "physick he honoured as a *profession,* but he despised it as a *trade;* however partial I may be to his memory, his friends will acknowledge this to be true, and his enemies will not venture to deny it"; Monro, *Remarks,* p. 36.

48. Ibid.

49. Monro, *Remarks,* pp. 35–36. Monro had confessed himself in his *Harveian Oration* (p. 4) of the previous year, "an unpolished speaker, unused to lecturing." His stance on the inappropriateness of lecturing as a means of imparting knowledge of insanity/medicine remained the orthodoxy at Bethlem well into the nineteenth century. John Haslam, apothecary to the hospital between 1795 and 1816, insisted in very similar terms on the empirical foundations of medical knowledge and the limited value of open theoretical disputation and communication, maintaining that the right approach to madness could only be learned from "experience." Hence, it "cannot be communicated . . . but . . . must perish with its possessor." John Haslam, *Observations on Madness,* 2nd ed. (London: Callow, 1809), p. 277, cited in Samuel Tuke, *Description of the Retreat, an Institution near York, for Insane Persons of the Society of Friends. Containing an Account of its Origin and Progress, the Modes of Treatment, and a Statement of Cases* (York: W. Alexander, 1813), p. 133. For discussion of the reasons for Haslam's insistence on the centrality of "experience," see Scull, MacKenzie, and Hervey, *Masters of Bedlam,* pp. 20–26.

50. Monro, *Remarks,* p. 10, emphasis in the original.

51. Ibid., emphasis in the original.

52. Ibid., pp. 3–4, emphases in the original.

53. Ibid., p. 4. Akihito Suzuki has shown that many seventeenth- and eighteenth-century physicians disagreed with *both* Monro and Battie on this point, arguing for "a combined disorder of both the faculty of making images and that of making judgment." See Suzuki, "Mind and Its Disease in Enlightenment British Medicine," pp. 247–52.

54. Monro, *Remarks,* p. 9. Monro is here alluding to John Locke's earlier division of the process of "perception" (that is, the acquisition, or processing, of a piece of knowledge about the external world into "sensation" and "judgement"). This twofold characterization of normal perception had been widely embraced by eighteenth-century philosophical writers, and it forms, as Akihito Suzuki has noted, a hidden subtext of the Monro-Battie debate. See his "Mind and Its Disease in Enlightenment British Medicine."

55. Monro, *Remarks,* p. 13.

56. Ibid.

57. Ibid., p. 16.

58. "Original madness," in Battiean terminology, was madness where the

seat of the disorder was "solely owing to an internal disorder of the nervous substance," whereas "consequential madness" was caused by any external event that placed unnatural pressure upon the nervous substance. A disorder that was purely internal to the nervous system was, ipso facto, beyond the reach of medical knowledge or art (Battie, *Treatise*, pp. 43–44).

59. Monro, *Remarks*, pp. 20–21.

60. Ibid., pp. 26, 34.

61. Ibid., p. 42.

62. Ibid., p. 43, emphasis in the original.

63. Ibid., pp. 42–43; Battie, *Treatise*, p. 79.

64. Monro, *Remarks*, pp. 49–50. Battie had incorporated precisely this passage, without identifying the "eminent practitioner," in his own *Treatise*, p. 68. Just to add a further complication, John Monro may have erred in concluding that the reference was to his father. Possibly Battie had been referring instead to George II's physician, Richard Mead, who had publicly set down "some rules for management of mad-folks, than which nothing conduces more to their cure." See his *Medical Precepts and Cautions*, reprinted in *The Medical Works of Richard Mead*, vol. 2 (London: Hitch, 1762), p. 492.

65. Battie's stress on divining the etiology of madness as a starting point for cure is a constant theme of his *Treatise*, but see esp. pp. 73, 88. This was actually translated into practice at St. Luke's, where, in contrast to Bethlem, standard admission forms for the hospital required from the certifying practitioner some account of the "state of the Patient's Case" and "of the Methods (if any) used to obtain a Cure." See book in St. Luke's, Woodside archives, entitled *Considerations upon the Usefulness*, p. 14. For Monro's skepticism on these matters, see *Remarks*, pp. 15, 21–23, 33–34.

66. Battie, *Treatise*, pp. 75–77, 97–99; Monro, *Remarks*, pp. 50–51; Bryan Robinson, *Observations on the Virtues and Operations of Medicines* (London: J. Nourse, 1752), p. 145. Monro might also have cited the work of the Bethlem governor Nicholas Robinson, *A New System of the Spleen, Vapours, and Hypochondriack Melancholy Wherein all the Decays of the Nerves, and Lownesses of the Spirits, are Mechanically Accounted for . . .* (London: Printed for A. Bettesworth, W. Innys, and C. Rivington, 1729), esp. pp. 399–402. For Nicholas Robinson's election as a governor, see BCGM, 27 March 1755, p. 175.

67. Monro, *Remarks*, pp. 50–51.

68. Ibid.

69. Battie, *Treatise*, pp. 93–94.

70. Ibid., pp. 74–76; Monro, *Remarks*, p. 50.

71. See Battie, *Treatise*, pp. 97–99; Monro, *Remarks*, pp. 50–51; Cheyne, *English Malady*, p. 206; Hunter and Macalpine, Introduction to facsimile edition, p. 14.

72. Monro, *Remarks*, pp. 38, 40.

73. Ibid., p. 40.

74. Monro, *Remarks*, p. 38; Battie, *Treatise*, pp. 84–85.

75. Ever the pragmatist, though, while stressing that "attendants [should n]ever be suffered to behave otherwise" to their patients than with "the greatest

tenderness and affection," Monro doubted that it was always "possible to prevent" ill treatment from keepers. Monro, *Remarks*, p. 38.

76. Battie, *Treatise*, pp. 28, 32, 75; Monro, *Remarks*, pp. 1, 4, 5, 8, 31, 45, 47. These complex admixtures were by no means unusual. The Enlightenment was characterized by an ambivalent attitude to the "ancients" and "moderns," typified by a somewhat contradictory enthusiasm for the theories of antiquity coupled with a concurrent concern to expose such theories to a thoroughgoing rational and empirical criticism.

77. Monro, *Remarks*, e.g., pp. 12–13.

78. Battie's support for "prohibition" laws against alcohol as a preventative measure, however, was rather less orthodox and may suggest sympathies with the religious radicals. See *Treatise*, pp. 49, 52–54, 56, 58, 83, 90.

79. Monro, *Remarks*, pp. 38, 45; Battie, *Treatise*, pp. 84–85. This theory seems to have derived from the Greek medical doctrine of the therapeutic benefits of opposites and extremes.

80. Monro, *Remarks*, pp. 26–27; Richard Mead, *Medical Precepts and Cautions* (London: Brindley, 1751), pp. 79, 90–91; Mead, "Medica Sacra," *The Medical Works of Richard Mead*, p. 619; Andrew Scull, *The Most Solitary of Afflictions: Madness and Society in Britain, 1700–1900* (London and New Haven: Yale University Press, 1993), p. 37; Thomas Arnold, *Observations on the Nature, Kinds, Causes, and Prevention, of Insanity,* 2nd ed., vol. 1 (London: Printed for Richard Phillips, 1806), pp. 155–56; Joseph Mason Cox, *Practical Observations on Insanity . . . To which are Subjoined Remarks on Medical Jurisprudence, as it Relates to Diseased Intellect,* 3rd ed. (1804; London: Printed for R. Baldwin and Thomas Underwood by E. Bryan, 1813), pp. 4–5.

81. Battie, *Treatise*, pp. 65–67, 96–97.

82. Ibid., p. 73.

83. Ibid., pp. 37, 42.

84. Ibid., pp. 71–72.

85. Ibid., pp. 59, 67; compare Monro, *Remarks*, pp. 24–25.

86. Haller to Tissot, 3 Dec. 1759, reprinted in *Albrecht von Haller's Briefe an August Tissot* (Bern: Huber, 1977), p. 87. His low opinion of Battie is reiterated in a subsequent letter, 17 Dec. 1759, p. 90. (We owe these references to Akihito Suzuki.)

87. [Tobias Smollett], "Dr. Battie's *Treatise on Madness,*" *Critical Review* 4 (1757), pp. 509–16; [Smollett], "Remarks on Dr. Battie's *Treatise of* [sic] *Madness,*" *Literary Review* 5 (1758), pp. 224–28. Smollett considered both Monro and Battie to be "men very eminent in their profession, especially in that branch of it on which they treat," and though "rivals in fame . . . hitherto the contest is conducted with spirit and decorum, free from personal abuse, and abounding with matter of real utility" (*Literary Review* 5 [1758], p. 224). Smollett freely plagiarized passages from both books in his 1762 novel *Sir Launcelot Greaves* (in chap. 23 especially), a work that was serialized originally in *The British Magazine* during 1760–61. Hunter and Macalpine were evidently the first to remark on this borrowing. See Ida Macalpine and Richard A. Hunter, "Tobias Smollett, M.D. and William Battie, M.D," *Journal of the History of Medicine and Allied*

Sciences 11 (1956), pp. 102–03; Macalpine and Hunter, "Smollett's Reading in Psychiatry," *Modern Language Review* 51 (July 1956), pp. 409–11.

88. Smollett objects that Monro misrepresents Battie's claim that "original madness does not shorten life . . . [in a way] we do not think just"; and he suggests that Monro is sometimes given to an excess of filial piety in defending his father—a minor offense that he considers entirely understandable. *Literary Review* 5 (1758), pp. 226, 228.

89. On the question of defining madness, for instance, Monro "indeed proves in our *judgments,* that Dr. Battie's *imagination* was not clear. . . . We agree with [Monro] . . . that Dr. Battie has expended much learning and pains to prove some things that we knew before . . . and in endeavouring to explain many things, that we have not a much clearer explanation of, than we had before his explanation." Monro "very sensibly" objects to Battie's division of madness into "original" and "consequential" forms. Smollett also approvingly notes that Monro "observes, that though the management of mad people is of the greatest moment, yet Dr. Battie has discussed that point with great brevity, though so diffuse in others of little importance. Our author makes up this deficiency by several judicious observations and directions . . . perhaps . . . the most valuable part of his ingenious performance" ([Smollett], "Remarks," pp. 226–27).

90. Crowther, *Practical Remarks on Insanity,* esp. pp. 87–90, 110–112, 128–29. Despite adopting a veneer of the language of "moral regimen," Crowther regularly snipes at Pinel in this work. He cites John Monro by way of objecting to Pinel's claim that the English were "silent" on the subject of moral management. He also disputes Pinel's claim that cold bathing commonly resulted in paralysis, asserting that this never occurred at Bethlem.

91. Haslam, *Observations on Insanity,* p. vii.

92. William Pargeter, *Observations on Maniacal Disorders,* ed. Stanley W. Jackson (London: For the author, 1792; London and New York: Routledge, 1988), pp. 49, 115, 133–34.

93. Alexander Crichton, *An Inquiry into the Nature and Origin of Mental Derangement . . .* (London: Printed for T. Cadell Jun. and W. Davies, 1798), pp. 157, 162.

94. George Man Burrows, *Commentaries on the Causes, Forms, Symptoms, and Treatment, Moral and Medical, of Insanity* (London: Underwood, 1828), pp. 65–66. With even greater vigor than Monro, Burrows was to champion the efficacy of medical means in every case, concerned as he was that the contemporary fashion for moral approaches to insanity was running away with itself. See his *An Inquiry into Certain Errors Relative to Insanity; and their Consequences; Physical, Moral, and Civil* (London: Printed for Thomas and George Underwood, 1820), pp. 150–51.

95. Francis Willis, *A Treatise on Mental Derangement. Containing the Substance of the Gulstonian Lectures, for May, 1822* (London: Longman, Hurst, Rees, Orme, and Brown, 1823), p. 48.

96. Willis quotes Monro's definition of "High Spirits," saying that he prefers it "to any that I might otherwise have thought fit to offer"; ibid., pp. x, 46–47; Monro, *Remarks,* p. 7.

97. Munk, *Roll*, vol. 2, pp. 183–85.

98. Burrows, *Commentaries*, p. 539:

All authors agree in ascribing the frequency of relapse to too early removal. Dr John Monro went further, and coincided with Mead in thinking, that "the danger of relapse being always great, every thing prescribed for the cure, such as medicines, diet, exercise, &c. should, when it is effected, be continued at intervals for a considerable time after recovery". This is very judicious advice; but it will be very difficult indeed to persuade the patient or his friends of the additional security to be derived from adopting it.

99. Ibid., pp. 639–41.

100. Cox, *Practical Observations on Insanity*, pp. 108–09.

101. Ibid., p. 105; Willis, *Treatise on Mental Derangement*, pp. 136–39. See also Monro, *Remarks*, p. 50; George Nesse Hill, *An Essay on the Prevention and Cure of Insanity; with Observations on the Rules for the Detection of Pretenders to Madness* (London: J. & J. Haddock for Longman, Hurst, Rees, Orme & Brown, 1814), p. 295; Haslam, *Observations on Insanity*, p. 328; William Saunders Hallaran, *An Enquiry into the Causes Producing the Extraordinary Addition to the Number of Insane, Together with Extended Observations on the Cure of Insanity* (Cork: Edwards & Savage, 1810), p. 52.

102. On the other hand, most British authors seem to have disagreed with Monro's negative opinion as to blisters, Willis, Hallaran, Cox, Haslam, and Hill being among those who believed them "very serviceable" remedies. Willis, *Treatise on Mental Derangement*, p. 140; Monro, *Remarks*, p. 47.

103. *Gentleman's Magazine* 33 (1763), pp. 20–21.

104. Battie, *Treatise*, pp. 5–6; Willis, *Treatise on Mental Derangement*, passim.

105. Joel Peter Eigen, *Witnessing Insanity: Madness and Mad-Doctors in the English Court* (New Haven and London: Yale University Press, 1995), p. 138, identified Dr. Ainsley's testimony in the 1812 trial of Thomas Bowler as "the first time a medical witness at the Old Bailey invoked delusion to characterize a prisoner's mental state."

106. Crichton, *Inquiry*, pp. xx, xxiii; James Cowles Prichard, *A Treatise on Insanity and Other Disorders Affecting the Mind* (London: Sherwood, Gilbert, and Piper, 1835), chap. 2, pp. 12–50, 382.

107. The following discussion is heavily indebted to Akihito Suzuki's "Mind and Its Disease in Enlightenment British Medicine," pp. 221–25.

108. See the debate on these issues in Hunter and Macalpine, "William Battie, M.D., F.R.S., Pioneer Psychiatrist," *The Practitioner* 174 (1955), pp. 208–15; Hunter and Macalpine, Introduction to the facsimile edition, pp. 7–21; Hunter and Macalpine, *Three Hundred Years of Psychiatry*, pp. 402–16. For a more or less faithful following of the Hunter and Macalpine line, see Neville C. Oswald, "Baker, Battie and Huxham: Three Eighteenth Century Physicians from the South Hams," *Reports and Transactions of the Devonshire Association for the Advancement of Science* 112 (1980), pp. 117–26.

109. Leigh, *British Psychiatry*, p. 51.

110. Ibid., pp. 51–54.

111. Klaus Doerner, *Madmen and the Bourgeoisie: A Social History of In-*

sanity and Psychiatry (Oxford: Basil Blackwell, 1986); trans. from the original *Burger und Irre* (1969), pp. 39–46, esp. 39, 43.

112. George S. Rousseau, "Science," *The Eighteenth Century,* ed. Pat Rogers (London: Methuen, 1978), pp. 153–207; Rousseau, "Psychology," *The Ferment of Knowledge,* ed. George S. Rousseau and Roy Porter (Cambridge: Cambridge University Press, 1980), pp. 143–210.

113. Dora Weiner, "The Origins of Psychiatry: Pinel or the Zeitgeist?" *Zusammenhang Festschrift für Marielene Putscher,* ed. Otto Bauer and Otto Glandien (Köln: Wienand Verlag, 1984), pp. 617–31.

114. Stanley Jackson, Introduction to the facsimile edition of William Pargeter, *Observations on Maniacal Disorders* (London: Routledge, 1988).

115. Roy Porter, *Mind-Forg'd Manacles* (London: Athlone, 1987), pp. 128–29, 192–93, 206–08.

116. Allan Ingram, *The Madhouse of Language: Writing and Reading Madness in the Eighteenth Century* (London and New York: Routledge, 1991), pp. 44–49. See also pp. 51, 57, 71–72, 75, 94, 105, 168, 173. See also Allan Ingram, ed., *Patterns of Madness in the Eighteenth Century: A Reader* (Liverpool: Liverpool University Press, 1998), p. 120, where he says even more anachronistically of Monro and his *Remarks:* "Monro's publication is much less significant than Battie's. . . . Few writers, and no psychiatrists, have ever produced a document that so blatantly spells out on every page its own reluctance to exist. As such Monro's *Remarks* stands as the headstone to eighteenth-century orthodox psychiatry's refusal to take the mad seriously." By contrast, "Battie's work" is erroneously distinguished as "the most important influence on the treatment of madness in the eighteenth century before the founding of the York Retreat in 1792"; ibid., p. 112.

117. Akihito Suzuki, "Mind and Its Disease in Enlightenment British Medicine," pp. 263–64: "Late eighteenth-century nosologists . . . paid more and more attention to the faculty of judgement in . . . explaining madness. Boissier de Sauvages, William Cullen, Thomas Arnold, and many others were departing from the Cartesian [and Battiean] characterisation of madness as illusion. . . . They were . . . Monro's allies, in the sense that they took wrong judgement as the most important symptom of madness." For detailed evidence in support of these claims, see ibid., pp. 269–328.

118. Perfect, *Methods of Cure,* p. 2.

119. Ibid., p. 9.

120. Baker was actually born in the same parish, Modbury, in Devon; was to publish on the colic in Devonshire (1767), and was chosen as one of the censors by Battie during his presidency in 1764. See Oswald, "Baker, Battie and Huxham."

121. Andrew Harper, *A Treatise on the Real Cause and Cure of Insanity* (London: Stalker & Walker, 1789).

122. Arnold, *Observations,* p. lix.

123. Hardinge to Barnard, in Nichols, *Literary Anecdotes,* vol. 8, part 4, p. 552.

124. William Perfect, *Cases of Insanity and Nervous Disorders, Successfully Treated* (Rochester: For the author, 1780); Perfect, *Select Cases in the Different*

Species of Insanity, Lunacy, or Madness, with the Modes of Practice as Adopted in the Treatment of Each (Rochester: Printed and sold by W. Gillman; London: Printed and sold by J. Murray & J. Dew, 1787); Perfect, *Annals of Insanity* (London: For the author, 1801). The fifth and last edition of this work was published in 1809. For a brief analysis of Perfect and his writings, see Hunter and Macalpine, *Three Hundred Years of Psychiatry*, pp. 501–05.

125. Philippe Pinel, *A Treatise on Insanity*, trans. D. D. Davis (Sheffield: Cadell & Davies, 1806); J. E. D. Esquirol, *Mental Maladies. A Treatise on Insanity*, trans. E. K. Hunt (Philadelphia: Lee & Blanchard, 1845); (Karl Wiegand) Maximilian Jacobi, *On the Construction and Management of Hospitals for the Insane* . . . , trans. by John Kitching, with introductory observations, &c., by Samuel Tuke (Berlin: 1834; London: J. Churchill, 1841); Joseph Guislain, *Traite sur l'aliénation mentale et sur les hospices des aliénés* (Amsterdam: J. Van der Hey, 1826); Étienne-Jean Georget, *De la folie: Considérations sur cette maladie* (Paris: Crevot, 1820; New York: Arno Press, 1976); Georget, *De la physiologie du système nerveux et spécialement du cerveau* . . . (Paris: J. B. Bailliere, 1821).

126. William Cullen, *First Lines in the Practice of Physic* (Edinburgh: Elliot, 1784); Cullen, *Nosology: Or, a Systematic Arrangement of Diseases, by Classes, Orders, Genera, and Species* (Edinburgh: Creech, 1800); Cox, *Practical Observations on Insanity;* Hallaran, *An Enquiry.*

127. Samuel Tuke, *Description of the Retreat, an Institution near York, for Insane Persons of the Society of Friends* (York: Alexander, 1813); John Ferriar, *Medical Histories and Reflections* (London: Cadell & Davies, 1795); Prichard, *A Treatise on Insanity.*

128. E.g., see the description of St. Luke's in *European Magazine* 6 (1784), p. 424. For more detailed comparison of Bethlem and St. Luke's, see Andrews, "Bedlam Revisited," pp. 314–18; Jonathan Andrews, Asa Briggs, Roy Porter, Penny Tucker, and Keir Waddington, *The History of Bethlem* (London and New York: Routledge, 1997), pp. 250, 277–78, 373.

129. See, e.g., St. Luke's Hospital for Lunatics, "The Physicians' Report and Statistical Tables for the year 1853," *Report of the General Committee of St. Luke's Hospital for the year 1853* (London: H. Teape and Son, 1854), pp. 7–8.

130. For Sir Alexander Morison's pioneering efforts on this front, see Scull, MacKenzie, and Hervey, *Masters of Bedlam*, pp. 137–39.

131. For more on the latter case, see chapter 4.

132. For more on this inquiry, see chapter 5.

133. Monro's 1766 case book (hereafter CB), reprinted in Andrews and Scull, *Customers and Patrons*, p. 5.

134. CB, pp. 50–54.

135. For more on this case, see chapter 5.

136. This account was part of Erskine's long speech in defense of another of George III's failed assassins, James Hadfield, in 1800. See "In behalf of James Hadfield," *The World's Orators*, vol. 8 (New York: Putnam, 1900), pp. 25–71; Henry Peter (Lord) Brougham, "English Orators—Erskine," *Works*, 11 vols. (London and Glasgow: R. Griffin & Co., 1855–61), vol. 7, pp. 209–55, vol. 11, pp. 1281–356; Morris, *The Hoxton Madhouses* (Cambridge: Goodwin Bros.,

1958), note 30; Ida Macalpine and Richard Hunter, *George III and the Mad-Business* (London: Allen Lane/Penguin, 1969), pp. 314–15.

137. Morris, *Hoxton Madhouses*.

138. In fact, Bethlem's place as a bastion of reaction would endure for longer still, cemented by John's successful perpetuation of the Monro family dynasty. As the investigations that swirled around the 1815–16 Select Committee on Madhouses would reveal, his son Thomas saw himself as little more than a loyal follower of his father's tried and tested practice. Thomas's admission that "he knew no better" method of proceeding, which came amid a welter of ironic self-incriminations, served in that very different environment as an indictment of what were now perceived to be outmoded "Habits and Opinions." Hands-off medical management and routine seasonal bleedings, purgings, vomitings, and bathings, long practiced at Bethlem, were portrayed as the very quintessence of medical nihilism, and the symbolic sanction for the neglect and abuse of patients.

139. Hunter and Macalpine, *Three Hundred Years of Psychiatry*, p. 403. Having retired to some extent from the fray, Battie was nonetheless not completely out of the picture. He remained an influential presence as a governor to St. Luke's, while Bethlem's archives demonstrate that during the 1760s and early 1770s he continued to be a very active governor there also, whether merely attending and voting at court and grand committee meetings (sometimes alongside Monro), helping to rewrite the rules governing the apothecary's post in 1772, or conveying the news to the alderman, Walter Rawlinson, that he had been elected as president in 1773. See BCGM, e.g., 1 April 1762, 25 July 1765, 9 July 1772, pp. 13, 142, 359, 383.

CHAPTER 3

1. Anon., *Bethlem A Poem* (7 May 1744), printed and sold for three pence to visitors to the hospital, and purporting to have been written by a patient.

2. Henry Fielding, *Amelia*, ed. Martin C. Battestin (1752; Oxford: Clarendon Press, 1993), pp. 138–39.

3. Theophilus Evans, *A History of Modern Enthusiasm, From the Reformation to the Present Times* (London: Printed for the author; and sold by W. Owen; and W. Clarke, 1757).

4. Samuel Foote, *The Minor, A Comedy* (London: For the author, 1760).

5. William Pargeter, *Observations on Maniacal Disorders*, p. 31. The "eminent physician" Pargeter referred to may well have been John Monro.

6. Burrows, *An Inquiry*, p. 186.

7. For general introductions to literature on the relationship between madness, reason, and religion in the early modern period, on which much of the following discussion is based, see, e.g., Porter, *Mind-Forg'd Manacles*, pp. 24–25, 41–42, 62–81, 264–68; Christopher Hill, *The World Turned Upside Down: Radical Ideas during the English Revolution* (London: Temple Smith, 1972; Harmondsworth: Penguin, 1991); Hill, *Change and Continuity in Seventeenth-Century England* (London: Weidenfeld and Nicolson, 1974; New

Haven and London: Yale University Press, 1991); George Rosen, "Enthusiasm: 'a dark lanthorn of the spirit,'" *Bulletin of the History of Medicine* 42 (1968), pp. 393–421; Michael Heyd, "Medical Discourse in Religious Controversy: The Case of the Critique of 'Enthusiasm' on the Eve of the Enlightenment," *Medicine as a Cultural System,* ed. Michael Heyd and Hans-Joerg Rheinberger, special issue of *Science in Context* 8.1 (Spring 1995), pp. 133–57; Michael Heyd, *Be Sober and Reasonable: The Critique of Enthusiasm in the Seventeenth and Early Eighteenth Centuries* (New York: E. J. Brill, 1995); Michael Mac-Donald, "Popular Beliefs about Mental Disorder in Early Modern England," *Münstersche Beiträge zur Geschichte und Theorie der Medizin,* ed. Wolfgang Eckhart and Johanna Geyer-Kordesch (Munster: Burgverlag, 1982), pp. 148–73; MacDonald, "Religion, Social Change and Psychological Healing in England, 1600–1800," *The Church and Healing,* ed. W. Shiels (Oxford: Basil Blackwell, 1982), pp. 101–25; MacDonald, "Insanity and the Realities of History in Early Modern England," *Lectures on the History of Psychiatry,* ed. R. M. Murray and T. H. Turner, the Squibb Series (London, Gaskell/The Royal College of Psychiatrists, 1990), pp. 60–77. For a less satisfying contextual discussion of the relationship between madness and religion in this period, see, e.g., N. P. Weeks, "Reconciling Scientific and Religious Discourse about Madness during the Age of Reason: Lessons for Today?" *Nursing Management* 3.2 (April 1996), pp. 95–101.

8. A brief definition seems necessary here for those readers unfamiliar with this term. Relatively narrowly defined by contemporaries, "enthusiasm" tended to mean excessive zeal or ardor in the prosecution of religio-political views, yet it could also more widely implicate any putatively passionate, mistaken, or foolish opinion, notion, or set of beliefs, taken to extremes by its proponent(s), or else any particular viewpoint that one did not agree with.

9. Henry More, *Enthusiasmus Triumphatus: Or, A Discourse of the Nature, Causes, Kinds, and Cure, of Enthusiasme* (London: Printed by J. Flesher, and sold by W. Morden, 1656); More, *Enthusiasmus Triumphatus. Abridgments. Enthusiasm Explained: Or, a Discourse on the Nature, Kind and Cause of Enthusiasm. With Proper Rules to Preserve the Mind from being Tainted with it . . .* (London: Printed for T. Gardner, 1739); Meric Casaubon, *A Treatise Concerning Enthusiasm, as it is an Effect of Nature: But is Mistaken by Many for Either Divine Inspiration, or Diabolical Posession* (London: Johnson, 1655). See also Henry Wharton, *The Enthusiasm of the Church of Rome Demonstrated in Some Observations upon the Life of Ignatius Loyola* (London: Printed for Richard Chiswell, 1688); George Lavington, *The Enthusiasm of Methodists and Papists Compar'd* (London: Printed for J. and P. Knapton, 1749); Samuel Roe, *Enthusiasm Detected, Defeated. With Previous Considerations Concerning Regeneration, the Omnipresence of God, and Divine Grace, &c.* (Cambridge: Printed for the author, by Fletcher and Hodson and sold by S. Crowder, J. Dodsley and M. Hingeston, 1768); Thomas Morgan, *Enthusiasm in Distress: Or, an Examination of the Reflections upon Reason, in a Letter to Phileleutherus Britannicus* (London: Printed for John Morley, 1722); Samuel Fancourt, *Enthusiasm Retorted . . .* (London: Printed by J. Humfreys, for Richard Ford, 1722);

Joseph Warton, *The Enthusiast: Or, the Lover of Nature. A Poem* (London: Printed for R. Dodsley; and sold by M. Cooper, 1744); Richard Kingston and John Morphew, *Enthusiastick Impostors no Divinely Inspir'd Prophets: Being an Historical Relation of the Rise, Progress, and Present Practices of the French and English Pretended Prophets . . .* (London: Sold by J. Morphew, 1707); John Allen, *The Enthusiast's Notion of Election to Eternal Life Disproved . . .* (Oxford: Printed for S. Parker, and D. Prince, and sold by J. Fletcher; London: 1769).

10. See, e.g., Ole Peter Grell, Jonathan I. Israel, and Nicholas Tyacke, eds., *From Persecution to Toleration: The Glorious Revolution and Religion in England* (Oxford: Clarendon Press, 1991); David Hempton, *Religion and Identity: Religious and Political Cultures in Britain and Ireland Since 1700* (Cambridge: Cambridge University Press, 1996).

11. See, e.g., Michael Heyd, "Robert Burton's Sources on Enthusiasm and Melancholy: From a Medical Tradition to Religious Controversy," *History of European Ideas* 5 (1984), pp. 17–44; Lawrence Babb, *Sanity in Bedlam: A Study of Robert Burton's Anatomy of Melancholy* (East Lansing: Michigan State University Press, 1959; Westport, Conn.: Greenwood Press, 1977); Stanley W. Jackson, "Robert Burton and Psychological Healing," *Journal of the History of Medicine and Allied Sciences* 44 (1989), pp. 160–78; Jackson, *Melancholia and Depression: from Hippocratic Times to Modern Times* (New Haven and London: Yale University Press, 1986); Porter, *Mind-Forg'd Manacles,* p. 21.

12. Earlier than Burton, the St. Bart's physician and (latterly) Anglican priest Timothy Bright had offered "consolation" to those with an "afflicted conscience," and his *A Treatise of Melancholie . . .* (London: Vautrollier, 1586) was among the books in John Monro's library. So too was Richard Baxter's *The Signs and Causes of Melancholy. With Directions Suited to the Case of those who are Afflicted with it. Collected out of the works of Mr. Richard Baxter . . . by Samuel Clifford* (London: Printed for S. Cruttenden and T. Cox, 1716). Monro, *Bibliotheca Elegantissima Monroiana,* nos. 424, 595.

13. Lawrence Babb, *The Elizabethan Malady: A Study of Melancholia in English Literature from 1580 to 1642* (East Lansing: Michigan State University Press, 1951); Veida Skultans, *English Madness: Ideas on Insanity 1580–1890* (London, Boston and Helley: Routledge and Kegan Paul, 1979), pp. 17–25; Porter, *Mind-Forg'd Manacles,* pp. 21–22, 28–29.

14. See, e.g., Günther Gawlick, "The English Deists' Contribution to the Theory of Toleration," *Studies on Voltaire and the Eighteenth Century* 152 (1976), pp. 823–35; Robert E. Sullivan, *John Toland and the Deist Controversy* (Cambridge, Mass.: Harvard University Press, 1982); J. A. Leo Lemay, ed. *Deism, Masonry, and the Enlightenment: Essays Honoring Alfred Owen Aldridge* (Newark: University of Delaware Press; London: Associated University Presses, 1987).

15. See, e.g., Edmund Hickeringill, *A Speech Without-doors . . . Proposed to . . . the Convention of Estates Assembled at Westminster, Jan. 22, 1688/9: Concerning I. Bigotism, or Religious Madness. II. Tests, and the Present Test in Particular. III. Penal Laws in Matters of Religion. IV. The Necessity of Changing*

and Recanting our Opinions in Religion. V. Restraint of the Press (London: Printed by George Larkin . . . , 1689).

16. Thanks to Steve King for this point. For examples of more traditional theological interpretations of dreams and visions, see Thomas Tryon, *A Treatise of Dreams and Visions . . . To Which is Added, a Discourse of the Causes, Natures and Cure of Phrensie, Madness or Distraction* (London: 1689); Rev'd David Simpson, *A Discourse on Dreams and Night-visions: With Numerous Examples Ancient and Modern* (Macclesfield: 1791); Malcolm Macleod, *Macleod's History of Witches &c: The Majesty of Darkness Discovered: in a Series of Tremendous Tales, Mysterious, Interesting, and Entertaining, of Apparitions, Witches, Augers, Magicians, Dreams, Visions, and Revelations, in Confirmation of a future State, & the Superintendency of a Divine Providence, by the Agency of Spirits and Angels* (London: Printed by and for I. Roach . . . , 1793). See also John Aubrey, *Miscellanies, viz. I. Day-fatality. II. Local-fatality. III. Ostenta. IV. Omens. V. Dreams. VI. Apparitions. VII. Voices. VIII. Impulses. IX. Knockings. X. Blows Invisible. XI. Prophesies. XII. Marvels. XIII. Magick. XIV. Transportation in the Air. XV. Visions in a Beril, or Glass. XVI. Converse with Angels and Spirits. XVII. Corps-candles in Wales. XVIII. Oracles. XIX. Exstasie. XX. Glances of Love. Envy. XXI. Second-sighted Persons* (London: Printed for Edward Castle . . . , 1696). Other contemporary literature, however, drew enthusiasm, madness, and medicine into a closer relation with such phenomena. For perhaps the earliest example, which predated the Restoration, see Alexander Ross, *Apocalypsis: Or, The Revelation of Certain Notorious Advancers of Heresie: Wherein their Visions and Private Revelations by Dreams, are Discovered to be most Incredible Blasphemies, and Enthusiastical Dotages . . .* , translated from Latin by John Davies, 2nd ed. (London: Printed for John Saywell . . . , 1688). This was a literature that culminated, perhaps, with William Newnham's *Essay on Superstition: Being an Inquiry into the Effects of Physical Influence on the Mind in the Production of Dreams, Visions, Ghosts, and other Supernatural Appearances* (London: J. Hatchard and son . . . , 1830).

17. See, e.g., Michael V. Deporte, *Nightmares and Hobbyhorses: Swift, Sterne, and Augustan Ideas of Madness* (San Marino, Calif.: Huntington Library, 1974).

18. See, e.g., W. M. Spellman, *The Latitudinarians and the Church of England, 1660–1700* (Athens and London: University of Georgia Press, 1993); Martin I. J. Griffin, Lila Freedman, and Richard Henry Popkin, *Latitudinarianism in the Seventeenth-Century Church of England* (Leiden: Brill, 1992); Richard W. F. Kroll, Richard Ashcraft, and Perez Zagorin, *Philosophy, Science, and Religion in England, 1640–1700* (Cambridge: Cambridge University Press, 1992); John Constable, *Deism and Christianity Fairly Consider'd, in Four Dialogues. To Which is Added a Fifth upon Latitudinarian Christianity. And Two Letters to a Friend upon a Book Intitled, The Moral Philosopher* (London: Printed by J. Hoyles, 1739).

19. Once again Steve King deserves our thanks for alerting us to this issue. See, e.g., Judith Jago, *Aspects of the Georgian Church: Visitation Studies of the Diocese of York, 1761–1776* (Madison, NJ: Fairleigh Dickinson University Press;

London: Associated University Presses, 1997); William Gibson, *The Achievement of the Anglican Church, 1689–1800: The Confessional State in Eighteenth Century England* (Lampeter and Lewiston, NY: Edwin Mellen Press, 1995).

20. Michael MacDonald, "The Secularization of Suicide in England 1660–1800," *Past & Present* 111 (May 1986), pp. 50–100; Michael MacDonald and Donna T. Andrew, "The Secularization of Suicide in England 1660–1800," *Past & Present* 119 (May 1988), pp. 158–170; Michael MacDonald, "The Medicalization of Suicide in England: Laymen, Physicians, and Cultural Change, 1500–1870," *Framing Disease: Studies in Cultural History,* ed. Charles E. Rosenberg and Janet Golden (New Brunswick, N.J.: Rutgers University Press, 1992), pp. 85–103; Michael MacDonald and Terence R. Murphy, *Sleepless Souls: Suicide in Early Modern England* (Oxford: Clarendon, 1990).

21. See, e.g., Thomas Lester Canavan, "Madness and Enthusiasm in Burton's *Anatomy of Melancholy* and Swift's *Tale of a Tub,*" Ph.D. diss., Columbia University, 1970.

22. For what remains an excellent synthesizing discussion of these themes, see Porter, *Mind-Forg'd Manacles,* pp. 62–81. See also Porter, "The Rage of Party: A Glorious Revolution in English Psychiatry?" *Medical History* 29 (1983), pp. 35–50.

23. See, e.g., Anon. [Brother Lunatic], *The Enthusiastic Infidel Detected: Being a Trial of a Moral Philosopher before the Grand Senate of Bedlam on a Statute of Lunacy, for Publishing a Rhapsody Intitled, The Resurrection of Jesus Considered, in Answer to the Trial of the Witnesses, by a Brother Lunatic* (London: Printed for Charles Corbett, 1743); Richard Brown, *The Case of Naaman Considered: A Sermon Preached Before the University of Oxford, at St. Mary's, on Sunday, October 12, 1740* (Oxford: Printed at the Theatre for Richard Clements, & sold by C. Rivington, J. and P. Knapton, and J. Roberts, 1741); Brown, *Job's Expectation of a Resurrection Considered. Three Sermons, etc.* (Oxford: Richard Clements, 1747).

24. Roy Porter, "Foucault's Great Confinement," *History of the Human Sciences* 3.1 (1990), 47–54.

25. Of course, one can overdo the portrayal of contested spheres here, and this argument is not intended to deny that the real power of Methodism resided in its stepping into areas where neither doctors nor the Anglican clergy were well represented. Thanks again to Steve King for pointing this out.

26. For a recent study of the links existing and drawn between Catholicism and Methodism in the eighteenth century, see David Butler, *Methodists and Papists: John Wesley and the Catholic Church in the Eighteenth Century* (London: Darton, Longman & Todd, 1995). For one of many contemporary diatribes against the virtually synonymous madness of the two religions, see, e.g., Lavington, *Methodists and Papists Compar'd.*

27. For a good working definition of "insensibility," best used to describe late eighteenth-century "opposition to the principles and values of Enlightenment," or less usefully and coherently, perhaps, to characterize "subversive tendencies within the age of Enlightenment itself," see John W. Yolton et al., *The Blackwell Companion to the Enlightenment* (Oxford: Basil Blackwell, 1991), pp. 108–10.

28. Thomas Monro (1764–1815) of Magdalen College, Oxford, *Essays on Various Subjects* (London: Printed by J. Nichols & sold by G. G. J. & J. Robinson, 1790), essay 12, pp. 111–20, esp. pp. 117–18. He was one of many trenchant contemporary critics of stoicism.

29. See, e.g., Isabel Rivers, *Reason, Grace, and Sentiment: A Study of the Language of Religion and Ethics in England, 1660–1780* (Cambridge: Cambridge University Press, 1991); John Mullan, *Sentiment and Sociability: The Language of Feeling in the Eighteenth Century* (1988; Oxford: Clarendon Press, 1990); Mackenzie, *The Man of Feeling*.

30. See, e.g., James Boswell, *The Hypochondriak*, ed. Margery Bailey (Stanford: Stanford University Press, 1928); Roy Porter, "'The Hunger of Imagination': Approaching Samuel Johnson's Melancholy," *The Anatomy of Madness*, ed. William F. Bynum, Roy Porter, and Michael Shepherd, vol. 1 (London: Tavistock, 1985), pp. 63–88.

31. See, e.g., Edward Young, *The Complaint: Or, Night-thoughts on Life, Death, and Immortality* (London: Printed for R. Dodsley and sold by M. Cooper, 1744); Thomas Gray, *An Elegy Wrote in a Country Church Yard: The Eton Manuscript & the First Edition, 1751*, reproduced in facsimile with an introduction by Alastair MacDonald (Ilkley, Yorkshire: Scolar Press, 1976); Robert Blair, *The Grave, A Poem* (London: Printed at the Cicero Press by Henry Fry for Scatcherd & Whitaker, 1787).

32. W. Wale, ed., *George Whitefield's Journals: To Which is Prefixed his "Short Account" and "Further Account"* (London: Henry J. Drane, 1905), pp. 261–67; *George Whitefield's Letters. For the Period 1734–42* (Edinburgh: The Banner of Truth Trust, 1976), letters 13, 273, 295, 497; Curnock, *The Journal of the Reverend John Wesley*, vol. 2, 17 Sept. 1740, 22 Feb. 1750, 12 May 1759.

33. For a useful general discussion of these issues, see Roy Porter, *Mind-Forg'd Manacles*, pp. 62–81.

34. Curnock, *The Journal of the Reverend John Wesley*, vol. 2, 17 Sept. 1740; Hunter and Macalpine, *Three Hundred Years of Psychiatry*, pp. 422–23.

35. Letter from Susannah Wesley to John Wesley, 19 Dec. 1746, Methodist Church, London, Colman Collection, reprinted in Hunter and Macalpine, *Three Hundred Years of Psychiatry*, p. 423; complaining of "poor Mr. MacCune" falling into the hands of "that wretched fellow Monroe," despite the fact that "by what I hear, the man is not Lunatick, but rather under strong convictions of Sin; and hath much more need of a Spiritual, than Bodily Physician. . . . Monroe last night sent him to a madhouse at Chelsea, where he is to undergo their usual methods of Cure in case of real Madness. . . ."

36. J. Phelps, *The Human Barometer, or, Living Weather-Glass; a Philosophick Poem* (London: 1743), p. 21. See also John Rich, *The Spirit of Contradiction. A New Comedy of Two Acts [and in prose]. By a Gentleman of Cambridge [i.e. J. Rich]* (London: 1760); *The Necromancer; or, Harlequin Doctor Faustus* was performed at the Theatre Royal in Lincoln's Inn Fields in 1723 and 1731. For published editions, see, e.g., Rich, *A Dramatick Entertainment, Called the Necromancer; or, Harlequin Doctor Faustus . . .* , as performed at the Theatre Royal in Lincoln's Inn Fields, 4th and 9th eds. (London: Printed and sold by

T. Wood, 1724 and 1731). For a satire on the latter, see Thomas Merrivale, *The Necromancer; or, Harlequin Doctor Faustus: a Poem; Founded on the Gentile Theology* (London: Printed and sold by J. Roberts in Warwick-lane, 1724) [dedicated to the pantomime *The Necromancer; or, Harlequin Doctor Faustus*, produced by John Rich at Lincoln's Inn Fields Theatre, 20 Dec. 1723].

37. See, e.g., *LEP*, no. 5997 (10–12 April 1766), p. 3, col. 3. "Wednesday afternoon, about five o'clock, the Quack Doctor that daily exhibits in Moorfields, cut off and dressed upon his stage, in a few minutes, a Wen from a man's face, which was said to weigh near nine pounds. There was a prodigious number of spectators present. . . ."

38. Anon., *British Frenzy: Or, the Mock-Apollo. A Satyr* [with special reference to the harlequinades of John Rich] (London: J. Robinson, 1745).

39. See, e.g., William Rufus Chetwood, *A General History of the Stage . . . with Memoirs of Most of the Principal Performers . . . for these Last Fifty Years . . .* (London: Printed for W. Owen, 1749); *The British Stage, or, The exploits of Harlequin: A Farce* (London: Printed for T. Warner, 1724), burlesque of Thurmond's *Harlequin Doctor Faustus* and Rich's *The Necromancer; or, Harlequin Doctor Faustus*, designed as an after-entertainment for the audiences of these plays.

40. Note also the scatological double entendre behind the word "stool."

41. *Bethlem A Poem* (1744), allegedly "By a Patient"; see Andrews, "Bedlam Revisited," appendix 2b, p. 556.

42. The playwright and man-about-town Samuel Foote, whose 1760 farce *The Minor* had launched a furious pamphlet war with supporters of Whitefield and Wesley, hastened to cement the association: "The force and miserable effects of Whitefield's mystical doctrines are obvious enough. *Bedlam* loudly proclaims the power of your preacher, and scarce a street in town but boasts its tabernacle; where some, from interested views, and others—unhappy creatures! Mistaking the idle offspring of a distempered brain for divine inspiration, broach such doctrines as are not only repugnant to Christianity, but destructive even to civil society." *A Letter from Mr Foote to the Reverend Author of Remarks, Critical and Christian, on 'The Minor'* (London: For the author, 1760). *The Minor*, a bawdy farce lampooning Whitefield, opened in July 1760 at the author's own little theater in the Haymarket (see *Lloyd's Evening Post*, 14 July 1760). Transferred in November after its successful first run to David Garrick's Theatre Royal in Drury Lane, it played to large and fashionable audiences, notwithstanding efforts by the Methodists' chief aristocratic patron, the countess of Huntingdon, to secure its suppression. Foote himself played all three of the play's characters, "Shift," "Smirk," and "Mrs Cole" (a prostitute given to canting about "the new Birth"), in a broad-ranging assault on "the Itinerant Field Orators, who are at declared enmity with common sense, and yet have the address to poison the principles, and, at the same time, to pick the pockets of half our industrious fellow-subjects." Whitefield was the particular target of Foote's ire, savagely burlesqued as the hypocritical and money-grubbing "Dr. Squintum," a characterization soon picked up in popular ballads and spread through vicious caricatures mass-produced for popular consumption.

43. See the contemporaneous attack by the Baptist minister on the Wesley-ites, John Macgowan, *The Foundry Budget Opened; Or, the Arcanum of Wes-leyanism Disclosed* (Manchester: Button, 1780; London, 1780). This was a re-ply to Walter Sellon, *A Defence of God's Sovereignty Against the Impious and Horrible Aspersions Cast Upon it by Elisha Coles, in his Practical Treatise on that Subject,* new ed., in *The Works of the Rev. W. Sellon,* vol. 2 (London: 1814). Coles's *A Practical Discourse of God's Sovereignty: With Other Material Points Deriving Thence* (London: Ben. Griffin for E. C., 1678) went into its 14th edition in 1762. For the continuous association of the Methodists with the foundry, see, e.g., Ralph M. Spoor, *Illustrated Hand-book to City Road Chapel, Burying-ground, and Wesley's House; with Notices of the Foundry and Bunhill Fields Burying-ground* (with a historical preface by G. J. Stevenson) (London: Wesleyan Conference Office, 1881).

44. See, e.g., Hunter and Macalpine, introduction to the facsimile edition, p. 11; C. N. French, *The Story of St. Luke's Hospital* (London: William Heine-mann, 1951), pp. 11–13. Among St. Luke's governors were prominent religious sectarians such as the Methodist Peter Dobree, who recommended nine patients for admission to St. Luke's in 1753; the great supporter of evangelicals and rich banker John Thornton (1720–90), who recommended twenty-one patients to St. Luke's in 1753–54 and twenty-six in 1758; and his son, the Clapham sect leader and banker Henry Thornton (1760–1815). Also on the St. Luke's board was Bonnell Thornton (1724–68), a.k.a. "the Rev. Busby Birch," the satirical writer who contributed to an Oxbridge student periodical in which Christopher Smart was a guiding hand. He was also joint author, with George Colman (1732–94), of *The Connoisseur* (1757), a magazine with rather puritanical, dis-senting sympathies, which was critical of the practice of visiting at Bethlem. Bonnell Thornton recommended five patients to St. Luke's in 1752. (Sir) Henry Cheere (1703–81), the Clapham sculptor and friend of the Thorntons', who sent his own son to a dissenting academy, was also on St. Luke's board, recom-mending seventeen patients in 1755. All of these men were significantly involved in philanthropic undertakings with a particularly dissenting flavor in the second half of the eighteenth century, many of them medical in nature. The Thorntons were close friends of William Wilberforce and of the onetime mentally deranged poet William Cowper (who himself wrote for *The Connoisseur*). (Thanks to the archivist Robert Leon for allowing the authors access to the list he has compiled of recommending governors at St. Luke's, and to Matthew Craske for helping to identify and further draw our attention to the sectarian involvement at St. Luke's.) See Christian (i.e., Peter Dobree), *Prayers, Thanksgivings and Med-itations to Assist the Devout Christian in his Preparation for and Attendance at the Lord's Supper . . .* (London: J. Mechell, 1746); Standish Meacham, *Henry Thornton of Clapham, 1760–1815* (Cambridge, Mass.: Harvard University Press, 1964); John Thornton, *The Love of Christ the Source of Genuine Phi-lanthropy . . . Occasioned by the Death of J. Thornton, etc.* (London: 1791); SLGCM, passim.

45. French, *Story of St. Luke's,* pp. 11, 13.

46. *LEP,* no. 3590 (23–25 Oct. 1750).

47. See Rev. L. Tyerman, *The Life and Times of the Rev. John Wesley, M.A., Founder of the Methodists,* vol. 2, 3rd. ed. (London: Hodder and Stoughton, 1876), pp. 364–65.

48. Lewis, *Correspondence,* vol. 9, pp. 398–99 and note 22. According to Walpole, Whitefield subsequently sought to exploit the Ferrers case as a moral exemplum in his sermons, apparently as a parable of the fate awaiting the heartless. We have, however, been unable to trace any record of these sermons in the preacher's published works.

49. Quoted in Rev. L. Tyerman, *The Life of the Rev. George Whitefield,* vol. 2 (New York: Randolph and Company, 1877), p. 426.

50. E.g., George Whitefield, *Twenty-three Sermons on Various Subjects. To Which are Added Several Prayers,* new ed. (London: Printed by W. Strahan and Sold at the Tabernacle near Upper Moorfields & at Hoxton, 1745), sermon 11, "Intercession every Christian's duty," pp. 175–90, esp. p. 184.

51. Whitefield, *Twenty-three Sermons,* sermon 18, "The Wise and Foolish Virgins," p. 325.

52. See Scull, *The Most Solitary of Afflictions,* pp. 175–78, on which we draw freely in what follows.

53. For a late seventeenth-century example of a "melancholic" who placed precisely such a set of religious interpretations on her sufferings, see Hannah Allen, *A Narrative of God's Gracious Dealings with that Choice Christian Mrs. Hannah Allen . . . Reciting the Great Advantages the Devil Made of her Deep Melancholy . . .* (London: Wallis, 1683).

54. See Henry D. Rack, "Doctors, Demons and Early Methodist Healing," *The Church and Healing,* ed. W. J. Sheils (Oxford: Blackwell, 1982), pp. 137–52; Ian Bostridge, *Witchcraft and Its Transformations 1650–1750* (Oxford: Clarendon Press, 1997); James Sharpe, *Instruments of Darkness: Witchcraft in England 1550–1750* (London: Hamish Hamilton, 1996); Owen Davies, "Methodism, the Clergy, and the Popular Belief in Witchcraft and Magic," *History* 82 (1997), pp. 252–65.

55. See John Wesley, *The Journals of John Wesley,* ed. Ernest Rhys (London: Everyman, 1906), e.g., vol. 1, pp. 190, 210, 363, 412, 551; vol. 2, pp. 225, 461, 489.

56. Lines from "The Mechanic Inspir'd: or, the Methodist's Welcome to Frome: A Ballad," *Poems on Various Subjects, with Some Essays in Prose, Letters to Correspondents, &c. and a Treatise on Health,* by Samuel Bowden (Bath: For the author, 1754). Box was a small West Country madhouse that had apparently existed since some time in the seventeenth century.

57. Among John's books were Meric Casaubon, *The Vindication or Defence of Isaac Casaubon Against those Impostors that Lately Published an Impious and Unlearned Pamphlet, Intituled The Originall of Idolatries, &c. Under his Name* (London: Printed by Bonham Norton, and John Bull, 1624); George Whitefield, *A Compleat Account of the Conduct of Mr Whitefield* (1739; unfortunately, we have been unable to locate publication details for this work); Whitefield, *A Journal of a Voyage from London to Savannah in Georgia. In two Parts . . .* (London: Printed for James Hutton, 1738); Whitefield, *A Continuation of the Reverend Mr Whitefield's Journal, from his Arrival at London, to his*

Departure from Thence on his Way to Georgia (London: Printed by W. Strahan, and sold by James Hutton, 1739); Whitefield, *A Short Account of God's Dealings with G[eorge] W[hitefield]* . . . *from his Infancy to the Time of his Entering into Holy Orders* (London: 1740); *The Quaker and Methodist Compared. In an Abstract of George Fox's Journal. With a Copy of his Last Will and Testament, and of the Reverend Mr. George Whitefield's Journals* . . . (London: Printed for J. Millan, 1740). Monro, *Bibliotheca Elegantissima Monroiana,* nos. 70 and 1359. John's library also contained many of the leading early modern English works on the "demoniacs" of the Old (and New) Testament—the authenticity of whose putative diabolical possession and miraculous dispossession had been repeatedly challenged by medical writers and Anglican divines, while concurrently being vigorously defended by a number of metropolitan and provincial and low churchmen, nonconformists, and Catholics.

58. *LEP,* no. 5969 (28–30 Jan. 1766), p. 3, col. 2.

59. von la Roche, *Sophie in London,* p. 170.

60. William Black, *A Dissertation on Insanity: Illustrated with Tables, and Extracted from Between two and three Thousand Cases in Bedlam* (London: Ridgway, 1810), pp. 18–19. This was a further, much enlarged edition of an earlier work by Black, *A Comparative View of the Mortality of the Human Species, at all Ages; and of the Diseases and Casualties by which they are Destroyed or Annoyed* (London: Dilly, 1788).

61. Haslam had thanked the Methodists (ironically) for providing him with so many patients, declaring "that the whole of their doctrine is a base system of delusion, riveted on the mind by terror and despair, and there is also good reason to suppose, that they frequently contrive, by the grace of cordials to fix the waverings of belief, and thus endeavour to dispel the gloom and dejection which these hallucinations infallibly excite." The *Annual Medical Register* had thoroughly approved of his "bold and manly" views, instructing "the disciples and advocates of methodism" to "read this and tremble." See Haslam, *Observations on Madness and Melancholy,* pp. 266–67; *The Annual Medical Register for the Year 1808–9,* vol. 2 (London: Printed by J. Mayes for John Murray, 1810), pp. 170–80, 306–07, esp. p. 179.

62. Pargeter, *Observations on Maniacal Disorders,* p. 134.

63. Ibid., pp. 31, 34, 35.

64. Ibid., pp. 32, 36. Pargeter, for example, spoke of one patient whose "misfortunes originated in [being] . . . publicly reproved by a clergyman for sleeping during divine service, which gave him so much offence that he seceded from the Church, and attached himself to the *Methodists; these deluded people* soon reduced him to the unhappy state in which I found him." On visiting another woman in a state of religious mania, Pargeter observed—in a somewhat Hogarthian way—copies of *"Wesley's Journal, Watt's Hymns the Pilgrim's Progress,* and *the Fiery Furnace of Affliction"* by her bedside, and was told by her husband that her mind had been turned by a Methodist preacher who "had much infested the parish." Of another patient who was said to have "followed the Methodists," Pargeter commented "that his behaviour since he had embraced the tenets of that sect, became gradually morose—he wandered from home by himself—would scarcely give an answer when spoken to, and his re-

pose by night was greatly interrupted." See ibid., pp. 31–37, 79–80, and the quotation at the opening of this chapter.

65. For Cox's discussion of Haslam and his own elaborate, if still somewhat cautious, defense of Methodism and attack on the "illiberal" bigotry and sectarianism of its detractors, see Cox, *Practical Observations on Insanity,* pp. 25–28. For Haslam's scathing commentary on Cox, and his mocking dismissal of the Evangelicals, see his *Observations on Madness and Melancholy,* pp. 303, 307, 330–31, 340–41; and his pamphlet, *A Letter to the Metropolitan Commissioners in Lunacy* (London: Whittaker, Treacher, 1830), pp. 4–5, 17–18.

66. Crowther, *Practical Remarks on Insanity,* pp. 80–85.

67. Ibid., p. 81.

68. For a useful, if old-fashioned, biography of Cruden, on which we have drawn for some of the details that follow, see Edith Oliver, *Alexander the Corrector: The Eccentric Life of Alexander Cruden* (London: Faber and Faber; New York: Viking, 1934). See also *DNB* entry on Cruden.

69. Oliver, *The Eccentric Life,* p. 33.

70. Cruden himself preferred a Scottish analogy: "it will be found that those who meddled with Alexander, touched a thistle which hurt themselves." Cruden, *Adventures,* part 1, p. 16.

71. For information on Derby, see, e.g., George Edward Cokayne, *The Complete Peerage of England, Scotland, Ireland, Great Britain, and the United Kingdom,* vol. 4 (London: St. Catherine Press, 1916), p. 216; William Pollard, *The Stanleys of Knowsley: A History of that Noble Family, Including a Sketch of the Political and Public Lives of the Right Hon. the Earl of Derby, K.G. . . .* (Liverpool: E. Howell, 1868).

72. Cruden's correspondence with Lord Derby is preserved in the Bodleian Library; Bodleian MS Rawl. C793 (16).

73. Ibid., letter dated 1729, fol. 17.

74. Reginald Blunt, *The Wonderful Village: A Further Record of Some Famous Folk and Places By Chelsea Reach* (London: Mills and Boon, 1918), p. 46. For some years in the aftermath of this debacle, Cruden worked as a private tutor in the Isle of Man, an employment that just possibly was secured with Derby's assistance. But by 1732 he had returned to London, setting himself up in business with a bookseller's shop at the Royal Exchange.

75. E.g., Alexander Cruden, *Cruden's Complete Concordance to the Old and New Testaments* (Peabody, Mass.: Hendrickson Publishers, 1984). Cruden's *Concordance* was first published in 1737 and reached its 42nd edition in 1879.

76. Cruden, *Adventures,* part 1, p. 4.

77. Cruden was not the only zealot to receive Queen Caroline's patronage. She also tendered her support, for example, to William Whiston (1667–1752), M.A., the apocalyptic prophet, clerk, and former follower of Isaac Newton, who was charged with heresy, thrown out of Cambridge University, and tried in the 1730s for defaming and denying the Holy Trinity. See, e.g., William Whiston, *Memoirs of the Life and Writings of Mr. William Whiston. Containing Memoirs of Several of his Friends also* (1713; London: Printed for the author, and sold by Mr. Whiston; and Mr. Bishop, 1749–50). Whiston quickly lost his patronage from polite society after styling himself as a Jewish prophet. Notably he was also

a defender of the authenticity of the demoniacs: William Whiston, *An Account of the Dæmoniacks, and of the Power of Casting out Dæmons* . . . (London: Printed for John Whiston, 1737). Thanks to David Nash for alerting us to some of these facts.

78. Alexander Cruden, letters to Sir Hans Sloane, British Museum, Manuscripts Dept., Additional MS4041.

79. Alexander Cruden, *A Verbal Index to Milton's Paradise Lost. Adapted to Every Edition but the First, Which was Publish'd in Ten Books Only* (London: Sold by W. Innys and D. Browne, 1741).

80. See Alexander Cruden, *A Compendium of the Holy Bible . . . To Which is Prefixed, a Brief Account of the History and Excellency of the Scriptures* (London, J. Lewis, 1750), and Cruden's entry in old *DNB*. See also Matthew Henry, *An Exposition of the Historical Books of the Old Testament* . . . (London: Printed for T. Parkhurst, J. Robinson, and J. Lawrence, 1708); Henry, *An Exposition of the Five Poetical Books of the Old Testament* . . . (London: Printed by T. Darrack, for T. Parkhurst, J. Robinson, and J. Lawrence, 1710). This book was later retitled as a devotional *Commentary*, but, unfortunately, we have been unable to locate the precise edition of Henry's *Commentary* that Cruden worked on.

81. The Board of Green Cloth invigilated over the district within the verge (or ca. fifteen miles) of the royal court and sent a substantial number of similar offenders to Bethlem. See Cruden, *Adventures*, part 3, p. 64; Jonathan Andrews, "The Politics of Committal to Early-Modern Bethlem," *Medicine in the Enlightenment*, ed. Roy Porter (Amsterdam: Rodopi, 1995), pp. 1–63. See also chapter 6.

82. Alexander Cruden, *The London Citizen Exceedingly Injured, or a British Inquisition Display'd . . . Addressed to the Legislature, as Plainly Shewing the Absolute Necessity of Regulating Private Madhouses* (London: Cooper and Dodd, 1739), reprinted in Ingram, *Voices of Madness*, p. 26.

83. The origin of Wightman's connection with Cruden remains obscure. Cruden claimed in the title-page of *The London-Citizen*, that he was "a mere Stranger." Wightman appears to have been a prominent Edinburgh merchant (see note 103, below) and a writer on religion and moral philosophy, strongly influenced by the ideas of the Scottish Enlightenment. His experiences with Cruden seem to have only encouraged his rather derogatory views of religious enthusiasm. For Wightman's political, philosophical, and religious views and interests, see, e.g., Robert Wightman, *A Specimen of Peculiar Thoughts upon Sublime, Abstruse and Delicate Subjects: Written Occasionally, in Monsieur Paschel's Manner . . . Intended as an Introduction to a Book, Entituled, Hidden Things Unveil'd, or, The Unseen World Uncovered; Wherein Natural Religion, Enthusiasm and Self-love, . . . are Explicated . . .* (Edinburgh: s.n., 1738); Wightman, *Private Letters [by Philotheus and Theophilus] Adapted to Publick Use, Written on Occasion of the As[semb]ly's Taking Cognisance of P[ro]f[esso]r [Archibald] C[ampbel]l's Writings . . .* (Edinburgh: 1736). Philotheus (fl. 899) was the Roman logician and author of the *Kletorologion*. Campbell, D.D. (1691–1756), St. Andrews Professor of Divinity and Ecclesiastical History, was a rather unorthodox bastion of the Scottish Presbyterian Church and a key

Christian philosopher and theologian of the Scottish Enlightenment, with whom (like Wightman) Cruden must surely have been familiar. (Cruden, of course, had been brought up a strict Presbyterian and was violently opposed to the secession of 1733 in the Scottish Church, but it was mostly toward the English Church that he looked after migrating to London.)

84. Throwing oneself on the mercy of the Lord Mayor was a relatively common recourse for those seeking protection against false imprisonment in this period. The mayor was not only representative head of city government and upholder of the legal rights and freedoms of its citizens; he was also a virtual non-officio member (and mayors were regularly also presidents) of the Bridewell and Bethlem Court of Governors. Therefore, this seems a thoroughly prudent way for Cruden to have sought to avoid confinement in Bethlem.

85. Cruden, *The London-Citizen*, title page, pp. 23, 74.

86. Ibid., p. 33.

87. Ibid., p. 38, emphasis in the original.

88. Ibid. When Cruden subsequently learned of James Monro's views, he was most indignant at the misrepresentation of his theological position. He was, he averred, "no Stoick, but believed in the Promise and Providence of God to be delivered in the use of Means" (i.e., rather than simply submitting to fate, Cruden believed it was his duty to employ such means as God permitted to come to hand to effect his release from the madhouse).

89. Unfortunately, none of these letters appear to have survived, and there is no record at Bethlem of any letter received from Cruden.

90. Cruden, *The London-Citizen*, especially pp. 39, 41–42, 47–49, 60, 68; Cruden, *Mr Cruden Greatly Injured*, p. 14.

91. Cruden, *Mr Cruden Greatly Injured*, p. 6.

92. Possibly the Robert Innes, A.M., who was author of *Miscellaneous Letters on Several Subjects in Philosophy and Astronomy: Wrote to the Learned Dr. Nicholson* . . . (London: Printed for S. Birt, 1732), or else related to the Robert Innes who received his M.D. thesis in 1753 from Edinburgh University, Robert Innes, *Dissertatio medica inauguralis, de ileo quam annuente summo numine* . . . (Edinburgh: Hamilton, Balfour, & Neill, 1753).

93. Possibly Joseph Rogers (1677–1753), who wrote *An Essay on Epidemic Diseases; and more Particularly on the Endemial Epidemics of the City of Cork, such as Fevers and Small-pox* . . . (Dublin: W. Smith, 1734), or else the Stamford practitioner who invented the "oleum arthriticum."

94. Cruden, *The London-Citizen*, pp. 42, 63; Munk, *Roll*, vol. 2, pp. 62–66, 97.

95. Cruden, *The London-Citizen*, p. 51.

96. Around 29 May; ibid., p. 54.

97. Cruden, *Mr Cruden Greatly Injured*, p. 24.

98. The action was ultimately moved to and decided in the Court of Common Pleas.

99. Ibid., p. 74. This trial occurred on 17 July 1739 and Monro and co. were defended by William Round, attorney. The only record of this trial we have been able to find outside of Cruden's account tells us very little about the case. See Cruden, *Mr Cruden Greatly Injured*, and PRO, Court of Common Pleas Pro-

thonotory Rolls and Docket Rolls, CP 40.3499, "Special issue in Assault & imprisonment; Jenkin for Cruden; Round for Wright & others," 674. Searches through other trial records at the PRO, including Affidavits CP3.11 and CP3.12; and Posteas Series CP41.53 and 54, have proved unavailing.

100. Cruden, *Mr Cruden Greatly Injured,* p. 21.

101. James had also been (unsuccessfully) sued once before this, by the Bethlem patient Thomas Leigh, the hospital's governors supporting their doctor against the charge. Leigh's suit was filed in the King's Bench in 1742 and the hospital filed bail and defended the action on Monro's behalf. See Bridewell General Committee Minutes, 22 Oct. 1742, p. 126.

102. Cruden, *Mr Cruden Greatly Injured,* pp. 34–35.

103. See ibid., p. 25, where Cruden claims that Wightman "went home to Edinburgh with Dr Monro's Son." In his usual hearsay style, Cruden alleged that "a noble Lord, well known in the House of Peers . . . had some knowledge of Wightman, and calls him a Madish sort of Man . . . notorious in Scotland for his wild Projects," including running the city of Edinburgh "into Debt" through his Leith pier project. Possibly, this peer was the earl of Hopeton, who had formerly been engaged with Wightman in a suit over a trading contract. See *Information for Robert Wightman and others against the Earl of Hopeton* (Scotland: s.n., 1730): "In the year 1722, The Earl of Hopeton entered into a contract with some merchants in Holland. . . . In the year 1723, his Lordship also made a contract with the said Robert Wightman and others." Wightman seems to have been related to John Wightman, also an Edinburgh merchant, and both were clearly prominent in trading and political intriguing in Edinburgh. See, e.g., Alexander Stevenson, *Copy Bill of Suspension, Preston &c., Against Wightman &c.* (Edinburgh: No publisher, 1721) (copy in King's College Library, Special Collections, University of Aberdeen, Thomson 1/20).

104. Cruden, *Adventures,* part 1, pp. 5–6.

105. Ibid., pp. 8–9. "Little Chelsea" was a detached hamlet consisting of a handful of farms and houses strung out along the road to Fulham, on the northwestern edge of "Great Chelsea," where Duffield's madhouses were located.

106. Ibid., p. 12.

107. Ibid., p. 14.

108. Ibid., p. 18.

109. Ibid., p. 22.

110. See especially Cruden's account of Monro's visits on 14, 18, 21, 25 and 27 Sept., ibid., pp. 14, 18, 20, 22–23, 24–25.

111. Ibid., p. 18.

112. Ibid., p. 22. It was, however, a purely tactical retreat: once released, Cruden gave voice to his conviction that he was a chosen one: "God," he informed his readers,

doth great and mighty wonders in his Providence, which is always righteous yet often mysterious, and he by his secret power and wisdom can bring about great and valuable purposes by seeming contrary means. . . . The Corrector is of opinion that his confinement and sufferings were emblematical and typical of something good and great designed by Providence for him; and has great reason of thankfulness that God greatly supported him, and turned his prison into a palace. (p. 39)

113. Ibid., part 2, p. 21.

114. Ibid., p. 22.

115. Subsequently, Cruden alleged, Isabella had designs on securing her brother's prompt admission to St. Luke's, but her plans were foiled as there were fifteen prospective patients on the admissions list ahead of him—a circumstance Cruden promptly attributed to divine intervention on his behalf. The baroque admission procedures Henry Fielding had complained about (see note 8 of chapter 2) thus had inadvertently kept him from being "dragged to that dishonourable place . . . No person could have a greater dread of it than the Corrector." Ibid., pp. 35–36.

116. E.g., on Monday, 1 October, he recorded that "the Corrector took his purging draught prescribed by Dr. Monro"; ibid., p. 25.

117. Ibid., pp. 27–28.

118. Ibid., p. 33, emphasis in the original.

119. Ibid., p. 34.

120. See Cruden's own verbose account of the court proceedings, *The Second Part of the Adventures of Alexander the Corrector, Giving an Account of a Memorable, or Rather Monstrous, Battle Fought, or Rather Not Fought, in Westminster Hall February 20 1754* (London: Cooper, 1754), passim. Attempts to locate the original records for this trial at the PRO have also proved fruitless; see PRO, King's Bench Judgement Books, CP47.39, and Affidavits, CP3.19 and CP41.84–87, 1754–55.

121. Cruden, *Adventures,* part 2, p. 28.

122. Ibid., part 1, pp. 14, 22.

123. Ibid., p. 21.

124. Ibid.

125. Ibid., part 2, p. 31.

126. Such a conceit obviously derived in part from Cruden's deep-rooted Calvinist conviction that as one of God's elect, he was destined for divinely ordained glory. However, the specifics of this latest scheme may possibly have been suggested by another contemporary critic of the morals of the nation, the novelist and magistrate Henry Fielding. One of Fielding's alter egos in his *Covent Garden Journal* beginning in January 1752 was "Sir Alexander [*sic*] Drawcansir, Knt. Censor of Great Britain," who served as "General" of a paper army in a series of mock-heroic wars. The follies and fashions of the capital, with its swarms of "Bawds, Whores, Thieves, Cullies, Fools and Drunkards," its ill-bred "People of Fashion," and legions of placemen and corrupt politicians, provided Fielding with an endless parade of examples with which to mock the delusions and dunces of the Augustan age. Fielding's interventions drew widespread attention in the contemporary press, and Sir Alexander Drawcansir and his classical lineage must assuredly have come to Alexander Cruden's attention. Cruden's Quixote, however, meant to tilt at a multitude of windmills in deadly earnest.

127. Cruden, *Adventures,* part 2, pp. 3–4.

128. Ibid., title page.

129. Cruden, *Adventures,* part 3, p. 64.

130. Cruden, *Adventures,* part 3, p. 4.

131. Ibid., p. 5.

132. Ibid., p. 8, emphasis in the original.

133. Ibid., p. 7, emphasis in the original.

134. Ibid., pp. 5–6.

135. Ibid., p. 7, emphasis in the original.

136. Alexander Cruden, *Alexander the Corrector's Humble Address and Earnest Application to Our Most Gracious King . . . Shewing the Necessity of Appointing a Corrector of the People* (London: For the author, 1755), pp. 4, 16, emphasis in the original.

137. Ibid., p. 7, emphasis in the original.

138. Ibid., p. 10, emphasis in the original. See also British Library Add. Ms. 32,853, fols. 129–30; and his petition to the duke of Newcastle, enclosing draft legislation to appoint him as Corrector, British Library Add. Ms. 32,861, fols. 238–39.

139. The king's levée was a formal reception held daily at St. James's Palace. Male members of the general public, provided they were known to someone at court, were permitted to attend, though no one could speak to the king unless spoken to. In Horace Walpole's words, "that was always thought High Treason." In agonies of frustration, Cruden pestered assorted courtiers to intervene in his behalf.

140. Cruden, *Adventures*, part 3, p. 50.

141. Alexander Cruden, *Memorial Concerning Elizabeth Canning Humbly Offered to His Majesty's gracious Consideration*. This memorial, which includes a portrait of Elizabeth Canning, and letters supporting it, is held at the Bodleian, Smith Newsb. C7, fols. 9–10.

142. For other works on Canning, see, e.g., Anon., *The Case of Elizabeth Canning Fairly Stated* (London: 1753).

143. Cruden, *Adventures*, part 3.

144. Cruden, *The London-Citizen*, pp. 33, 45, 48.

145. Ibid., pp. 25, 29, 43–46, 49–54; Cruden, *Mr Cruden Greatly Injured*, pp. 4, 7; Cruden, *Adventures*, part 1, title page.

146. For references to restraint, see especially Cruden, *The London-Citizen*, pp. 30–32, 34, 36, 37, 38; Cruden, *Adventures*, part 1, pp. 8, 13.

147. Between 8 and 19 April, for example, apart from Monro and Wightman, Cruden received at least twenty-one visits, although a few of these were from those Cruden regarded as far from friends. By contrast, between 6 and 18 May Cruden had no visitors at all, besides the madhouse servants and its proprietor, Wright. For visitors admitted and excluded from him in 1738 and 1753, see Cruden, *The London-Citizen*, pp. 25, 31–32, 34, 36, 37, 39, 40–41, 51–52; Cruden, *Adventures*, part 1, pp. 22, 24.

148. Cruden, *Adventures*, part 1, p. 19.

149. For his garden and parlor privileges at both institutions, see Cruden, *The London-Citizen*, pp. 32–34, 36, 38–39, 47; Cruden, *Adventures*, part 1, pp. 14, 22.

150. Cruden, *The London-Citizen*, p. 33; Cruden, *Adventures*, part 1, p. 18.

151. Cruden, *Mr Cruden Greatly Injured*, part 1, p. 24.

152. Cruden, *Adventures*, part 2, pp. 22, 29–30.

153. Cruden, *The London-Citizen,* pp. 33, 45, 48, 71; Cruden, *Adventures,* part 1, p. 18.

154. Cruden, *Adventures,* part 1, p. 18.

155. Ibid.

156. Ibid.

157. Cruden, *The London Citizen,* pp. 36, 42; Cruden, *Mr Cruden Greatly Injured,* p. 28.

158. Cruden, *The London-Citizen,* p. 28.

159. Cruden, *Mr Cruden Greatly Injured,* p. 24.

160. Cruden, *Adventures,* part 1, p. 23.

161. Thanks to David Nash for drawing to our attention some of the issues behind Cruden's particular choice of national identity.

162. Cruden, *Mr Cruden Greatly Injured,* p. 24.

163. Cruden, *The London-Citizen,* p. 61. Never one to lightly coat his brush, Cruden repeated this claim in various forms again and again in his publications; see ibid., p. 68 and Cruden, *Mr Cruden Greatly Injured,* p. 35.

164. Cruden, *The London-Citizen,* pp. 30, 33, 44; Cruden, *Mr Cruden Greatly Injured,* pp. 4, 6.

165. Cruden, *Adventures,* part 1, pp. 14, 18, 20, 24. As early as 1667 at Bethlem, the physician had been instructed on his appointment to "be careful to see and speake with every lunatike before hee p[re]scribeth any physicke for him from tyme to tyme" (BCGM, 26 June 1667, p. 53). A century later, it was still recognized as a contemporary commandment for good medical practice that, as Smollett's Protestant chaplain put it in *The Adventures of Roderick Random,* "no physician will prescribe for his patient until he knows the circumstances of his disease." However, these and other sources suggest that the very opposite was not uncommonly patients' actual experience and that doctors often failed not only to see their patients but also to make thorough inquiries into their histories and situations. Just as Cruden had censured James Monro, Smollett's Dr. Mackshane was censured by Roderick for "never once enquiring about me, or even knowing where I was" (Tobias Smollett, *The Adventures of Roderick Random,* ed. Paul-Gabriel Boucé [London: 1748; Oxford: Oxford University Press, 1979], chap. 34, pp. 191–92). Yet, knowing the circumstances of a case was not always understood as requiring that a patient be seen. Numerous busy eighteenth-century physicians, with lots of patients to attend to, were accustomed to offering their opinions on a case in a verbal or written form on the basis of information provided by relations, as their clients were more or less accustomed to receiving them. For example, William Perfect records a number of case he consulted on by letter in his *Select Cases,* pp. 169–83, 304–18, 324–35. See also Joan Lane, "'The doctor scolds me': The Diaries and Correspondence of Patients in Eighteenth-Century England," *Patients and Practitioners: Lay Perceptions of Medicine in Pre-industrial Society,* ed. Roy Porter (Cambridge: Cambridge University Press, 1985), pp. 205–48, esp. p. 227.

166. Cruden, *Mr Cruden Greatly Injured,* p. 4; Cruden, *The London-Citizen,* pp. 52, 56.

167. Cruden, *Adventures,* part 2, pp. 23, 29.

168. Ibid., p. 21.

169. Ibid., p. 22, "the dishonourable criminals have never paid him."

170. Cruden described his various sojourns at Oxford and Cambridge in another of his addresses published in 1756 (this time, addressed to all the inhabitants of Britain and dedicated to the princess dowager of Wales), but directly inspired by the Lisbon earthquake and the war with France, which the Corrector predictably interpreted as providential signs, further legitimating his ongoing crusade. See Alexander Cruden, *The Corrector's Earnest Address to the Inhabitants of Great Britain* (London: The Author, 1756). See also *DNB*, pp. 250–51.

171. Letters from J. Neville to Dr. Cox Macro, in British Museum, Manuscripts Dept., Additional MS 32557, dated 18 July 1755.

172. Benjamin Rush, *Travels Through Life. The Autobiography of Benjamin Rush*, ed. George W. Corner (Princeton: Princeton University Press, 1968), p. 63.

173. Nichols, *Literary Anecdotes*, vol. 9, part 4, p. 628.

174. Alexander Cruden, *The History of Richard Potter, a Sailor and Prisoner in Newgate, who was Tried at the Old-Bailey in July 1763, and Received Sentence of Death for Attempting, at the Instigation of Another Sailor, to Receive Thirty-five Shillings of Prize-money Due to a Third Sailor. Containing an Account of his Being Convinced of Sin and Converted in the Cells of Newgate, etc.* (London: G. Keith, etc., 1763).

175. Alexander Cruden, *The Corrector's Instructions to the Deputy-Correctors for the Reformation of the People* (Aberdeen? For the author, 1770).

176. Parry-Jones, *The Trade in Lunacy*, p. 223.

177. Hunter and Macalpine, *Three Hundred Years of Psychiatry*, p. 358. At the other extreme, Oliver, Cruden's biographer, was perhaps overly prepared to take the Corrector at his word. See Oliver, *The Eccentric Life*, passim.

178. Dale Alfred Peterson, ed., *A Mad People's History of Madness* (Pittsburgh: University of Pittsburgh Press, and London: Feffer and Simmons, 1982), pp. 48–49.

179. Roy Porter, *A Social History of Madness: Stories of the Insane* (London: Weidenfeld and Nicolson, 1987), pp. 126–35. See, also, Porter, *Mind-Forg'd Manacles*, pp. 80, 139, 142, 149–50, 158–59, 260, 262–63, 269–70.

180. Allan Ingram, *The Madhouse of Language: Writing and Reading Madness in the Eighteenth Century* (London and New York: Routledge, 1991), pp. 6, 12, 26, 117–20, 122, 128–29, 141–42, 156, 158, 164, 174; Ingram, *Voices of Madness*, pp. xvi–xviii, 23–74.

181. Bethlem Admission Registers, p. 184. In 1738, there were attempts to establish Cruden's settlement in the parish of St. Christopher le Stocks in Cornhill, where his shop at the Royal Exchange was located, and in Southgate, where he had friends, although he was actually resident in lodgings at White's-Alley, Chancery Lane, in Holborn and worked in the printing office at Wild Court, just south of Holborn. Cruden, *The London-Citizen*, pp. 26–27, 48–49, 65.

182. Alexander Cruden, letters to Sir Hans Sloane, British Museum, Manuscripts Dept., Additional MS 4041.

183. Cruden, *The London-Citizen*, pp. 47–53.

184. Cruden, *Adventures*, part 1, pp. 24–25.

185. Ibid., pp. 34–37; ibid., part 3, p. 7.

186. Cruden, *Mr Cruden Greatly Injured,* p. 5.

187. Ibid.

188. Lewis, *Correspondence,* vol. 34, HW to Mary Berry, 17 April 1794, p. 95. It is possible that Walpole meant Thomas here, as John had died two years earlier, but this seems unlikely.

CHAPTER 4

1. Lewis, *Correspondence,* vol. 24, HW to Mann, 9 April 1778, p. 372.

2. Ibid., HW to Sir Edward Walpole, 25 April 1777, p. 125.

3. Jonathan Swift, *The Legion Club* (a satire on the Irish House of Commons) (London: 1736), *The Poems of Jonathan Swift,* ed. Harold Williams, 2nd ed., vol. 3 (Oxford: Clarendon, 1958), pp. 827–39, quotes on pp. 831, 837.

4. See the discussion in Scull, MacKenzie, and Hervey, *Masters of Bedlam,* pp. 137–38, 143–49.

5. N. Jewson, "Medical Knowledge and the Patronage System in Eighteenth-Century England," *Sociology* 12 (1974), pp. 369–85.

6. Munk, *Roll,* vol. 2, pp. 127, 207–09.

7. For Jebb, see ibid., pp. 262–64. For Orford's illness, see references below, and also Lewis, *Correspondence,* vol. 36, appendix 6, pp. 331–36.

8. We discussed the origins and development of Monro's links with the Walpole family in chapter 1, but it seems worth noting here that Monro's association is also reflected in his library, which included Walpole's *Catalogue of Royal and Noble Authors,* 2 vols. (1759); Walpole's *Anecdotes of Painting in England,* and his *Catalogue of Engravers,* 5 vols. (Strawberry Hill, 1762), and *Aedes Walpolianae: A Description of the Pictures at Houghton Hall* (1752). See Monro, *Bibliotheca Elegantissima Monroiana,* nos. 469, 1689, 1788.

9. Lewis, *Correspondence,* vol. 39, HW to the Hon. H. S. Conway, 30 Aug. 1773, pp. 172–73.

10. Ibid., vol. 23, HW to Mann, 15 Aug. 1773, p. 505; cited in vol. 36, appendix 6, p. 333.

11. Ibid., vol. 23, HW to Mann, 31 Dec. 1773, p. 540; vol. 36, appendix 6, p. 334. The day previous to this, Orford's ability to write "three letters with coolness and clearness" had been seen as a sign of his return to reason. Evidently he was then told not to write any more in the belief that this would help preserve his mental calm. See vol. 23, 30 Dec. 1773, p. 539.

12. Ibid., vol. 23, HW to Mann, ca. 19 May 1773, p. 482; vol. 36, appendix 6, p. 332.

13. As well as "an ointment of sulphur and hellebore" applied on the advice of his groom, Orford also had a consultation with Dr. Robert James (1703?–76), who had prescribed his fever powders for him. But Orford apparently failed to tell James that he had already been dosed with other some "quack drops," namely "a violent antimonial medicine, which sweated him immoderately," and he also ignored James's advice "to keep at home," returning "into the country"; ibid., vol. 36, HW to Mann, 17 Feb. 1773, p. 332, and vol. 23, p. 460.

14. Ibid., vol. 23, HW to Mann, 28 March 1774, p. 560; vol. 36, appendix 6, p. 334.

15. Ibid., vol. 23, HW to Mann, 19 Jan. 1774, p. 546; also cited in ibid., vol. 36, p. 334.

16. Ibid., vol. 24, HW to Mann, 28 April 1777, p. 264.

17. See *The Diary of Joseph Farington,* ed. Kenneth Garlick and Angus Macintyre, vol. 2, 26 May 1796 (New Haven and London: Yale University Press, 1978), p. 558. He had voiced similar sentiments on other occasions, writing to Mann on 14 May 1777, for example, that "in my private opinion, he [Orford] has been mad these twenty years and more. On his coming of age, I obtained a fortune [i.e., a prospective wife] of one hundred and fifty-two thousand pounds for him: he would not look at her." Lewis, *Correspondence,* vol. 24, HW to Mann, 14 May 1777, p. 301. What else but madness, after all, could possibly prompt a rational Englishman to reject, sight unseen, so self-evidently eligible a match?

18. Garlick and Macintyre, *Diary of Joseph Farington,* p. 559. Sir Henry was perhaps the ancestor of another Henry Oxenden, a patient kept in near-continuous restraint at Ticehurst Asylum in the 1850s. See Ticehurst Asylum Medical Journal, 1843–53, 5 Sept. 1853; Ticehurst Asylum Case Book, vol. 2, pp. 123–24. There is a larger irony surrounding the question of Orford's ancestry and his genetic links (or absence thereof) to Horace Walpole: many contemporaries noted that

> latterly Sir Robert [Walpole] and his wife did not live happily together, and [there was a general belief that] Horace, the youngest, was not the son of the great Prime Minister of England, but of Carr, Lord Hervey. . . . Horace was born eleven years after the birth of any other child that Sir Robert had by his wife; in every respect he was unlike a Walpole and in every respect, figure and formation of mind, very like a Hervey. Lady Mary Wortley divided mankind into men, women and Herveys. . . . Walpole was certainly of the Hervey class. [Yet] we have no evidence whatever that a suspicion of spurious parentage ever crossed the mind of Horace Walpole. His writings, from youth to age, breathe the most affectionate love for his mother, and the most unbounded filial regard for Sir Robert Walpole. (Peter Cunningham, introduction, *Letters of Horace Walpole,* quoted in Mason, *Horace Walpole's England,* p. vii)

19. Garlick and Macintyre, *Diary of Joseph Farington,* p. 559.

20. Pargeter, *Observations on Maniacal Disorders,* p. 37.

21. Ibid.

22. Lewis, *Correspondence,* vol. 24, HW to Mann, 28 April 1777, p. 295.

23. Ibid., pp. 293–94. See also vol. 36, HW to Sir Edward Walpole (henceforth EW), 21 April 1777, p. 118.

24. Ibid., vol. 36, HW to EW, 21 April 1777, p. 118.

25. Ibid., vol. 24, HW to Mann, 28 April 1777, p. 295.

26. Walpole's attitude to Orford was complicated by the fact that, in addition to his role in his nephew's madness, he had "two families dependent on myself afflicted with the [same] calamity," circumstances that must have placed further onus on the dangers to the family name and further taxed Walpole's emotional resources and patience. See ibid., vol. 31, HW to Mary Hamilton, 7 Oct. 1783, p. 208 and note 6.

27. E.g., ibid., vol. 24, Mann to HW, 16 May 1777, p. 303.

28. E.g., ibid., HW to Mann, 9 April 1778, p. 373.

29. Ibid., vol. 23, HW to Mann, 27 April 1773, p. 476; also cited in ibid.,

vol. 36, appendix 6, p. 332. Two months later, he complained to the Reverend William Mason about the troubles he faced dealing with his "mad and ruined" nephew:

> All Lord Orford's affairs are devolved upon me, because nobody else will undertake the office. I am selling his horses, and buying off his matches. . . . Mr Manners, who was the son of Lord William, who was the son of Beezlebub, deserves to be crucified. He was so obliging the other day to . . . tell me he should seize the pictures at Houghton [the Orford family estate]—I sent for a lawyer to exorcise him . . . what vicissitudes have I seen in my family! (Ibid., vol. 28, HW to the Reverend William Mason, 28 June 1773, pp. 92–93)

30. Ibid., vol. 24, HW to Mann, 28 April 1777, p. 294.

31. Ibid. Two weeks later, he claimed that "had I remained charged with his affairs six months longer on his last illness, he would have been five thousand a-year richer than the day he fell ill. My reward was, not to see him for three years." Ibid., vol. 24, HW to Mann, 14 May 1777, p. 301.

32. Ibid., vol. 36, HW to EW, 21 April 1777, p. 118.

33. Ibid., vol. 36, HW to EW, 21 April 1777, p. 118, including notes 4–6; ibid., vol. 24, HW to Mann, 28 April 1777, pp. 293–94 and notes 10–11. Martha Turk was the daughter of Orford's housekeeper in Green Street, Grosvenor Square. She had several children by Orford, but all died, and although she was bequeathed property in Orford's will, she died before him. See Garlick and Macintyre, *Diary of Joseph Farington,* vol. 2, 19 Jan. and 26 May 1796, pp. 476, 558–59.

34. Walpole's correspondent Horace Mann was similarly prone to disregarding the sayings and doings of the insane, although this could sometimes be to their advantage in politically charged contexts—as when Mann passed over Mr. St. John's cursing of the king and "a strange treasonable letter" because the latter was "outrageous and rebelliously mad, quite mad, and so not worth any notice." See Lewis, *Correspondence,* vol. 19, Mann to HW, 4 Jan. 1746, p. 191, note 7.

35. Ibid., vol. 36, HW to EW, 21 April 1777, p. 118.

36. Ibid., vol. 24, HW to Mann, 9 April 1778, p. 372.

37. Ibid.

38. Ibid., vol. 36, HW to EW, 21 April 1777, pp. 117–18.

39. Ibid., p. 119.

40. Ibid., p. 120.

41. Ibid., HW to EW, 22 April 1777, p. 120.

42. Tim Mowl, *Horace Walpole: The Great Outsider* (London: John Murray, 1996). Disappointingly, this study pays hardly any attention to Walpole's involvement with his nephew's illness.

43. Lewis, *Correspondence,* vol. 24, HW to Mann, 2 May 1777, p. 296.

44. Ibid., vol. 36, HW to EW, 21 April 1777, p. 119.

45. Ibid., vol. 32, HW to Lord Ossory, 22 April 1777, p. 350; also cited in vol. 36, p. 119, note 10.

46. Ibid., vol. 36, HW to EW, 21 April 1777, p. 119, note 10.

47. See, e.g., mention of the letter he wrote to Sir Edward Walpole in ibid., vol. 24, HW to Mann, 19 July 1777, p. 319.

48. E.g., ibid., vol. 36, HW to Mann, 28 April 1777, p. 294.

49. It is not surprising that Jebb, having attended Orford in his previous attack, was the first London doctor to personally attend on the scene and offer a diagnosis—declaring, despite an initial failure to get Orford to show his tongue, that he was without "understanding," and had a slight fever, without delirium. The lack of any exciting cause seems to have persuaded both Walpole and Jebb that Orford's madness was "constitutional." See ibid.

50. Ibid., HW to Mann, 17 July 1777, p. 316. This was a verdict Walpole represented as a lesson for Orford's other physicians and "the faculty not [to] pronounce in a hurry again," he having repeatedly felt that they had tended to speak too soon of Orford's recovery, as he certainly felt Battie and Jebb had done in 1773–74.

51. Ibid., HW to Mann, 27 March 1778, pp. 367–68.

52. Ibid., vol. 42, appendix 4, p. 498. Walpole's letter to the *Public Advertiser* was first printed on 28 August 1767 and signed "Toby."

53. Ibid.

54. E.g., ibid., vol. 36, HW to EW, 25 April 1777, pp. 122–24.

55. Ibid., p. 124.

56. Ibid., p. 125.

57. E.g., ibid., vol. 24, HW to Mann, 9 April 1778, p. 372.

58. E.g., ibid., vol. 36, 21 April 1777, HW to EW, p. 119; and vol. 24, HW to Mann, 9 April 1778, p. 372.

59. Ibid., vol. 34, HW to Lady Ossory, 23 Nov. 1791, p. 130.

60. Ibid., vol. 24, HW to Mann, 9 April 1778, pp. 372–73. Mann gave the same opinion of Orford's own mother: "She never pretended to have any extraordinary tenderness for him, or that he ever gave her cause for it," such a sentiment requiring "more cultivation than blood alone gives"; ibid., Mann to HW, 28 April 1778, p. 376.

61. Ibid., vol. 36, HW to EW, 25 April 1777, p. 123; vol. 25, HW to Mann, 11 Feb. 1881, p. 126.

62. Ibid., vol. 25, HW to Mann, 11 Feb. 1781, pp. 126–27.

63. Ibid., vol. 24, HW to Mann, 27 March 1778, p. 367.

64. It seems worth remarking here that, while Bethlem patients were discharged throughout Monro's physicianship as "cured" rather than as "recovered," as Battie preferred to term it at St. Luke's, Monro's evident preference in his case book and private practice for terms such as "well" and "better" implies a degree of reticence in taking personal credit when patients recovered.

65. Lewis, *Correspondence*, vol. 24, HW to Mann, 9 April 1778, p. 372.

66. Ibid., HW to Mann, 27 March 1778, pp. 367–68.

67. Ibid., HW to Mann, 28 April and 18 June 1777, pp. 295, 310. See also ibid., Mann to HW, 16 May 1777, p. 303; vol. 25, HW to Mann, 6 Feb. 1780, p. 11.

68. Ibid., vol. 24, HW to Mann, 9 April 1778, p. 372. Orford was colonel of the Norwich Militia 1758–91. Later in life, reflecting on this period more soberly and with more than a decade having passed since his nephew's last attack, Walpole seems to have forgotten, or revised, his earlier negativity about Orford's mental fitness for such duties. Indeed, he trumpeted the accuracy of

Monro's prognostic skill by emphasizing the "strongest proof" that was provided within a week of the mad-doctor having "pronounced him sane" in his
"marching to Norwich at the head of the militia," something that Walpole had
sought to stop and had been commanded to prevent by the king. In citing these
events, Walpole sought to reassure Lady Ossory that George III's recent recovery
was likely to be similarly "perfect." Ibid., vol. 34, HW to Lady Ossory, 28 Feb.
1789, pp. 47–48 and notes 6–7.

    69. Ibid., vol. 26, HW to Mann, 28 April 1777, p. 295.

    70. Ibid., vol. 24, HW to Mann, 27 March 1778, p. 368.

    71. Ibid., vol. 34, HW to Lady Ossory, 23 Nov. 1791, p. 129. Thomas
Monro was to attend Orford alongside Drs. William Norford (1715–93) and
John Ash (1723–98), and Walpole had also had recourse on this occasion to
Francis Willis (1718–1807), the reverend doctor who attended George III during his first alleged attack of insanity in 1788. This attendance was scarcely less
contentious than the former, Dr. Norford being, according to Walpole, subjected to a series of insults and injuries. After Orford's death, both Monro and
Norford encountered considerable difficulty getting paid by the executors. Walpole claimed that Orford's steward Cony "prevented" it and also blamed Cony
for Orford's death, allegedly the result of "forcibly carrying him, against his
consent, from Brandon to Houghton, in the height of his fever." Walpole lost no
time in sacking Cony once Orford was deceased. See ibid., vol. 16, HW to John
Pinkerton, 26 Dec. 1791, p. 314, note 5; vol. 42, HW to Lady Bristol, 3 April
1792, pp. 355–56.

    72. Ibid., vol. 34, HW to Lady Ossory, 23 Nov. 1791, p. 132.

    73. Ibid., p. 129; and vol. 42, HW to Lady Bristol, 3 April 1792, p. 355.

    74. Speaking to Farington in 1796, Walpole was "fully convinced that the
late Lord Orford fell a martyr to bad management at the commencement of
his last illness"; Garlick and Macintyre, *Diary of Joseph Farington*, vol. 2,
26 May 1796, p. 558.

CHAPTER 5

    1. William Belcher's description of his confinement in a Hackney madhouse,
from which he was liberated with the support of John Monro's son Thomas, in
his pamphlet *An Address to Humanity: Containing, a Letter to Dr. Thomas
Monro; a Receipt to Make a Lunatic, and Seize his Estate; and a Sketch of a True
Smiling Hyena* (London: The Author, 1796), reprinted in Ingram, *Voices of
Madness*, pp. 127, 131, 132, 134.

    2. Pargeter, *Observations on Maniacal Disorders*, p. 123, emphasis in the
original.

    3. Evidence of Charity Thom, explaining the circumstances under which
Dame Byzantia Clerke or Cartwright wrote her will while under confinement
in Dr. William Battie's care during 1775, in the 1793 case of *Cartwright v
Cartwright*, 1 Phillmore Ecclesiastical 90, 161 ER 923, in the *English [Law] Reports*, CD ROM version. It would be rather outside of the scope of our remit in
this book to discuss this interesting case in any more detail.

4. See Neil McKendrick, John Brewer, and J. H. Plumb, *The Birth of a Consumer Society: The Commercialization of Eighteenth-Century England* (Bloomington: Indiana University Press, 1982); Roy Porter, *English Society in the Eighteenth Century* (London: Penguin, 1982).

5. Battie undertook Williams's care at a Kensington house soon after his return to England from Hamburg in February 1758, the patient having become deranged a few months after leaving St. Petersburg the previous year. He improved and was released after five weeks of care under Battie, but from March 1759, Williams was under treatment once again for the same complaint, this time by John Monro. By the end of July, he was being lodged in Lord Bolingbroke's house at Chelsea, but despite some amelioration of his condition, he never fully recovered and remained in confinement until his death on 2 Nov. 1759; Lewis, *Correspondence,* vol. 33, HW to Lady Ossory, 19 Dec. 1778, pp. 77–78 and notes 10–12.

6. See the discussion in Scull, MacKenzie, and Hervey, *Masters of Bedlam,* pp. 137–38, 143–49.

7. For documentation, see Peter Rushton, "Lunatics and Idiots: Mental Disability, the Community, and the Poor Law in North-East England 1600–1800," *Medical History* 24 (1980), pp. 34–50; Rushton, "Idiocy, the Family and the Community in Early Modern North-east England," *From Idiocy to Mental Deficiency,* ed. David Wright and Anne Digby London (London and New York: Routledge, 1996), pp. 44–64; Jonathan Andrews, "Identifying and Providing for the Mentally Disabled in Early Modern London," ibid., pp. 65–92; Andrews, "'Mad and Poor and Cannot Otherwise Be Provided For': Lunacy, Bedlam, and the Old Poor Law," unpublished paper; Akihito Suzuki, "Lunacy in Seventeenth and Eighteenth-Century England: Analysis of Quarter Sessions Records, Part I," *History of Psychiatry* 2 (1991), pp. 437–56; Suzuki, "Lunacy in Seventeenth and Eighteenth-Century England: Analysis of Quarter Sessions Records, Part II," *History of Psychiatry* 3 (1992), pp. 29–44; Suzuki, "The Household and the Care of Lunatics in Eighteenth-Century London," *The Locus of Care,* ed. Peregrine Horden and Richard Smith (London: Routledge, 1998), pp. 153–75; A. Fessler, "The Management of Lunacy in Seventeenth-Century England, An Investigation of Quarter-Sessions Records," *Proceedings of the Royal Society of Medicine* 49 (1956), pp. 901–07; E. G. Thomas, "The Old Poor Law and Medicine," *Medical History* 24 (1980), pp. 1–19.

8. See Scull, *The Most Solitary of Afflictions.*

9. Porter, *Mind-Forg'd Manacles,* p. 164. Charlotte MacKenzie has suggested that from another point of view, "the trend towards confinement away from home can be seen as part of the aspirations to gentility which accompanied increased spending power.... Gentrifying clergy and farmers [for instance] who remodelled their houses, so that they could eat and sleep in rooms that were segregated from those used by servants and labourers, may also have chosen to distance themselves from the uncontrolled behaviour of their disturbed relations." *Psychiatry for the Rich: A History of Ticehurst Private Asylum* (London: Routledge, 1992), p. 20.

10. Joseph Jean Hecht, *The Domestic Servant Class in Eighteenth-Century*

England (London: Routledge and Kegan Paul, 1980); Peter Earle, *A City Full of People: Men and Women of London, 1650–1750* (London: Methuen, 1994), pp. 38–54, 123–30.

11. Suzuki, "The Care of Lunatics," pp. 155–56. Suzuki's paper provides substantial evidence of how these factors worked out in practice. For the further arguments explaining the rise of the asylum, see, e.g., Scull, *The Most Solitary of Afflictions,* esp. pp. 19–45.

12. For some details on the use of madhouses by London parishes in the eighteenth century, see Andrews, "Bedlam Revisited," pp. 497–99.

13. *The Distress'd Orphan, or Love in a Mad-house,* 2nd ed. (London: Printed for J. Roberts, 1726), p. 35. The book appeared anonymously, but was actually by the prolific Eliza Fowler Haywood or Heywood (1693?–1756), editor of *The Female Spectator,* 4 vols. (London: T. Gardner, 1744–46). Her first novel was *Love in Excess; or, the Fatal Enquiry. A Novel* (London: Printed for W. Chetwood and R. Francklin, and sold by J. Roberts, 1719), and she was also known as the author of quasi-pornographic texts. She was one of Pope's targets in the *Dunciad,* where her sexual favors are offered as a prize in a urinating contest between the booksellers. One of her later novels, *The History of Miss Betsy Thoughtless,* 4 vols. (Dublin: Printed for Oliver Nelson, 1751), was a reworking of the story of Betty Careless, a dissolute bagnio keeper whose name Hogarth had depicted scratched on the banister rails of his Bedlam scene in *The Rake's Progress.* Other late eighteenth-century novels by women with madhouse themes include Mary Wollstonecraft's *Maria; or, the Wrongs of Women* (1798) and Charlotte Smith's *The Young Philosopher* (1798).

14. *The Distress'd Orphan,* p. 39.

15. Ibid., pp. 39–40.

16. Ibid., p. 37.

17. Ibid., pp. 52, 58.

18. Ibid., pp. 40–43, 50.

19. Ibid., p. 42.

20. Ibid., pp. 41–42. The 1790 edition of this novella attached it more explicitly to the literature of sentiment and sensibility, including an additional letter from Annilia further emphasizing "the horrors of a mad-house, which words cannot describe" and quoting Stern's *Sentimental Journey.* See *The Distress'd Orphan, or Love in a Mad-house,* 4th ed. (London: Printed for J. Roberts, 1790). For excellent studies of this genre of literature, see, e.g., John Mullan, *Sentiment and Sociability,* and Everett Zimerman, "Fragments of History and *The Man of Feeling* from Richard Bentley to Walter Scott," *Eighteenth-Century Studies* 23.3 (Spring 1990), pp. 283–300.

21. See Jonathan Andrews, "'In her Vapours [or] Indeed in her Madness'? Mrs Clerke's Case: An Early Eighteenth-Century Psychiatric Controversy," *History of Psychiatry* 1 (1990), pp. 125–43.

22. Coverture meant a woman's person (and her property) being legally bound over, according to her marital contract, to her husband's keeping and protection. See Elizabeth Foyster, "Wrongful Confinement in Eighteenth-Century England: A Question of Gender?" unpublished paper delivered at University of Wales, Bangor, conference, July 1999, "Social and Medical Represen-

tations of the Links between Insanity and Sexuality," passim. We are greatly indebted to Dr. Foyster for permitting us to quote from this paper.

23. Anon., *A Full and True Account of the Whole Tryal, Examination, and Conviction of Dr. James Newton, who Keeps the Mad House at Islinstton [sic], for Violently Keeping and Misusing of William Rogers . . . by his Wife's Orders . . .* (London: Printed by J. Benson, 1715).

24. Tobias Smollett, *The Adventures of Launcelot Greaves* (London: Coote, 1762). Smollett, as we shall see, borrowed heavily from Monro in constructing his images of treatment in a madhouse.

25. Daniel Defoe, *Augusta Triumphans* (London: Roberts, 1728).

26. Robert Baker, *A Rehearsal of a New Ballad-opera Burlesqu'd, Call'd The Mad-house. After the Manner of Pasquin. As it is now Acting at the Theatre-Royal in Lincoln's-Inn-Fields. By a Gentleman of the Inner-Temple* (London: Printed for T. Cooper, 1737).

27. See Ingram, *Voices of Madness;* Anon., *Proposals for Redressing Some Grievances Which Greatly Affect the Whole Nation* (London: Johnson, 1740); Anon., "A Case Humbly Offered to the Consideration of Parliament," *Gentleman's Magazine* 33 (1763), pp. 25–26.

28. Pargeter, *Observations on Maniacal Disorders*, p. 123, emphasis in the original.

29. See especially the testimony recorded in the House of Commons, *Report, together with the Minutes of Evidence;* and J. W. Rogers, *A Statement of the Cruelties, Abuses, and Frauds, Which Are Practised in Mad-Houses*, 2nd ed. (London: For the author, 1816).

30. The point was first made in Parry-Jones's pioneering study, *Trade in Lunacy*. It has subsequently been amplified by such scholars as Roy Porter in *Mind-Forg'd Manacles* and Leonard Smith in "Eighteenth-Century Madhouse Practice: The Prouds of Bilston," *History of Psychiatry* 3 (1992), pp. 45–52.

31. Thomas Willis, *Two Discourses Concerning the Soul of Brutes* (London: Dring, Harper, and Leigh, 1684), p. 206. See, for example, William Cowper's description of his breakdown and treatment (1763–65) by Nathaniel Cotton, in his *Memoir of the Early Life of William Cowper, Esq., Written by Himself* (London: Edwards, 1816); and the more self-interested claims of the Reverend Lewis Southcomb about his successful treatment of patients without resort to those "tormenting Means . . . which tend to the giving of Pain and Uneasiness." Southcomb described his clientele as mostly drawn from the ranks of the marginally disturbed, not those who "have been really mad, but very frequently . . . such as have been madly dealt with withal before I have ever known them." See *Peace of Mind and Health of Body United* (London: Cowper, 1750), pp. 57, 61, 70.

32. Benjamin Faulkner, *Observations on the General and Improper Treatment of Insanity: With a Plan for the More Speedy and Effectual Recovery of Insane Persons* (London: For the author, 1790).

33. Addington jun. also became a governor of Bethlem. See *Report from the Committee Appointed to Examine the Physicians Who Have Attended his Majesty, During his Illness, Touching the State of his Majesty's Health* (London: 1788), p. 13.

34. Lewis, *Correspondence,* vol. 32, HW to Lady Ossory, 15 Aug. 1776, p. 315; Hunter and Macalpine, *Three Hundred Years of Psychiatry,* p. 402.

35. The fees sought from affluent families could be enormous: Richard Hunter and Ida Macalpine reprint a letter of Battie's dated 3 March 1763 in connection with the treatment of a Miss Marriott. Battie sets forth charges of £749 18s. od., and requests that the recipient "pay that summe immediately," closing with a reminder that "your answer is desired by the return of the post." See *Three Hundred Years of Psychiatry,* p. 403; also, Munk's *Roll,* vol. 2, pp. 139–43, entry on William Battie.

36. MacKenzie, *Psychiatry for the Rich,* p. 14.

37. See the case book (hereafter CB), reprinted in Andrews and Scull, *Customers and Patrons,* passim.

38. However, in the first case that was heard, which the committee dismissed as unfounded, "many Witnesses of Weight and Authority" were referred to, but not specified by name, so the committee probably interviewed nearer twenty witnesses. See *A Report from the Committee, Appointed . . . to Enquire into the State of the Private Madhouses in this Kingdom . . .* (London: J. Whiston etc., 1763). See also *The History, Debates, and Proceedings of Both Houses of Parliament of Great Britain from the Year 1743 to the Year 1774* (London: Debrett, 1792), pp. 125–26. For an example of the agitation that laid the groundwork for this inquiry, see, e.g., "Thoughts on Private Mad-Houses, or A Case Humbly Offered to the Consideration of [Parliament], & c.," *Royal Magazine* 8 (Jan. 1762), pp. 27–29.

39. *A Report from the Committee,* p. 5 and passim.

40. Mrs. Hawley's case was separately covered by the *Annual Register* for 1763, which provided a detailed and relatively faithful summary of the 1763 *Madhouses Enquiry* (vol. 6, pp. 56, 158–59), during which, it asserted, "many acts of oppression have been discovered." Hawley had been in Turlington's Chelsea madhouse from 5 Sept. to 4 Oct. 1762, as the *Annual Register* put it, "on pretence of insanity," and four of those five persons accused of falsely confining her were indeed convicted in the ensuing King's Bench trial.

41. See Robert Turlington, *By Virtue of the King's Patent . . . Turlington's Balsam of Life is Prepared and Sold by the Patentee . . . The Efficacy and Virtues of Which . . . are Exemplified . . . in this Book* (London: For the author, 1748). This association between the peddling of specific, antimaniacal or quack medicines and the mad-business is one that is encountered relatively commonly in this period; see, e.g., Hunter and Macalpine, *Three Hundred Years of Psychiatry,* pp. 198–99, 293–95.

42. *A Report from the Committee,* p. 7.

43. Ibid., pp. 7–9.

44. Ibid., pp. 9–10.

45. Ibid., p. 10.

46. Ibid.

47. For this case, see *[The] English [Law] Reports,* vol. 97, p. 741; Anon., *The Laws Respecting Women* (1777), pp. 74–75, quoted in Bridget Hill, *Eighteenth-Century Women: An Anthology* (London, Boston, and Sydney:

George Allen and Unwin, 1984), pp. 146–47; Parry-Jones, *Trade in Lunacy,*
p. 224, note 2. It was probably to this case that the *Annual Register* of 26 Feb.
1761 referred (vol. 6, p. 76) as a "shocking instance" of the abuses of private
madhouses. Like many journalistic accounts, it veered toward melodrama and
inaccurate reportage, claiming that the confinement was precipitated by "an
unnatural father, in order to gratify his cruel disposition, and to cut off his
[sane and] only daughter from her birth-right," her death only being averted
by "a providential accident" leading her friends to discover "the place of her
confinement."

48. See Eigen, *Witnessing Insanity,* p. 163. Thanks once more are due to Liz
Foyster for insights freely offered into King's Bench habeas corpus proceedings.

49. *A Report from the Committee,* p. 9.

50. Ibid., p. 11.

51. Ibid., p. 10.

52. Ibid.

53. See, e.g., G. F. Russell Barker, ed., *Memoirs of the Reign of King
George III* (London: Lawrence & Bullen, 1894), pp. 192–93 and note 1.

54. See *Annual Register,* vol. 14 (1771), pp. 78–79. Evidently, Mrs. Leggatt,
whose case was heard before the Surrey Quarter Sessions at Southwark on
26 Feb. 1771, had been confined by her husband, who employed the ruse of "an
airing to Kingston" to waylay her. The keeper was found guilty on all charges.

55. *Five Letters on Important Subjects. First Printed in a Public Paper, now
Collected and Revised* (London: Printed for W. Owen, 1772), letter 4, pp. 21–
27. This was the more than likely the work of a High Church Anglican cleric,
the author variously styling himself "A Citizen of London," "A Respecter of the
Clergy," and being "well known to Dr Hayter Bishop of London," while he was
also highly critical of the writings of the Quakers.

56. Ibid., p. 22.

57. Ibid., p. 23.

58. Ibid., pp. 23–26.

59. Porter, *Mind-Forg'd Manacles,* pp. 151–52.

60. Nonetheless, although the Act said nothing about pauper lunatics, occasionally provincial and metropolitan madhouses took it upon themselves to require a certificate from the parish clergyman providing information as to the
individual's pauper status and lunacy. Under the auspices of the Old Poor Law
local ministers continued to play an important role in providing certificates of
settlement and other information about the sick poor. See, e.g., Hunter and
Macalpine, *Three Hundred Years of Psychiatry,* pp. 452–56, 468, fig. 97.

61. E.g., Nichols, *Literary Anecdotes,* vol. 8, part 4, p. 507, note to vol. 4,
p. 611.

62. Miles left the Painter-Stainers Company twenty guineas in his will
(which was witnessed by three members at Painters Hall), for the purchase of a
silver coffee pot and waiter for them to remember him by. For a fuller discussion
of his will, see note 67, below.

63. For more information on the madhouses at Hoxton, see Arthur David
Morris, *The Hoxton Madhouses* (March, Cambridge: Goodwin Bros., 1958);

Parry-Jones, *Trade in Lunacy,* pp. 36, 39, 43, 225; *House of Commons Mad-houses Enquiry* (1815), 1st–4th reports, esp. pp. 10, 25, 30–32, 42–43, 81–84, 92–94, 99–101, 118, 144–45, 153–54, 160, 171–75.

64. See Hunter and Macalpine, *Three Hundred Years of Psychiatry,* pp. 452, 790, fig. 159; *Fourteenth Annual Report of the Commission in Lunacy to the Lord Chancellor* (London: HMSO, 1860), p. 21; Parry-Jones, *Trade in Lunacy,* p. 39.

65. See Scull, *The Most Solitary of Afflictions,* p. 21. On his death, the older Miles had bequeathed the house to the management of his widow and thereafter to his son, (Sir) Jonathan Miles, who had been born there (see below). Miles's madhouse was the second largest of the metropolitan madhouses of the period. By 1815, the establishment of this kingpin of madhouse entrepreneurs was accommodating 486 patients in six separate buildings, although the number of inmates declined subsequently. Most patients came from the lower classes, "three-quarters of them being paupers," and almost one third (136) of the total were (predominantly) low-ranking naval cases. For this motley crew, a medical attendant was employed at £150 per annum. For further details, see Parry-Jones, *Trade in Lunacy,* pp. 43, 60, 67–68; Hunter and Macalpine, *Three Hundred Years of Psychiatry,* p. 525; *House of Commons Madhouses Enquiry* (1815), 1st report, p. 75; 3rd report, pp. 171–73.

66. For these cases, see CB, pp. 1, 2, 20, 37, 38, 39, 65, 67, 68, 79, 89, 108, 111, 114. Of the sixteen patients in the case book who went to Hoxton, nine were men and seven women, reversing the gender balance found generally in the case book, where female cases were significantly predominant. This might be seen to confirm evidence from other sources that institutional confinement in both public and private asylums tended to be resorted to more often in male than in female cases. However, if we include all cases mentioned in the case book who were sent to any private madhouses, we arrive at a less striking male:female ratio of 12:14.

67. Public Record Office, P.C.C. Prob. 11/984, fol. 193. Miles's will not only testifies to the enormous profits of his business, but also suggests much about the origins and character of that enterprise and its interrelationship with other family concerns and occupations. He appointed Richard Woodhouse of Fulham, Middlesex, Gent., and Michael Pearson, an apothecary of Norton Falgate near Bishopsgate Street, London, as Trustees (the latter very likely the apothecary who served Hoxton House), bequeathing twenty guineas to them. He left most of the rest of his estate, including a substantial quantity (at least £1,000 worth) of 3 percent annuities, to his daughter Augusta Miles (or Preston), by his wife Margaret Preston, and (in trust) to his son Jonathan Miles (or Preston), who was three years old in 1772 when John was writing his will. Not entirely sure he could trust his wife to bring up his son as he would have wished, Miles further stipulated that, should the trustees be dissatisfied, Jonathan was to be maintained and educated by them out of a sum of £70 a year. John's sister was Susannah Simpson, wife of Merchant Simpson, a nurseryman and seedsman in "Wisbich" (i.e., Wisbech), Isle of Ely, Cambridge, and they had four nieces, Mary, Susannah, Elizabeth, and Ann, who are also mentioned in Miles's will. Miles's extensive property in the four counties of London, Middlesex, Essex,

Herts., and Northampton, most of which he bequeathed in trust to Jonathan, comprised lands, messuages, and tenements, etc., in Charles's Square, Hoxton; other lands and tenements (mainly comprising his madhouse) in Hoxton Town; a moiety or interest in the White Hart Inn, at Romford, Essex, then in the possession of one John Atkinson; a house, yard, and premises opposite the Loom Pond in Romford; two cottages or houses and lands (comprising or entailing a farm) in Hornchurch, Essex; a moiety in Gains Farm in Hornchurch; a farm at Halgrave, Northampton; Bedhall farm in or near North Mimms, Herts.; and a farm at Uppminster. In addition, as well as the profits of Miles's business and most of his household goods, a share of the profits from some of the above properties was to go toward supporting his widow during her lifetime once Jonathan had taken over the business. Other lands and premises in Pitfield Street, St. Leonard Shoreditch, he directed to be sold and laid out for the purchase of 3 percent annuities, the interest of which was to go to his daughter and her family. Miles's executors were John Atkinson and James Stretton of Bethnal Green, Middlesex, Gent., and each received twenty guineas in his will. Among the household goods and utensils Miles left his widow were his "Brewing Slaughtering Butchering and Boileing Utensils" from his two Hoxton houses, probably used to prepare food for the patients.

68. For Miles's testimony before this inquiry, see *House of Commons Madhouses Enquiry* (1815), 3rd report, pp. 171–75.

69. Scull, MacKenzie, and Hervey, *Masters of Bedlam,* pp. 16–17; *House of Commons Madhouses Enquiry* (1815), 1st report, p. 30; 3rd report, pp. 171–74.

70. Morris, *The Hoxton Madhouses;* William Alexander Devereux Englefield, *History of the Painter-Stainers Company of London* (London: Chapman & Dodd, 1923). The ambitious Jonathan Miles also unsuccessfully contested the parliamentary seat of Tregony, Cornwall, in 1806, investing ca. £10,000 in the bid.

71. The Admiralty contract was to admit and "cure" deranged "officers, seamen, and marines belonging to His Majesty's Naval Service." See *Papers Relating to the Management of Insane Officers, Seamen, and Marines, Belonging to His Majesty's Naval Service* (London: 1814).

72. For information on these farms, see note 67, above.

73. See *House of Commons Madhouses Enquiry* (1815), 1st report, p. 30. This evidence highlights the key relationship between farming and the history of the asylum, a history that may be perceived to link the farming and feeding of the mad poor and the mad-trade in the eighteenth century to the asylum farms of the nineteenth century and the "funny farms" of the twentieth century.

74. Scull, MacKenzie, and Hervey, *Masters of Bedlam,* pp. 16–17; *House of Commons Madhouses Enquiry* (1815), 1st report, p. 30; 3rd report, pp. 171–75.

75. See *House of Commons Madhouses Enquiry* (1816), pp. 65–67, evidence of James Veitch, surgeon at Miles's madhouse. Veitch testified that on 27 June 1815, the establishment contained 180 seamen, soldiers, and marines, 104 of whom had been transferred from Bethlem.

76. CB, pp. 66–67.

77. CB, pp. 47–48, 114.

78. CB, p. 20.

79. CB, pp. 6–7, 47–48.

80. See CB, pp. 4, 115, and references. Quite possibly, the reference here is to the Dutchman Isaac De Vic. His will is dated 7 Jan. 1772, and was proved on the oaths of his sons Isaac and Henry 9 Aug. 1773. See PCC Prob. 11/990, q.n. 327.

81. Parry-Jones, *Trade in Lunacy,* pp. 33–39, 95.

82. Morris, *The Hoxton Madhouses.*

83. For cases sent/recommended to Duffield's, see CB, pp. 31–34, 50–54, 56–58, 106–08, 123–24.

84. John Bowack, *The Antiquities of Middlesex* . . . (London: Printed by W. Redmayne for S. Keble, D. Browne, A. Roper, R. Smith, and F. Coggan, 1705–06).

85. See, e.g., Reginald Blunt, *The Wonderful Village* (London: Mills and Boon, 1918).

86. For the Duffields' wills, see PCC Prob. 11/869, q.n. 315; 11/1308, q.n. 392. Michael Duffield senior, who died in 1761, was brother to Elizabeth Inskip, widow, who received an annuity of twenty guineas in his will and whose son, Peter Inskip, ran another Chelsea madhouse. Michael senior's will is dated 10 May 1760 and was proved on 25 Sept. 1761. His bequests to his son Michael not only reveal substantial family wealth, but suggest that Duffield junior was having marital problems that his father was attempting to heal (or else to punish) posthumously. The legacies included an annuity of fifty-two guineas and the residue of his personal estate left to Michael junior, and an annuity of £80, paid in trust to his nephews (Samuel Duffield and Thomas Newton) for his son's wife, Mary's, "Sole and Separate Use," and an extra £20 annuity paid in trust to Mary for his nephews, provided Michael and Mary "shall choose to live and cohabit together." On the same condition, Mary and Michael junior were also to be permitted to reside gratis in any of Michael senior's houses in Gloucester Street, St. George the Martyr, Middlesex. Both were finally left £10 each for mourning. The other major bequests were £3,000 left to the granddaughter, Catherine Duffield (or, in the event of her death, to her brother Michael), while all messuages (dwellings and outbuildings) and lands were left to the grandson, Michael Duffield (or, in the event of his death, to his sister Catherine), while the grandchildren's support and his grandson's education "in an handsome Genteel manner" were also to be provided for out of his estate. Michael senior's disapproval for his son seems not only to have reduced the level of bequests made to the latter, but even to have caused him to exclude his son from the role of executor, a task that was left to his grandson and to a Thomas Newton. Perhaps it was this blight over his full inheritance that helped to impel Michael junior into the madhouse business.

87. Little Chelsea was at this time a detached hamlet consisting of a couple of farms and a few houses dotted along the road to Fulham, at the northwestern boundary of the main riverside village of Great Chelsea.

88. CB, pp. 1, 7, 43, 53–54, 117.

89. See Andrews, "Bedlam Revisited," table 4a, p. 321; Bethlem Auditor's Accounts, 1752–68.

90. See Andrews et al., *The History of Bethlem,* pp. 265–70; and BCGM,

19 Jan. 1753, p. 97, "Ordered that Dr John Monro, Physitian to these Hospitals, have the same Salary as his Father had."

91. For cases definitely or probably sent to Bethlem, see CB pp. 17, 38, 41, 44, 80–81, 107–08.

92. CB, p. 117.

93. CB, pp. 7–8.

94. CB, pp. 86–89.

95. CB, pp. 1–2.

96. CB, pp. 50–54.

97. Foyster, "Wrongful Confinement."

98. Ibid., p. 5, and B. Rizzo, "John Sherratt, Negociator," *Bulletin of Research in the Humanities* 86.4 (1985), pp. 413–21. Sherratt had also been of assistance to the poet Christopher Smart, who had been confined in St. Luke's during a bout of derangement and who wrote about his experiences there in his poem *Jubilate Agno*. Smart published an epistle addressed to Sherratt in ca. 1763. See Christopher Smart, *Poems by Mr Smart. Viz. Reason and Imagination, a Fable. Ode to Admiral Sir George Pocock. Ode to General Draper. An Epistle to John Sherratt*, Esq. (London: Printed for the author, 1763). See also Elizabeth Rivers, *Out of Bedlam: XXVII Wood Engravings* (Glengeary, Ireland: Dolmen Press, 1956).

99. Eigen states that over half of the 331 allegedly mad prisoners he has identified during 1760–1843 "made some statement in their defence during their trial"; *Witnessing Insanity*, p. 163.

100. For this case see *[The] English [Law] Reports*, vol. 97, pp. 875–56, also reproduced in CD ROM version published by Juta Hart Law Publishers; Parry-Jones, *Trade in Lunacy*, p. 224, note 3. Peter McCandless has likewise argued for the nineteenth century that clear-cut cases of false confinement are difficult to substantiate, and that the frequency of conspiracies has been exaggerated; "Liberty and Lunacy: The Victorians and Wrongful Confinement," *Madhouses, Mad-Doctors and Madmen: The Social History of Psychiatry in the Victorian Era*, ed. Andrew Scull (Philadelphia: University of Pennsylvania Press, 1981), pp. 339–61.

101. *Annual Register* (1771), vol. 14, p. 86.

102. For information on this case, see *Rex v Coate Loft* 73, 98 ER 539, *[The] English [Law] Reports*, CD ROM version.

103. The outcome of both of these cases was, once again, a compromise separation between husband and wife, with a financial settlement and somewhat inequitable agreement over access to children.

104. See *Rex v Coate Loft*.

105. For biographical information and details of other cases adjudicated by Mansfield, see, e.g., Edmund Howard, *Lord Mansfield* (Chichester: Barry Rose, 1979); John Campbell, *The Lives of the Chief Justices of England from the Norman Conquest to the Death of Lord Mansfield* (London: John Murray, 1849); William David Evans, *A General View of the Decisions of Lord Mansfield in Civil Causes* (London: J. Butterworth, 1803); *Reports of Cases Argued and Adjudicated in the Court of King's Bench: During the Time Lord Mansfield Presided in that Court . . . 1756 . . . to . . . 1772* (London: W. Clarke, 1812).

106. See, e.g., William Murray, Lord Mansfield, *The Thistle: A Dispassionate Examine of the Prejudice of Englishmen in General to the Scotch Nation; and Particularly of a late Arrogant Insult Offered to all Scotchmen by a Modern English Journalist,* 2nd ed. (London: H. Carpenter, 1747); Anon., *A Candid and Impartial Discussion of the False Reasonings, Gross Misrepresentations, and Studied Fallacies of two late Pieces: the Former [i.e., "The Thistle," signed: Aretine, i.e., William Murray, Lord Mansfield] Written to Vilify the Inhabitants of one End of this Island; and the Latter [i.e., an answer to "The Thistle"]* . . . (London: M. Cooper, 1747). Interestingly, as solicitor general during the 1750s, Mansfield had taken a significant part in the Schomberg case, referred to in chapter 2, in which both Battie and Monro (as, respectively, president and censor at the College of Physicians) were so intimately involved. This may well have been the first occasion on which he encountered Monro. Mansfield's evident support for Schomberg suggests that he was far from always in agreement with Monro. See, e.g., Sir William Browne, *A Vindication of the Royal College of Physicians: In Reply to the Speech of the Solicitor General [i.e., the Hon. W. Murray, afterwards Lord Mansfield] on Opening the Petition and Appeal of Doctor Isaac Schomberg . . . to the . . . Visitors of the College* (London: W. Owen, 1753).

107. See *Rex v Coate Loft.*

108. CB, pp. 106–08.

109. Library of the Royal College of Physicians, London, MS C.362.2; F. H. W. Sheppard, ed. *Survey of London. Volume XXVIII. Parish of Hackney (Part I). Brooke House a Monograph* (London: Athlone Press, 1960), pp. 52–64.

110. *The English [Law] Reports,* vol. 97, King's Bench Division, *Rex versus William Clarke, keeper of a private madhouse at Clapton* (1762), available in CD ROM, *Rev v Clarke* 3 Burrow 1362, 97 ER 875; also cited in *Survey of London Volume XXVIII: Brooke House, Parish of Hackney* (London: Athlone Press, 1960), pp. 65, 86, and in Parry-Jones, *Trade in Lunacy,* p. 224, note 3. Evidently keen to minimize his business connections with Clarke, Monro described him in 1762 as the man "who keeps a private mad-house, and is accustomed to have the care of such unfortunate persons." While offering evidence in Clarke's defense, Monro was careful to stress that he had merely "recommended" Mrs. Hunt to his care and that it was under Clarke's care (rather than his own) that she remained. As for the evidence suggesting his possible involvement as a silent partner, we find it significant that Monro became the madhouse's licensee as soon as the law required it, in 1774, even though the lease of the establishment continued to be held in the name of William Clarke, and its day-to-day management was carried on by Clarke and a Miss Mary Hawkins. Following Clarke's death in 1777 (with Miss Hawkins appointed as his executrix), the lease of the property passed to John Monro (ca. 1781), and together or singly, he and Miss Hawkins held the license for the madhouse till her death in 1790, when it was passed on to his son Thomas.

111. CB, pp. 6–7, 80, cases of Mrs. Alcock and Mr. Hamilton.

112. Bennett's name had been incorporated into Sayer's firm as early as 1775, although evidence given during the 1784 Chancery trial between the two men indicated that the partnership was only officially contracted in 1777. Sayer's

firm was responsible for printing the Carington Bowles's (1724–93) collection of maps of the English and Welsh counties (1775), and Thomas Jefferys's (d. 1771) *American Atlas* (1776), as well as Samuel Dunn's (d. 1774) astronomical and geographical map of the heavens and earth (1780). For another example of Bennett's collaboration with him, see Robert Sayer and John Bennett, *Sayer and Bennett's Enlarged Catalogue of New and Valuable Prints . . . [for 1775]* (London: P. Holland, 1970).

113. For the account of this case, which was heard before Sir Lloyd Kenyon on 21 June 1784, see *Sayer v Benet* 1 Cox's Chancery Cases 107, 29 ER 1084, in *[The] English [Law] Reports*, 1220–1866, CD ROM published by Juta Hart Law Publishers, and available at the PRO and other major libraries.

114. Oliver Beckett, *The Life and Work of James Ward, R.A., 1769–1859: The Forgotten Genius* (Lewes: Book Guild, 1995); Cecil Reginald Grundy, *James Ward, R.A. His Life and Works, with a Catalogue of his Engravings and Pictures* (London: Otto, 1909); James Northcote, *Conversations of James Northcote R.A. with James Ward, on Art and Artists*, ed. and arranged from the manuscripts and notebooks of James Ward by E. Fletcher (London: Methuen & Co., 1901); George Edwin Fussell, *James Ward, R.A: Animal Painter 1769–1859 and his England* (London: Michael Joseph, 1974); Julia Frankau, *Eighteenth Century Artists and Engravers. William Ward, A.R.A. James Ward, R.A. Their Lives and Works . . .* (London: Macmillan & Co, 1904); Frankau, *An Eighteenth-century Artist and Engraver: John Raphael Smith, his Life and Works* (London: Macmillan, 1902). See also William Young Ottley, *An Inquiry into the Origin and Early History of Engraving* (Bristol: Thoemmes, 1998).

115. The case seems another example of the vulnerabilities, rather than the authority, of expert medical testimony at this time. As Eigen has shown, medical testimony as to insanity tended to be assessed as scarcely any more weighty, or any less ambivalent, than lay testimony, although there are signs of a gradual refocusing of such testimony on the nature of lunacy itself, rather than on the actual individual being assessed. Eigen, *Witnessing Insanity,* esp. pp. 120, 135–36.

116. For this case of a sailor who had formerly been sent to Bethlem by the Commissioners for Sick and Hurt Seamen, see ibid., pp. 127–28, and note 44; OBSP, 1784, case 943, 8th sess., 1259. Relying on an inaccurate court transcript, Eigen spells Gozna's name incorrectly as "Gosner" here.

117. Eigen, *Witnessing Insanity,* p. 127. See also p. 27, fig. 1.4, and pp. 128, 136. Eigen calculated that medical participation in insanity trials increased from ca. 3 to 10 percent of cases in the early 1760s to ca. 16 to 17 percent by the 1770s and 1780s and 30 percent by 1810–19, but the sharpest rise was after 1830.

118. *Survey of London, Vol. XXVIII: Brooke House*, pp. 52–64.

119. 1758 Rate Book, Hackney Public Library.

120. E. S. de Beer, *The Diary of John Evelyn: Now Printed in Full from the Manuscripts Belonging to Mr. John Evelyn*, vol. 3 (Oxford: Clarendon Press, 2000).

121. *Survey of London, Vol. XXVIII: Brooke House*, p. 4.

122. Ibid., pp. 5–6.

123. Richard Paternoster, *The Madhouse System* (London: For the author, 1841), pp. 9, 30. This source is also cited in Parry-Jones, *Trade in Lunacy*, p. 100.

124. PRO PCC Prob. 11/1213, q.n. 32, fols. 256–58; Wills in the Family Records Centre, London.

125. According to Hunter and Macalpine, Battie had around 1751 "acquired premises in Islington Road for private patients," and had taken over the Clerkenwell house in 1754 from a Dr. Newton (d. 1750), probably the son of James Newton, who had been running it since the late seventeenth century. The establishment was evidently part of a leasehold estate situated in Wood's Close, off Islington Road, in the parish of Saint James's (or St. John), Clerkenwell, Middlesex. The Clerkenwell house subsequently passed to John Monro almost immediately on Battie's death in 1776, and after *his* death, the business was carried on by Thomas until 1803, when it was converted into a boarding school. See Hunter and Macalpine, *Three Hundred Years of Psychiatry*, pp. 200–01, 402.

126. See, e.g., Nichols, *Literary Anecdotes*, vol. 4, part 3, p. 609.

127. *Survey of London, Vol. XXVIII: Brooke House*, p. 66. See, also, Parry-Jones, *Trade in Lunacy*, p. 77, note 2.

CHAPTER 6

1. Jonathan Swift, *A Vindication of his Ex[cellenc]y the Lord C[artere]t* (London: Printed for T. Warner, 1730), *The Prose Works of Jonathan Swift*, ed. Herbert Davis, vol. 12 (Oxford: Basil Blackwell, 1955), p. 158.

2. Jonathan Swift, *Traulus* (1730), ll. 38–40, *The Poems of Jonathan Swift*, ed. Harold Williams, vol. 3 (Oxford: Clarendon, 1958), p. 797.

3. Henry Fielding, *The Life/History of Jonathan Wild the Great* (London: 1743; London: A. Millar, 1754).

4. This quote is taken from John Monro's assessment of the case of Margaret Nicholson before the Privy Council in 1786. See below and PRO PC2–131, fols. 357–88; Macalpine and Hunter, *George III and the Mad-Business*, p. 311.

5. See, e.g., the bill that was tabled for one of his lunatic ancestors, evidently his uncle; [25 March 1730] *An Act for Making Effectual an Agreement made Between Selina Countess Dowager Ferrers . . . Robert and George Shirley, Esqs. . . . and two Infant sons of the said Countess, and Lawrence Shirley, Esq. . . . in behalf of Himself and his four Infant sons, and of Henry Earl Ferrers a Lunatick, etc.* (London: 1730).

6. Alfred Bishop Mason, ed., *Horace Walpole's England As His Letters Picture It*, HW to Sir Horace Mann, 21 March 1758 (Boston and New York: Houghton Mifflin, 1930), p. 129.

7. Reverend Luke Tyerman, *The Life and Times of the Rev. John Wesley, M.A., Founder of the Methodists*, vol. 1, 3rd ed. (London: Hodder and Stoughton, 1876), vol. 1, p. 364. In his rage, Tyerman records, Ferrers "always carried pistols to bed with him, and often threatened to kill her before morning." A Mrs. Clifford had been his long-time mistress, since before his marriage, and had borne him several children. Presumably, this was the same woman he would en-

deavor vainly to see during his later confinement in the Tower of London, and en route to Tyburn. Ibid.

8. See King's Bench writ proceedings at the PRO, KB1/12. The case was seen as sufficiently precedent-setting to be entered in *The English [Law] Reports,* exemplifying how even membership of the peerage did not exempt one from the requirements of the law. We are extremely grateful to Elizabeth Foyster for so generously providing us with her own transcribed notes on these writs and for her comments on the wider significance of the Ferrers case.

9. See PRO King's Bench affidavits and proceedings, KB1/13, May/June 1757.

10. See PRO DL/C/554/073, 21 Jan. 1758, for London Consistory Court cause papers concerning the separation, and KB33/20/3 for printed act of separation. See also *Journal of the House of Lords* (1758), p. 381. By the eighteenth century, of course, the significance of the sanction of excommunication was sharply reduced, and the court's penalty would have had few consequences of any substance for Ferrers.

11. According to Lawrence Stone, Mary had taken the highly unusual, but ultimately unsuccessful, step of trying to get a divorce from her husband by private act of Parliament. Very few women indeed in this period obtained a divorce in this way, and the ground they cited was invariably adultery, not cruelty, as Mary's petition alleged. See Stone, *Road to Divorce: England 1530–1987* (Oxford: Oxford University Press, 1990), p. 318, note 50. We are grateful to Elizabeth Foyster for drawing our attention to this reference.

12. PRO CL/C/554/073 (once again, we are indebted to Elizabeth Foyster for sharing her transcripts of this case).

13. Johnson, a rather old gentleman, had been working faithfully for the Ferrers family for over thirty years, a point he made to the earl when desperately and vainly pleading for his life, and one that was emphasized in accounts of the crime in the press (see below). It seems to have been Johnson's management of a farm belonging to the earl that particularly grated on Ferrers, who testified: "I have long wanted to drive *Johnson* out of the Farm." Ferrers had allegedly been dissatisfied less with Johnson's accounts than with the fact that "he had been a tyrant, and he was determined to punish him." Reflecting more soberly on the crime to the chaplain as he awaited execution, Ferrers was recorded as stating that "he had met with so many crosses and vexations, that he scarce knew what he did; and solemnly protested that he had not the least malice towards him [Johnson]." *Royal Magazine* 2 (1760), pp. 106, 228, 230; *The Trial of Lawrence Earl Ferrers for the Murder of John Johnson . . . Before the House of Peers, in Westminster-Hall . . . On 16th, 17th and 18th April 1760* (London: Printed for Samuel Billingsley, 1760; Dublin: Printed for G. Faulkner, and H. Bradley), pp. 8–9.

14. Lewis, *Correspondence,* vol. 9, HW to George Montague, 28 Jan. 1760, p. 272.

15. "Unhappy Affair of the Earl Ferrers," *London Magazine* (April 1760), pp. 206–07. A virtually identical account was reproduced in the *Royal Magazine* 2 (1760), pp. 106–07.

16. *Royal Magazine* 2 (1760), p. 106.

17. Thomas Kirkland's (1722–98) first publications seem to have been *A Treatise on Gangrenes. In which the Cases that Require the use of the Bark . . . are Ascertain'd . . . and the Objections to its use in the Cure of Gangrenes Consider'd* (Nottingham: 1754) and *An Essay on the Methods of Suppressing Hœmorrhages from Divided Arteries* (London: Printed for R. and J. Dodsley, 1763). He was later to become a prolific author (although writing nothing on the Ferrers case), publishing on subjects as wide as, e.g., childbed fevers, the brain and nerves (1767, 1768/9 and 1774), fractures (1770 and 1771), "the kink-cough" (1774), the state of surgery (1783), amputation (1780), cattle disease (1783), and apoplectic and paralytic affections (1792).

18. We have relied here primarily on the voluminous documents relating to the case that are preserved in the House of Lords Record Office. These include records of the coroner's and grand jury hearings, the printed transcript of the trial itself, a variety of correspondence, and a bound volume of relevant materials (assembled in the mid-nineteenth century by W. D. Fellowes, secretary to the then Lord Great Chamberlain of England), which includes both printed and manuscript contemporary accounts of the case (Ref. 10/L/5/12, House of Lords Record Office). These sources have been supplemented by other trial and magazine literature on the case in the Bodleian Library.

19. The peers had received regular updates on the case over the preceding months. See *Journals of the House of Lords*, 7, 13, and 26 Feb., 17, 25, 28, and 31 March, and 1 April 1760, pp. 580, 584, 590–91, 607, 614, 619, 626, 629–31, 634.

20. Quoted by W. D. Fellowes in his introduction to his collection of papers dealing with the case, House of Lords Record Office, 10/L/5/12.

21. *Royal Magazine* 2 (1760), p. 215.

22. Many of these begging letters are preserved in the bound volume in the House of Lords Record Office, 10/L/5/12. Its compiler had originally planned to include a sample "ticket" in his scrapbook, but the surviving examples were consumed in the fire that burned down much of the Houses of Parliament. In their place, as exemplifying the style of the ticket used for the occasion, he inserted a ticket for the coronation of George IV!

23. *Royal Magazine* 2 (1760), pp. 215–16.

24. Ibid., p. 222.

25. Ibid., p. 223.

26. The most insightful discussion of the eighteenth-century criminal code remains Douglas Hay, "Property, Authority and the Criminal Law," *Albion's Fatal Tree: Crime and Society in Eighteenth Century England*, ed. D. Hay, P. Linebaugh, J. Rule, E. P. Thompson, and C. Winslow (New York: Pantheon, 1975), pp. 17–63.

27. Juries, for instance, often with the active connivance of the bench, frequently valued the property that had been stolen below the threshold that mandated the death penalty. See Peter Linebaugh, *The London Hanged: Crime and Civil Society in the Eighteenth Century* (London: Allen Lane/Penguin, 1991).

28. However, as Langbein and others have argued, the law was not always as much at the beck and call of the ruling classes as some would have it: there

were rather more than merely conspicuous exceptions to this rule in the eighteenth century, while an expanding section of the propertied middling classes were exerting an increasing influence on the way property and persons were to be protected, even from the excesses and recklessness of their social superiors. See, e.g., J. H. Langbein, "Albion's Fatal Flaw," *Past and Present* 99 (1983), pp. 96–120. Our thanks to Elizabeth Foyster for stressing this point to us.

29. T. B. Howell, *A Complete Collection of State Trials and Proceedings for High Treason and Other Crimes and Misdemeanours*, vols. 22–33 (London: R. Bagshaw: Longman & Co., 1809–26), quoted in Nigel Walker, *Crime and Insanity in England*, vol. 1 (Edinburgh: Edinburgh University Press, 1968), p. 59.

30. For good surveys of the development of this tradition, see, e.g., Nigel Walker, *Crime and Insanity in England*, vol. 1, chap. 1; Eigen, *Witnessing Insanity*, chaps. 2 and 3, esp. pp. 34–46.

31. Eigen, following Walker and other historians of forensic psychiatry, identified Monro's appearance at Ferrers's trial as the first by a medical witness, and took it as the starting point for his survey of mad-doctors in the English court. He calculated with reference to Old Bailey Sessions Papers "that between 1760 and 1843, medical participation increased from approximately one trial in ten . . . to one in two." He also emphasized that "the medical man in the insanity trial was an exceptional feature, at least until the second quarter of the nineteenth century," and that "the majority of defendants in the years 1760–1843 were acquitted without the services of a medical witness." *Witnessing Insanity*, pp. 24, 28.

32. *Trial of Lawrence Earl Ferrers*, pp. 29–31.

33. See *Trial of Lawrence Earl Ferrers*, pp. 35–42, evidence of Richard Phillips, Peter and Elizabeth Williams, Thomas Huxley, Wilhelmina Coates, and the two Shirleys.

34. Mason, *Horace Walpole's England*, HW to George Montague, 19 April 1760, pp. 140–41, emphasis in the original.

35. Walker, *Crime and Insanity*, pp. 60–62.

36. *Trial of Lawrence Earl Ferrers*, pp. 9–10.

37. Ibid., p. 8.

38. Ibid.

39. Lewis, *Correspondence*, vol. 8, HW to Mann, 7 May 1760, p. 396.

40. *Trial of Lawrence Earl Ferrers*, p. 49. For Monro's testimony, see pp. 42–43, and for the complete summation by the solicitor general, see pp. 45–50.

41. Ibid.

42. Ibid.

43. Ibid., p. 49.

44. Ibid., pp. 45–46.

45. Ibid., p. 62.

46. Ibid., p. 50.

47. Ibid., pp. 50–54.

48. Hand-written copy of Earl Ferrers's second speech to the House of Lords, House of Lords Record Office.

49. *Trial of Lawrence Earl Ferrers,* p. 55.

50. Manuscript preserved in House of Lords Record Office, 10/L/5/12. Ferrers's reaction to the sentence was the focus of equally minute attention elsewhere. In reporting on the case, the *Gentleman's Magazine* informed its rapt readership that "he received the sentence in a submissive attitude, with his head declined, and his eyes fixed on the ground. . . ." It noted, too, that some bystanders "imagined that" on hearing he was to be publicly dissected, "his lower jaw was agitated by some convulsive quivering" and he exclaimed, "God forbid." "Account of Earl Ferrers," p. 137.

51. *Trial of Lawrence Earl Ferrers,* p. 55.

52. Ibid.

53. Ibid., p. 138. A "german cousin" (more usually rendered as "cousin german") is a term for first cousin, sometimes used generically to designate a close relative.

54. Ferrers's case was compared in some detail by the *Royal Magazine* to that of Lord Stourton, executed under Elizabeth I for murder, who was given the choice of either a hempen or silken noose to be hanged with; *Royal Magazine* 2 (1760), pp. 106–07.

55. This was a far from eccentric act, for, as Hay et al. have pointed out, Tyburn malefactors often treated their executions as if they were on their wedding day, not merely because this was part of a ritualized gallows theater signifying dying the good death, but also as a kind of confidence trick and rite of passage for the soul into the next life; *Albion's Fatal Tree,* pp. 112–13.

56. Mason, *Horace Walpole's England,* HW to Sir Horace Mann, 7 May 1760, p. 141. According to the *Royal Magazine* 2 (1760), p. 230, there were two parties of horse-grenadiers and two of foot, divided more or less equally at the front and back of the procession.

57. "Account of Earl Ferrers," p. 138.

58. "A Full Account of the Execution of Laurence, Earl Ferrers, Viscount Tamworth, and Baronet," *The London Magazine* (May 1760), p. 262.

59. *Universal Magazine* 1 (May 1760), p. 259.

60. Ibid.

61. Ibid.

62. Ibid.

63. Mason, *Horace Walpole's England,* HW to Sir Horace Mann, 7 May 1760, p. 141. Other estimates put it at eight minutes.

64. Ibid., pp. 138–39.

65. Ibid., p. 139.

66. "A Full Account of the Execution of Laurence, Earl Ferrers," p. 263.

67. Mason, *Horace Walpole's England,* HW to Sir Horace Mann, 7 May 1760, p. 141. This version of events may be erroneous, however. The *Universal Magazine* ([May 1760], p. 260) claimed that reports that Ferrers had been left standing for some time on tip-toe had been "mistaken," asserting that the trap had merely failed to sink down as low as it was designed to do and had to be pressed down, but that the earl was still properly "suspended." Catering to its readers' evident interest in every morbid detail, the *London Magazine* reported that "his lordship was turned off about two minutes before twelve, and seemed

to die very easy; but his hands turned presently remarkably black." "A Full Account of the Execution of Laurence, Earl Ferrers," p. 263.

68. *Universal Magazine* (May 1760), pp. 260–61.

69. On the riots that often erupted after public hangings, as friends of the condemned sought to prevent bodies being handed over for the desecration that was public dissection, see Peter Linebaugh, "The Tyburn Riot against the Surgeons," in *Albion's Fatal Tree,* ed. Hay et al., pp. 65–117.

70. Mason, *Horace Walpole's England,* HW to Sir Horace Mann, 7 May 1760, pp. 141–42.

71. *Royal Magazine* 2 (1760), p. 232.

72. Mason, *Horace Walpole's England,* HW to Sir Horace Mann, 7 May 1760, p. 142.

73. The *London Magazine,* for example, took pains to point out that "from the time of his ascending the scaffold to his execution, was about eight minutes, during which his countenance never changed, nor did his tongue faulter" [*sic*]. "A Full Account of the Execution of Laurence, Earl Ferrers," p. 263.

74. Lewis, *Correspondence,* vol. 9, pp. 395–96.

75. Ibid., vol. 9, p. 397.

76. Ibid., p. 397 and note 16; *Trial of Lawrence Earl Ferrers,* p. 38. The earl's grandmother was Mary Washington, who married Robert Shirley, the first Earl Ferrers. Her third cousin, John Washington, emigrated to Virginia in 1756, and was the grandfather of George Washington, first president of the United States—still another member of this "very frantic race."

77. See especially Hay, "Property, Authority and the Criminal Law," p. 34.

78. *Royal Magazine* 2 (1760), pp. 225–27, 232.

79. *An Analysis of the Philosophical Works of Lord Bolingbroke, by the late Unfortunate Earl Ferrers, for his Private Entertainment; to Which is Prefixed, A Parallel of Earl Ferrers' Case, with that of Lord Santry, a Peer of Ireland, both Convicted of Murder: and a Sentimental Letter to a Friend* (London: Printed for J. Burd, 1760). The advertisement for this work stated that its object was "to clear the memory of a late noble peer from the many cruel aspersions so wickedly thrown out against him," asserting that when sober Ferrers "was an intelligent, benevolent, and valuable member of society." Ferrers seems to have written his abridgement for private circulation out of genuine admiration for Bolingbroke's doctrines, but also because he felt the latter's work was too expensive, long, and full of redundancies to merit publication.

80. Ibid., pp. x, xi.

81. Ibid., pp. xiv–xv.

82. For the developing role of mad-doctors in the eighteenth-century criminal courtroom, see Eigen, *Witnessing Insanity,* and Walker, *Crime and Insanity.* For the most sophisticated discussion of the evolution of medico-legal relations regarding insanity in the Victorian era, see Roger Smith, *Trial by Medicine: Insanity and Responsibility in Victorian Trials* (Edinburgh: Edinburgh University Press, 1981).

83. Claims in the press that she was the daughter of George Nicholson, a barber of Stockton-on-Tees, Durham, and was forty-eight years old appear to have been erroneous. Indeed, they represent the first of a deluge of apocryphal

reports about Nicholson that circulated wildly in a press so hungry for tidbits of information about her that it was plainly disposed to sensationalize her story and to give credit uncritically to gossip and idle speculation. The most reliable account of Nicholson seems to have been that by her former landlord, Jonathan Fiske, *The Life and Transactions of Margaret Nicholson; Containing not Only . . . her Attempt to Assassinate his Most Gracious Majesty; but also Memoirs of her Remarkable Life . . .* (London: Printed for J. Fiske, 1786), copy in Cambridge University Library Hunter Collection, d.78.1.

84. Fiske, *The Life*, pp. 8–9.

85. For the large literature of manuscript and other primary and secondary sources concerning Nicholson, on which our own account is also based, see BSCM entries detailed in notes below; Patricia H. Allderidge, "Criminal Insanity: Bethlem to Broadmoor," *Proceedings of the Royal Society of Medicine* 67 (1974), pp. 897–904; *DNB; European Magazine* 10 (Aug. 1786), pp. 117–20; *The Lady's Magazine* 17 (Aug. 1786), pp. 395–97; *Universal Magazine* 79 (Aug. 1786), pp. 94–96; Anon., *The Plot Investigated; or, a Circumstantial Account of the Late Horrid Attempt of Margaret Nicholson to Assassinate the King. With many Interesting Particulars of her Character and Family, and of the Cause of her First Petitioning His Majesty . . .* (London: Printed for the author and sold by Mr. Macklaw, 1786); Anon., *Authentic Memoirs of the Life of Margaret Nicholson, Who Attempted to Stab his Most Gracious Majesty . . . Likewise the Whole of her Examination before the Privy Council, etc.* (London: Printed for J. Ridgeway, 1786); Perfect, *Select Cases; GM* 56 (1786), pp. 708–11; Anon., *High Treason, Committed by Margaret Nicholson, Guilty of the . . . Crime of Endeavouring to Murder . . . George III . . . With an Account of her Examination, Life, and Transactions* (London: 1786); Sir Robert Adair, *Margaret Nicholson (A Political Eclogue)* (London: 1790; PRO PC2–131, fols. 357–88); Anon. (recently and credibly attributed to James Smyth, a former keeper), *Sketches in Bedlam; or Characteristic Traits of Insanity, as Displayed in the Cases of One Hundred and Forty Patients . . . now, or Recently, Confined in New Bethlehem, Including Margaret Nicholson . . . By a Constant Observer* (London, Sherwood, Jones, & Co., 1823), pp. 253–58; *Annual Register*, vol. 29 (1786), pp. 233–34; Amelia Gillespie Smyth, *Memoirs and Correspondence . . . of Sir Robert Murray Keith . . .* , ed. G. Smyth., vol. 2 (London: 1849), p. 189; William Eden Auckland, *The Journal and Correspondence of William, Lord Auckland . . .* , vol. 1 (London: R. Bentley, 1861), pp. 152, 389; Sir Nathaniel William Wraxall, *The Historical and Posthumous Memoirs of Sir N. W. Wraxall, 1772–1784*, ed. H. B. Wheatley (London: Bickers & Son, 1884), vol. 1, p. 295; vol. 4, p. 353; Frances Burney (afterward D'Arblay), *Memoirs of Doctor Burney . . .* , vol. 3 (London: Edward Moxon, 1832), pp. 45, 47; George Smeeton, *Biographia Curiosa; or, Memoirs of Remarkable Characters of the Reign of George the Third. With their Portraits* (London: J. Robbins & Co., 1822), p. 91; Macalpine and Hunter, *George III and the Mad-Business*, pp. 311–13.

86. Fiske, *The Life*, p. 18.

87. *Annual Register*, vol. 29 (1786), p. 233; *Universal Magazine* 79 (1786), p. 94.

88. *Universal Magazine* 79 (1786), p. 94.

89. Fiske, *The Life,* p. 11.

90. According to various accounts (including Fiske's, *The Life,* pp. 9–20, the *European Magazine,* 10 [1786], pp. 118, 120, and *The Plot Investigated,* pp. 10, 13), the households she had served in comprised those of a Mr. and Mrs./Miss Rice of Argyle Buildings/Mayfair; a Mr. Hopkins, grocer and porter to Lord Arundel, in Seymour Street, Portman Square; the hatter, Mr. Watson, in New Bond Street; a Mr. Taylor; a Mrs. Boothby in Upper Grosvenor Street; a Mrs. Beaumont; Lady Seabright, "a lady of quality" in Brudenel Street; the Scot, Mr. Paul[e], and his wife, where Fiske seems to have first made Meg's acquaintance playing cribbage; a Mr. White; and a tailor, whom she left after "bickerings arose." Penultimately, before she moved to Fiske's, she lived at Vere Street, Oxford Road, leaving within a year "upon friendly terms." The press alleged that it was while in Brudenel Street that Nicholson had the affair with the valet. However, Fiske said that the affair occurred in the household of Mrs. Boothby; *The Life,* p. 9.

91. *Universal Magazine* 79 (1786), p. 95.

92. *Lady's Magazine* 17 (1786), p. 395.

93. Ibid., pp. 35–36.

94. Ibid., p. 395.

95. Fiske, *The Life,* p. 37. According to the *European Magazine* (10 [1786], p. 117), "the knife only just touched the waistcoat" and "was so much worn, and so very thin, that when she thrust it against his Majesty's waistcoat, it bent.—A gentleman tried the point of it against his hand, when the knife bent almost double, without piercing the skin." The *Lady's Magazine* (17 [1786], p. 395) gave a similar, if briefer, description. Accounts vary significantly, however, some sources choosing to highlight the seriousness of the attempt and Nicholson's dangerousness, referring to her act as "diabolical" and characterizing her as a relatively determined "assassin." The *Universal Magazine* (79 [1786], pp. 94, 95), for example, described the knife as "worn very plain, but sharp on each side, and much sharpened, and very bright at the point," alleging that it "made a little cut, the breadth of the point, through the cloth" in the king's waistcoat. It asserted, furthermore, that the king only avoided being seriously wounded "by bowing as he received the paper . . . had not his Majesty shrunk in his side, the blow must have been fatal!" *The Plot Investigated* (p. 19) speculated that there would have been "fatal consequences . . . if the wretch had made use of her right hand instead of her left," while there was considerable attention paid in the press and during the examination as to how the knife had been sharpened before the attempt, a matter that obviously bore on the issues of premeditation and intent (see, e.g., ibid., p. 34). Most accounts spoke of the knife falling to the ground, and some only mentioned one thrust, but others— clearly more disposed to credit and publicize the most sensational versions of events—quoted bystanders as having seen her either strike or raise "her arm a second time," and claimed that the knife was "wrenched . . . out of her hand"; ibid., p. 94; *Lady's Magazine* 17 (1786), p. 395. The latter seems to have been the only account that represented Nicholson as having resisted arrest, alleging that "the disappointed assassin made some faint efforts to disengage herself, but finding resistance ineffectual, calmly submitted to superior force."

96. Apparently both were subsequently rewarded with a gratuity for their bravery, on the earl of Salisbury's order, the former receiving £200 and the latter £60; *European Magazine* 10 (1786), p. 120.

97. Ibid., p. 117.

98. Fiske, *The Life*, p. 36.

99. This was a sentence that was universally applauded, the *Lady's Magazine* (17 [1786], p. 397) typically distinguishing it as something rendered "indispensably necessary" by "the warmest affection and loyalty of all his majesty's subjects, and the most essential interests of the nation."

100. Some years before, "as the King was coming in his chair from Buckingham-house to St. James's a[nother] woman . . . made a blow at his Majesty with a knife, and broke the front glass of his sedan. Upon examination, she also appeared insane!" George had additionally been "assaulted some years since at a review on Wimbledon common, by a well-dressed man, who seized the bridle of the King's horse, and insisted 'upon his grievances being attended to.' He was immediately taken into custody, and on examination proved to be a Lieutenant out of his senses, who had left his regiment at Gibraltor, in consequence of the sentence of a court martial"; *European Magazine* 10 (1786), pp. 118–19.

101. *The Plot Investigated*, p. 20.

102. Ibid., pp. 17–18.

103. Ibid., p. 18.

104. Ibid., p. 16.

105. *European Magazine* 10 (1786), p. 118: "and appeared entirely unmoved by any representation of the atrocity of the crime."

106. Ibid. According to the more censorious account of Nicholson in the *Lady's Magazine* (17 [1786], p. 396), while in the guardroom, she had "bid them not trouble her with questions which she was not obliged to answer" and "maintained the same composure in the queen's antechamber." Here, although she did respond to the nobles who questioned her, she did so "in a contemptuous manner . . . [saying] that her motives would justify her actions; that she was not bound to answer persons who had no authority to examine her; and that before a judge, she was ready to make a proper defence."

107. *Lady's Magazine* 17 (1786), p. 396.

108. *Annual Register*, vol. 28 (1786), p. 233. According to the *Lady's Magazine* (17 [1786], p. 396), her words were a little different from this: pressed for a fuller response, she went on to state that "the King has no right to the crown; I have; and if I do not have justice, England will be in blood for a thousand generations."

109. *Universal Magazine* 79 (1786), p. 94.

110. *Annual Register*, vol. 28 (1786), p. 233; *European Magazine* 10 (1786), p. 118.

111. *European Magazine* 10 (1786), p. 118.

112. "There are intervals when lunatics assume reason, and are capable of conversing with a seeming rationality; but when close questioned as to a particular crime they may have committed, they then wander into the wild labyrinth of a distracted imagination and discover their insanity. Such a one MARGARET NICHOLSON appears to be." Ibid.

113. *Universal Magazine* 79 (1786), p. 94.

114. *Lady's Magazine* 17 (1786), p. 396.

115. Most sources merely reported that three further letters were found "about her pretended right to the Crown," addressed to Lord Mansfield, Lord Loughborough, and General Bramham. Fiske related that in addition, there were letters to her uncle and from her father and a lady in Gloucester Street; *The Life*, p. 38. The *Universal Magazine* (79 [1786], p. 94) gave a fuller, if more scornful, inventory of the contents of her apartments: "nothing more could be traced than scraps of paper, in which the names of Lord Mansfield and other persons of consequence appeared, with some disjointed writing, mentioning effects, and what she denominated 'Classics,' a term she did not seem to understand; all of which denoted a disordered state of mind." *The Plot Investigated* (p. 15) made it clear that her lodgings were searched on two separate occasions.

116. *The Plot Investigated*, p. 33; Fiske, *The Life*, p. 32.

117. Fiske, *The Life*, pp. 37–38.

118. E.g., *Annual Register*, vol. 29 (1786), pp. 233–34; *European Magazine* 10 (1786), p. 118.

119. Fiske, *The Life*, pp. 32–33.

120. A Mr. Paul[e], a pastry cook in Oxford Street, with whom she had previously lodged for five years, gave similar testimony to Fiske: he "declared that she was industrious" and that "he had not discovered the least appearance of insanity," and he thought her a "harmless and inoffensive woman." Fiske, *The Life*, pp. 33–34; *Annual Register*, vol. 29 (1786), pp. 233–34; *European Magazine* 10 (1786), p. 118; Macalpine and Hunter, *George III and the Mad-Business*, p. 311; *The Plot Investigated*, pp. 32–34. According to the *Lady's Magazine* (17 [1786], p. 396), both Fiske and Paul[e] had "joined in representing her as an inoffensive and industrious woman; they said they had never suspected her of insanity, but only remarked that they had frequently heard her talking to herself." The *Universal Magazine* (79 [1786], pp. 94–95) was more explicit, but probably less accurate, as to Fiske's testimony, quoting him as saying that "she always appeared a harmless character" and, although frequently seeming "in a state of absence," the only marks of insanity he had observed were "frequently moving her lips, as if talking, and appearing agitated, although in no conversation with any person."

121. Fiske, *The Life*, p. 46.

122. *European Magazine* 10 (1786), p. 118; *Lady's Magazine* 17 (1786), p. 396; *The Plot Investigated*, p. 34.

123. *The Plot Investigated*, pp. 32, 34.

124. Ibid., p. 21.

125. Fiske, *The Life*, p. 48.

126. *The Plot Investigated*, pp. 21–23. The judicial refusal to resort to torture after Felton's stabbing of the duke of Buckingham was alluded to as exemplary.

127. Ibid., pp. 37–39.

128. Apparently it was customary for the king on receiving a petition to deliver it to the Lord in Waiting to read and report its contents, but this custom had fallen into abeyance recently, and petitions generally were being delivered to

the Gentlemen Ushers or an inferior attendant, who "seldom" read them. Possibly, however, this version of events was a strategic elision, designed to shift any blame away from royalty and the higher officers, while concurrently permitting a gentle admonishment as to the proper responsibilities of the crown. Ibid., pp. 40–41.

129. *Lady's Magazine* 17 (1786), p. 396.

130. Fiske, *The Life*, pp. 8, 12.

131. Ibid., p. 12.

132. Ibid., p. 13.

133. *The Plot Investigated*, p. 48.

134. Fiske, *The Life*, p. 28.

135. *The Plot Investigated*, pp. 48–49.

136. *European Magazine* 10 (1786), p. 120; *The Plot Investigated*, pp. 50–52.

137. Fiske, *The Life*, pp. 9–10.

138. *The Plot Investigated*, p. 52.

139. Fiske, *The Life*, p. 14.

140. Ibid., p. 23.

141. Ibid., p. 45.

142. Ibid., p. 23.

143. Ibid., pp. 46–47. This outfit comprised two new shifts at 7/ each, two pairs of stockings at 3/6 a pair, a pair of 4/6 shoes, and a black quilted petticoat at 12/.

144. Ibid., pp. 21–22, 26–27.

145. Ibid., p. 47.

146. According to Fiske, Nicholson seldom mentioned her brother, who himself not only "never visited her" at Mr. Paul's, despite living nearby, but also "d[am]ned" and accused her of breaking a window that she claimed had been broken by his own child when she was taking it for a walk. Her sister, meanwhile, seems to have lived far away in Cumberland. Ibid., pp. 18, 22–24, 40.

147. Ibid., pp. 40, 47.

148. Ibid., pp. 23–24.

149. Ibid., pp. 27–29.

150. Ibid., pp. 29–30.

151. While some sources suggest that John Monro examined Nicholson alone for the first time, others record him attending with his son from the very start. Contrast, e.g., ibid., pp. 12–13; *Lady's Magazine* 17 (1786), p. 396; *Annual Register*, vol. 29 (1786), p. 234. Fiske claimed that Monro's son arrived shortly after Monro was sent for; *The Life*, p. 39.

152. *Annual Register*, vol. 29 (1786), p. 234, and see also subsequent note.

153. *European Magazine* 10 (1786), p. 118. The latter quoted Monro slightly differently: "such a discovery could not be made *immediately*," while the *Lady's Magazine* (17 [1786], p. 396), claiming that it was both Monros who had been summoned and who gave their opinions jointly from the start, quoted them as stating "that no certain opinion on that subject could be formed in less than three or four days."

154. Macalpine and Hunter, *George III and the Mad-Business* (p. 311),

claimed (on the authority of Fiske, *The Life*, p. 39) that this examination was conducted by "three elderly matrons" to determine her sex. According to the *Lady's Magazine* (17 [1786], p. 396) and *The Plot Investigated* (p. 10), however, Nicholson was inspected in a "private chamber" with the assistance of "two women belonging to the palace," the main (or only) reason being to see if she had any "weapon, or any information relative to the preceding attempt . . . upon her"—none being found.

155. Macalpine and Hunter, *George III and the Mad-Business*, p. 311; *European Magazine* 10 (1786), p. 119.

156. *European Magazine* 10 (1786), p. 119.

157. *Universal Magazine* 79 (1786), p. 95.

158. Ibid.

159. A. Aspinall, ed., *The Later Correspondence of George III* (Cambridge: Cambridge University Press, 1962), vol. 1, letter of Lord Sydney to George III, 3 Aug. 1786, p. 317.

160. Fiske, *The Life,* p. 46.

161. *European Magazine* 10 (1786), p. 119.

162. Ibid. According to the *Universal Magazine* (79 [1786], p. 95), it was while at the Coates's the previous day that Nicholson had first said "that although she had never been married," the judges "were her sons, and that they knew it; with various other things equally ridiculous."

163. Fiske, *The Life*, p. 17.

164. Ibid., p. 21.

165. *Universal Magazine* 79 (1786), p. 95.

166. Roy Porter, "The Prophetic Body: Lady Eleanor Davies and the Meaning of Madness," *Women's Writing: The Elizabethan to Victorian Period* 1.1 (1994), pp. 51–63.

167. *The Plot Investigated*, p. 17.

168. Ibid., pp. 27–28. The guard was increased to a sergeant, grenadiers, and four yeomen. George's conduct was excused by the ingratiating author as an "accident," or else "advisable," and yet there was also an implicit criticism and admonishment in the comment that "the Sovereign bears too exalted a mind, to have recourse to naked arms in the midst of his subjects."

169. Ibid., pp. 28–30. Plainly the author was sublimating the reactions of the crowd, with observations such as: ". . . a universal joy seemed to beam in their countenances."

170. *Universal Magazine* 79 (1786), p. 95.

171. *The Plot Investigated*, p. 31.

172. Ibid., p. 38.

173. Ibid., p. 31.

174. Ibid., p. 36.

175. Ibid., p. 38.

176. *Lady's Magazine* 17 (1787), p. 396.

177. According to the *Universal Magazine* (79 [1786], p. 95), these witnesses included "Ann Southey, who lodged in the next apartment to Nicholson" and who offered testimony almost identical to Fiske's. Fiske himself attended but was not questioned.

178. Ability to play cards appears to have featured as one of the tests for lunacy in other legal cases, and it may well have been a formulaic legal criterion for establishing insanity at the time. See, e.g., Foyster, "Wrongful Confinement."

179. PRO PC2–131, fols. 357–88; Macalpine and Hunter, *George III and the Mad-Business*, p. 311.

180. Fiske, *The Life*, p. 47.

181. *GM* 56 (1786), pp. 708–11; Bethlem Admission Registers.

182. Fiske, *The Life*, pp. 43–44; *European Magazine* 10 (1786), pp. 119–20.

183. Fiske, *The Life*, pp. 43–44.

184. Ibid.; *European Magazine* 10 (1786), p. 120.

185. *European Magazine* 10 (1786), p. 120; Macalpine and Hunter, *George III and the Mad-Business*, p. 312.

186. *European Magazine* 10 (1786), p. 120.

187. *Lady's Magazine* 17 (1786), p. 386.

188. BSCM, 12 Aug. and 2 Sept. 1786, 3 Feb. 1787.

189. Perfect, *Select Cases*, p. 196.

190. BSCM, 14 April 1787; Bethlem Admission Registers (BARs) and Bethlem Incurables Admission Registers (BIARs).

191. BSCM, 11 Aug. 1787.

192. BSCM, 12 March 1791, p. 5.

193. *Lady's Magazine* 17 (1786), p. 395.

194. See *The Plot Investigated*, esp. pp. 3–4.

195. Ibid., pp. 48–49; this was an explanation that, indeed, as the author rightly claimed, "the public prints have been wholly silent as to."

196. See Matthew Lewis, *Crazy Jane* (1793), cited in Elaine Showalter, *The Female Malady: Women, Madness and English Culture 1830–1980* (New York: Pantheon Books, 1985; London: Virago Press, 1987), p. 13; John Davy, *Crazy Jane: A Ballad, Sung by Mrs. Mountain . . . at Mr Raussini's Concerts, Bath,* words by G. M. Lewis; music by John Davy (London: Longman, Clementi & Co., 1799). Those verbal images were repeatedly taken up in artists' work over the ensuing decades, as in George Shepheard's 1815 painting. However, here the genre was in the realm of Ophelia-like naturalism, bucolic invocation, and pastoral wandering—Jane's attire an amalgam of wildflowers, garlands, patched robes, and tattered shawls—rather than the spinster-cum-trollop glamour and poverty-constrained pretensions of a city housemaid.

197. Our thanks to Sue Carter for urging us to analyze in more depth this dichotomized presentation of Nicholson, and for helpful suggestions about the ways in which her case was being constructed by contemporaries.

198. See Alan Hunt, *Governance of the Consuming Passions: A History of Sumptuary Law* (Basingstoke: Macmillan, 1996).

199. See, e.g., Mullan, *Sentiment and Sociability*; G. J. Barker-Benfield, *The Culture of Sensibility: Sex and Society in Eighteenth-Century Britain* (Chicago: University of Chicago Press, 1992); Frances Hodgson Burnett, *A Lady of Quality: Being a Most Curious, Hitherto Unknown History, as Related to Mr. Isaac Bickerstaff but not Presented to the World of Fashion Through the Pages of the Tatler, and now for the First Time Written Down* (London: F. Warne, 1896); William Alexander, *Picturesque Representations of the Dress and Manners of*

the English: Illustrated in Fifty Coloured Engravings, with Descriptions (London: Printed for John Murray by W. Bulmer & Co., 1814); Malcolm Andrews, *The Picturesque: Literary Sources and Documents* (Robertsbridge: Helm Information, 1994).

200. See, e.g., *A Genuine Account of the Life of John Rann, alias Sixteen-string Jack: Who was Executed November 30th. 1774, for a Robbery on the Highway, near Brentford; . . . some Curious Anecdotes of Miss Smith and Miss Roche . . .* (London: Bailey, 1774); Joseph Radley, *An Authentic Account of the life of Joseph Radley, an Notorious Highwayman . . . Who was Executed at Aylesbury [&etc.]* (Aylesbury: 1784).

201. See, e.g., *An Authentic Account of Forgeries and Frauds of Various Kinds Committed by that Most Consummate Adept in Deception, Charles Price: Otherwise Patch, many years a Lottery Office Keeper, in London and Westminster . . . with Which is Given as a Frontispiece, an Exact Representation of his Person, in the Disguise Which he Wore When he Negotiated his First Parcel of Counterfeit Bank Notes, in the year 1780, and Likewise his Portrait in his Usual Dress* (London: Printed for the editor and sold by G. Kearsley, 1786).

202. Terry Castle, *Masquerade and Civilisation: The Carnivalesque in Eighteenth-Century English Culture and Fiction* (London: Methuen, 1986).

203. I.e., Fiske, *The Life; The Plot Investigated; Authentic Memoirs.*

204. Perfect, *Select Cases.*

205. von la Roche, *Sophie in London,* pp. 169–70.

206. Ibid., p. 169.

207. Jacques de Cambry, *De Londres et de ses Environs* (Amsterdam: 1788), p. 60.

208. Sophie had also reported seeing her reading Shakespeare. Oddly enough, Margaret's intended victim, George III, engaged in the same activity during his own convalescence from madness in 1789—choosing, of all plays, *Lear* as his preferred text.

209. See Munk, *Roll,* vol. 2, p. 185; Joseph Strutt, *A Biographical Dictionary; Containing an Historical Account of all the Engravers, from the Earliest Period of the Art of Engraving to the Present Time . . . ,* 2 vols. (London: R. Faulder, 1785).

210. For a famous, if brief, discussion of this case, see Michel Foucault, *Discipline and Punish: The Birth of the Prison* (Harmondsworth, Middlesex: Penguin, 1977), trans. from *Naissance de la prison* (Paris: Editions Gallimard, 1975). See also W. H. Dilworth, *The Royal Assassins, Containing . . . II The Trial and Execution of R. F. Damiens for Stabbing Lewis XV . . . etc.* (London: Printed for W. Anderson, 1759); Jacques Delaye, *Louis XV et Damiens* (Paris: Gallimard, 1986); Dale K. Van Kley, *The Damiens Affair and the Unravelling of the Ancien Régime, 1750–1770* (Princeton: Princeton University Press, 1984); Anne Léo Zévaès, *Damiens le regicide* (Paris, 1933); Pierre Chevallier, *Les regicides: Clement, Ravaillac, Damiens* (Paris: Fayard, 1989). However, the real fuss about Anglo-French attitudes toward regicide broke out in the years following the execution of Louis XVI.

211. In France, besides the Damiens attempt, there was that of Clement, who stabbed Henry IV, and Raveillac, who poignarded Henry III. In addition,

the press mentioned two attempts on the king of Prussia; the 1771 attempt on the king of Poland; that of 1758 on the king of Portugal, Joseph I; and the 1695 attempt on King William at Turnham Green. See *European Magazine* 10 (1786), p. 119. See also *A Full, Clear, and Authorised Account of the Late Conspiracy in Portugal; the Horrid Attempt upon the Life of His . . . Majesty; and the . . . Execution of the Conspirators . . .* , trans. from the original Portuguese [etc.] (London: 1759).

212. Percy Bysshe Shelley and Thomas Jefferson Hogg, *Posthumous Fragments of Margaret Nicholson. Being Poems Found Amongst the Papers of that Noted Female who Attempted the Life of the King in 1786*, ed. John Fitzvictor (Oxford: T. Munday, 1810), p. 13.

213. The *Lady's Magazine* (17 [1786], p. 896) was plainly exaggerating to fuel the curiosity of its readership when claiming that Nicholson's crime was "of so extraordinary a nature, that no similar instance occurs in the whole annals of England." The last attempt had actually been that of James Sheppard (or Shepherd), a coach painter, in ca. 1718. Sheppard was executed for treason despite having been offered a reprieve, having refused to ask George I's pardon, and while many condemned him as a vicious non-juror, a number of contemporaries protested the execution on the grounds that he was insane. In another echo of the Nicholson case, the Newgate jailer was even to seek credit out of publishing an account of Sheppard. (Sheppard is not to be confused with the robber immortalized by Defoe, namely John or Jack Sheppard, 1702–24.) See, e.g., Brother Will (pseud.), *J- S-d's [James Shepherd's] Ghost: Being News from t'other Side the World. In a Letter from Newgate, from Brother Will to Brother Jack* (London: J. Peters 1718); Paul Lorrain (d. 1719), *A Narrative; or, the Ordinary of Newgate's Account of what Passed Between him and James Sheppard . . .* (London: Printed and sold by J. Morphew, 1718); *Observations on the Conspiracies of the Non-jurors; and their Spiriting-up Assassines and Murderers; Particularly James Shepherd . . .* (Edinburgh: 1718).

214. See, e.g., *High Treason: A Full Report of the Proceedings Against James Hadfield, at the . . . King's Bench . . . for Shooting at the King . . .* (Dublin: Printed by John Stockdale, 1800); *Sketches in Bedlam* (1823).

215. von la Roche, *Sophie in London*, p. 169.

216. Shelley and Hogg, *Posthumous Fragments of Margaret Nicholson*.

217. Ibid., "Advertisement."

218. Ibid., pp. 21–22.

219. *Sketches in Bedlam*, pp. 253–58; Macalpine and Hunter, *George III and the Mad-Business*, pp. 312–13. For good discussions of the authorship and content of the volume, see Patricia Allderidge, "Sketches in Bedlam," in *Proceedings of the First European Congress on the History of Psychiatry and Mental HealthCare, 's-Hertogenbosch, The Netherlands, 24–26 October 1990*, ed. Leonie de Goei and Joost Vijselaar (Rotterdam: Erasmus Publishing, 1993), pp. 76–82; Francis Schiller, "Haslam of 'Bedlam,' Kitchiner of the 'Oracles': Two Doctors under Mad King George III, and Their Friendship," *Medical History* 28 (1984), pp. 189–201.

220. *Annual Register*, vol. 29 (22 Aug. 1787), pp. 219–20.

221. Ibid., p. 220.

222. Ibid.

223. Ibid.

224. Ibid.

225. BSCM, 27 Sept. 1788.

226. Stone was admitted as an incurable on 27 Sept. 1788 and died on 14 Sept. 1805; BSCM, 8 Sept. 1787; BAR and BIAR.

227. BSCM, 12 and 19 Sept. 1761. For more on the Board of Green Cloth and political committals, see Andrews, "The Politics of Committal to Early-Modern Bethlem," pp. 6–63.

228. He was admitted on 26 Aug. 1780, his residence recorded as St. Catharine Coleman Street. His sureties were Thomas Gates of Monkwell Street and John Kirby of Wood Street, Counter, in London, and he was discharged cured but recommended to the care of a relation on 3 Nov. 1781. See Bethlem Admission Register.

229. BSCM, 14 July and 13 Oct. 1781.

230. *The Whole Proceedings upon the King's Commission of the Peace Oyer and Terminer, and Gaol Delivery for the City of London, & . . . for the County of Middlesex . . . in the Old Bailey on Wednesday 6th June 1780 and the Following Days,* no. 6, part 13, case 415 (London: Joseph Gurney, 1780), pp. 610–13; Walker, *Crime and Insanity,* p. 63.

231. Walker, *Crime and Insanity,* p. 63; Eigen, *Witnessing Insanity.*

232. Lewis, *Correspondence,* vol. 25, HW to Mann, 6 Feb. 1780, p. 11 and note 13.

233. Nichols, *Literary Anecdotes,* vol. 4, part 3, p. 609; 8, part 4, p. 507.

234. However, John being old and increasingly infirm, the majority of assistance was provided by Gozna, the Bethlem apothecary, and by Thomas Monro, "upon whom the principal medical department of Bedlam now devolves." See William Black, *A Comparative View of the Mortality of the Human Species, at all Ages; and of the Diseases and Casualties by which they are Destroyed or Annoyed* (London: C. Dilly, 1788); Black, *Dissertation on Insanity, Illustrated with Tables* (London: D. Ridgway, 1810; London: Smeeton, 1811), p. 11; Macalpine and Hunter, *George III and the Mad-Business,* pp. 298–99.

235. von la Roche, *Sophie in London.* See also Rosmaund Bayne-Powell, *Travellers in Eighteenth-Century England* (London: John Murray, 1951), p. 118.

236. See, e.g., César de Saussure, *A Foreign View of England in the Reigns of George I & George II. The Letters of Monsieur César de Saussure to his Family,* trans. and ed. Madame van Muyden (London: John Murray, 1902); Zacharias Conrad von Uffenbach, *London in 1710. From the Travels of Z. C. von Uffenbach* (extracted from *Herrn Zacharias Conrad von Uffenbach merkwürdige Reisen durch Niedersachsen, Holland und Engelland*), trans. and ed. W. H. Quarrell and Margaret Mare (London: Faber and Faber, 1934); Andrews, "Bedlam Revisited," chap. 2; Andrews et al., *The History of Bethlem,* chap. 13.

237. Lady Llanover, ed., *The Autobiography and Correspondence of Mary Granville, Mrs Delany* (London: Richard Bentley, 1862), p. 233.

238. Anon. [William Rowley, M.D.], *Important Facts and Opinions Relative to the King; Faithfully Collected from the Examination of the Royal Physicians . . .* (London: 1788), p. 30.

239. *House of Commons Sessional Papers of the Eighteenth Century,* vol. 66, *Report from the Committee Appointed to Examine the Physicians who have Attended his Majesty, During his Illness, Touching the Present State of his Majesty's Health . . . 13 Jan. 1789* (Wilmington, Del.: Scholarly Resources Inc., 1975), p. 89.

240. G. Hogge, ed., *The Journal and Correspondence of William, Lord Aukland* (London: R. Bentley, 1862), vol. 2, Anthony Storer to William Eden, 14 and 28 Nov. 1788, pp. 242, 246.

241. Countess of Minto, ed., *The Life and Letters of Sir Gilbert, First Earl of Minto from 1751 to 1806* (London: Longmans, Green & Co., 1874), 11 Nov. 1788, p. 233.

242. *House of Commons Sessional Papers,* pp. 8–9, 38; *Important Facts,* p. 30. Pepys was evidently well acquainted with Monro and accustomed to calling upon the mad-doctor when privately attending mental cases.

243. *Letters Relating to Illnesses of George III in 1789 and 1811–12,* Royal College of Physicians, London, MS, 3011/46–56, 46. Thomas Monro was paid £500 for attending George III in 1811–12, and was interested enough in the royal malady, and sufficiently devoted to his father, to provide the College with these letters relating to John's consultation and his own attendance on the king. For Warren's nomination and election as a governor, see chapter 1, note 18.

244. Ibid., 3011/48.

245. See note 243, above.

246. Pitt's father, the Right Honorable William Pitt (the elder), was elected a governor of Bethlem in 1757; BCGM, 22 Dec. 1757, p. 273.

247. See Willis, *Treatise on Mental Derangement,* p. 179, which states that his grandfather became joint physician with Dr. Petrie to a general hospital in Lincoln from 1769, attending there twice a week, and only subsequently began to specialize in cases of insanity.

248. Countess of Minto, ed., *Life and Letters of Sir Gilbert Elliot,* vol. 1, p. 252, letter dated 29 Dec. 1788, p. 252; John Mitford, *A Description of the Crimes and Horrors in the Interior of Warburton's Private Mad-House at Hoxton, Commonly Called Whitmore House . . .* (London: Benbow, 1825), p. 3.

249. Porter, *Mind-Forg'd Manacles,* p. 276.

250. E.g., Macalpine and Hunter, *George III and the Mad-Business,* pp. 114–15, 126, 323; Morris, *The Hoxton Madhouses.*

251. Given the frequency with which Monro also attended the Hoxton madhouses, it is unlikely that he was unacquainted with Willis and Warburton.

252. Countess of Minto, *Life and Letters of Sir Gilbert Elliot,* vol. 1, 16 Dec. 1788, p. 246.

253. Frank Mckno Bladon, ed., *The Diaries of Colonel the Hon. Robert Fulke Greville* (London: John Lane, 1930), 23 Jan. 1789, p. 185.

254. For a general discussion of this tradition, see Scull, *The Most Solitary of Afflictions,* pp. 64–77. Even mad-doctors like William Pargeter, who professed to embrace a milder approach, saw advantages in placidity and kindness,

and criticized the use of compulsion in the treatment of the insane (whom they claimed were "exceedingly timorous and easily terrified"), also stressed the need to "gain an ascendancy over them," and to employ anger, fear, shock, and absolutism in their management. Pargeter, *Observations on Maniacal Disorders*, pp. 49–60, 61, 94. The transition from an older coercive management or taming of the insane to the sense in which some late eighteenth-century figures began to speak of employing moral management to domesticate the mad was naturally an extremely complex phenomenon. Linguistic usage provides important evidence of this transformation. Etymologically, the word "management" derived from the Italian *maneggiare* and the French *management* or *ménage* (i.e., horsemanship). The word was originally used in the sense of handling or training animals, especially horses, and referred in particular to the disciplinary methods by which horses were accustomed to the bit and the bridle, and brought under the control of their human masters. When the term began to be extended to human beings, it was originally employed in closely related senses. Significantly, in the early part of the eighteenth century, "manage" retained the cluster of meanings of its original Italian and French derivation, but during the second half of the century, the standard meaning gradually began to undergo a subtle shift, and by the turn of the century the concept came to be used in the rather different sense of treating persons with indulgence or showing them consideration; or, alternatively, of using tact, care, and skill to manipulate the behavior of others. Analogously, the manager, once the wielder of a weapon or one who waged war, now became someone skilled in handling people and in administering a business. This is plainly crucial to understanding the shifting meanings that underlay apparently similar emphases on the importance of management in the treatment of the mad.

255. Bladon, *Greville*, 25 Jan. 1789, p. 190.

256. *House of Commons Sessional Papers*, vol. 66, pp. 37–38.

257. BSCM, 20 and 27 March 1784.

258. Thomas Monro was appointed assistant physician on 19 July 1787 and physician on 2 Feb. 1792. See BCGM; *GM* (1787).

259. See, e.g., *GM* (1791), p. 1237.

260. BSCM, 26 Dec. 1778.

261. For John Monro's will, see FRC PCC Prob. 11/1213, q.n. 32, fols. 256–58.

262. According to Dr. F. J. G. Jefferiss ("Extracts from a Biography of Dr Thomas Monro," *Dr Thomas Monro (1759–1833) and the Monro Academy* (London: Victoria and Albert Museum, 1976), John had six children by his wife, Elizabeth. Clearly not all were still living by the time of his death, John and Charlotte having died before him, and we have been unable to identify his sixth child.

263. Thomas was educated at Harrow and then at Oriel College Oxford, but where precisely he trained in medicine remains unclear, although his father plainly had a significant role in his medical education. Thomas certainly obtained his M.D. (1787) and his fellowship (1791) at the College of Physicians before his father's death. Dr. Jefferiss conjectured that he may well have trained at St. Bartholomew's Hospital, Thomas having mentioned his father attending

the annual governors' dinner there on several occasions. Dr. Jefferiss also related that his older brother Charles had been envious of Thomas, having "hated the law" and felt that he too would have preferred medicine, but "Thomas had been too quick for him." Thomas's own career as an aspiring doctor was far from dependable at this stage, however (as correspondence dating from 1787 in the family's possession reveals). At the time, he was courting Hannah Woodcock, the woman he was to marry the following year. Her father, Reverend Edward Woodcock of Bath, former vicar of Watford, initially opposed the match, however, on the grounds that Thomas's financial position was as yet insecure. Thomas wrote back underlining his "good prospects, as he was just about to become Assistant Physician to his father at Bethlem," and Woodcock then relented, granting his permission soon after Thomas's appointment in 1787. Thomas lived with his father until his marriage, when he moved briefly to Mitchell Place, Brompton, before taking over his father's house at 53 Bedford Square in 1790, when John retired in declining health to the country. In 1793, he moved once again, to 8 Adelphi Terrace. See ibid.

Select Bibliography

All primary source materials, and secondary material not cited in the bibliography but used in this book, may be found fully referenced in the notes to each chapter.

BOOKS, MONOGRAPHS, AND DISSERTATIONS

Allen, Elizabeth, T. L. Turk, and Sir Reginald Murley, eds. *The Case Books of John Hunter FRS.* London: Royal Society of Medicine, 1993.

Andrews, Jonathan. "Bedlam Revisited. A History of Bethlem Hospital c1633–c1770." Unpublished Ph.D. diss., University of London, 1991.

Andrews, Jonathan, Asa Briggs, Roy Porter, Penny Tucker, and Keir Waddington. *The History of Bethlem.* London: Routledge, 1997.

Andrews, Malcolm. *The Picturesque: Literary Sources and Documents.* Robertsbridge: Helm Information, 1994.

Babb, Lawrence. *The Elizabethan Malady: A Study of Melancholia in English Literature from 1580 to 1642.* East Lansing: Michigan State University Press, 1951.

———. *Sanity in Bedlam: A Study of Robert Burton's Anatomy of Melancholy.* East Lansing: Michigan State University Press, 1959. Westport, Conn.: Greenwood Press, 1977.

Bateson, Gregory, ed. *Perceval's Narrative: A Patient's Account of His Psychosis, 1830–1832.* Stanford, Calif.: Stanford University Press, 1961.

Bayne-Powell, Rosamund. *Travellers in Eighteenth-Century England.* London: John Murray, 1951.

Beer, E. S. de, ed. *The Diary of John Evelyn: Now Printed in Full from the Manuscripts Belonging to Mr. John Evelyn.* Vol. 3. Oxford: Clarendon Press, 2000.

Beier, Lucinda M. *Sufferers and Healers: The Experience of Illness in Seventeenth-Century England.* London and New York: Routledge and Kegan Paul, 1987.

Bostridge, Ian. *Witchcraft and Its Transformations 1650–1750.* Oxford: Clarendon Press, 1997.

Braslow, Joel. *Mental Ills and Bodily Cures.* Berkeley: University of California Press, 1997.

Buchanan, James H. *Patient Encounters: The Experience of Disease*, Charlottesville, Va.: University Press of Virginia, 1989.

Butler, David. *Methodists and Papists: John Wesley and the Catholic Church in the Eighteenth Century*. London: Darton, Longman and Todd, 1995.

Bynum, William F., and Roy Porter, eds. *Companion Encyclopedia of the History of Medicine*. Vol. 2. London: Routledge, 1993.

———, eds. *Medicine and the Five Senses*. Cambridge and New York: Cambridge University Press, 1993.

———, eds. *William Hunter and the Eighteenth Century Medical World*. Cambridge: Cambridge University Press, 1985.

Byrd, Max. *Visits to Bedlam*. Columbia: University of South Carolina Press, 1974.

Canavan, Thomas Lester. "Madness and Enthusiasm in Burton's *Anatomy of Melancholy* and Swift's *Tale of a Tub*." Unpublished Ph.D. diss., Columbia University, 1970.

Castle, Terry. *Masquerade and Civilisation: The Carnivalesque in Eighteenth-Century English Culture and Fiction*. London: Methuen, 1986.

Colley, Linda. *In Defiance of Oligarchy: The Tory Party, 1714–60*. Cambridge: Cambridge University Press, 1982.

———. *Britons: Forging the Nation, 1707–1837*. Pimlico, 1994. London: Vintage, 1996.

Deporte, Michael V. *Nightmares and Hobbyhorses: Swift, Sterne, and Augustan Ideas of Madness*. San Marino, Calif.: Huntington Library, 1974.

Digby, Anne. *Making a Medical Living: Doctors and Patients in the English Market for Medicine, 1720–1911*. Cambridge: Cambridge University Press, 1994.

Dingwall, Robert. *Aspects of Illness*. London: Martin Robertson, 1976.

Doerner, Klaus. *Madmen and the Bourgeoisie: A Social History of Insanity and Psychiatry*. Oxford: Basil Blackwell, 1986.

Dow, Derek A. *The Influence of Scottish Medicine: An Historical Assessment of Its International Impact*. Carnforth, Lancashire, England: Parthenon, 1988.

Earle, Peter. *A City Full of People: Men and Women of London, 1650–1750*. London: Methuen, 1994.

Eigen, Joel Peter. *Witnessing Insanity: Madness and Mad-Doctors in the English Court*. New Haven and London: Yale University Press, 1995.

Fissell, Mary E. *Patients, Power and the Poor in Eighteenth-Century Bristol*. Cambridge: Cambridge University Press, 1991.

Foucault, Michel. *Discipline and Punish: The Birth of the Prison*. Harmondsworth, Middlesex: Penguin, 1977. Trans. from *Naissance de la prison*. Paris: Editions Gallimard, 1975.

———. *Madness and Civilisation: A History of Insanity in the Age of Reason*. London: Tavistock, 1971. Trans. and abr. from *Histoire de la Folie à l'âge classique*. Paris: Librairie Plon, 1961.

French, C. N. *The Story of St. Luke's Hospital*. London: William Heinemann, 1951.

Gijsw, Marijke, ed. *Illness and Healing Alternatives in Western Europe*. London: Routledge, 1997.

Granshaw, Lindsay, and Roy Porter, eds. *The Hospital in History*. London and
   New York: Routledge, 1990.
Grell, Ole Peter, Jonathan I. Israel, and Nicholas Tyacke, eds. *From Persecution
   to Toleration: The Glorious Revolution and Religion in England*. Oxford:
   Clarendon Press, 1991.
Griffin, Martin I. J., Lila Freedman, and Richard Henry Popkin. *Latitudinarian-
   ism in the Seventeenth-Century Church of England*. Leiden: Brill, 1992.
Harrison, J. F. C. *The Second Coming: Popular Millenarianism, 1780–1850*.
   New Brunswick, N.J.: Rutgers University Press, 1979.
Hay, D. P. Linebaugh, J. Rule, E. P. Thompson, and C. Winslow. *Albion's Fatal
   Tree: Crime and Society in Eighteenth Century England*. New York: Pan-
   theon, 1975.
Hecht, Joseph Jean. *The Domestic Servant Class in Eighteenth-Century En-
   gland*. London: Routledge and Kegan Paul, 1980.
Hempton, David. *Religion and Identity: Religious and Political Cultures in Brit-
   ain and Ireland Since 1700*. Cambridge: Cambridge University Press, 1996.
Heyd, Michael. *Be Sober and Reasonable: The Critique of Enthusiasm in the
   Seventeenth and Early Eighteenth Centuries*. New York: E. J. Brill, 1995.
Hill, Bridget. *Eighteenth-Century Women: An Anthology*. London, Boston, and
   Sydney: George Allen and Unwin, 1984.
Hill, Christopher. *Change and Continuity in Seventeenth-Century England*.
   London: Weidenfeld and Nicolson, 1974. New Haven and London: Yale
   University Press, 1991.
———. *The World Turned Upside Down: Radical Ideas during the English
   Revolution*. London: Temple Smith, 1972. Harmondsworth: Penguin, 1991.
Hitchcock, Tim. *English Sexualities, 1700–1800*. Basingstoke: Macmillan,
   1997.
Hixson, William F. *Triumph of the Bankers: Money and Banking in the Eigh-
   teenth and Nineteenth Centuries*. Westport, Conn.: Praeger, 1993.
Hunt, Alan. *Governance of the Consuming Passions: A History of Sumptuary
   Law*. Basingstoke: Macmillan, 1996.
Hunter, Richard, and Macalpine, Ida. *Three Hundred Years of Psychiatry,
   1535–1860: A History Presented in Selected English Texts*. London and
   New York: Oxford University Press, 1963.
Ingram, Allan. *The Madhouse of Language: Writing and Reading Madness in
   the Eighteenth Century*. London and New York: Routledge, 1991.
———, ed. *Patterns of Madness in the Eighteenth Century: A Reader*. Liver-
   pool: Liverpool University Press, 1998.
———, ed. *Voices of Madness: Four Pamphlets, 1683–1796*. Thrupp and
   Stroud, Gloucestershire: Sutton, 1997.
Ingrassia, Catherine. *Authorship, Commerce, and Gender in Early Eighteenth-
   Century England: A Culture of Paper Credit*. Cambridge and New York:
   Cambridge University Press, 1998.
Jackson, Stanley W. *Melancholia and Depression: From Hippocratic Times
   to Modern Times*. New Haven: Yale University Press, 1986.
Kleinman, Arthur. *The Illness Narratives: Suffering, Healing and the Human
   Condition*. New York: Basic Books, 1988.

Knox, R. A. *Enthusiasm.* Oxford: Oxford University Press, 1950.

Kroll, Richard W. F., Richard Ashcraft, and Perez Zagorin. *Philosophy, Science, and Religion in England, 1640–1700.* Cambridge: Cambridge University Press, 1992.

Leigh, Denis. *The Historical Development of British Psychiatry.* Oxford: Pergamon, 1961.

Lewis, W. S. *Horace Walpole's Correspondence.* 48 vols. New Haven: Yale University Press, 1954, and London: Oxford University Press, 1937–83.

Linebaugh, Peter. *The London Hanged: Crime and Civil Society in the Eighteenth Century.* London: Allen Lane/Penguin, 1991.

Loudon, Irvine S. L. *Medical Care and the General Practitioner, 1750–1850.* Oxford and New York: Clarendon Press. Oxford University Press, 1986.

Lunbeck, Elizabeth. *The Psychiatric Persuasion: Knowledge, Gender, and Power in Modern America.* Princeton: Princeton University Press, 1994.

Macalpine, Ida, and Richard Hunter. *George III and the Mad-Business.* London: Allen Lane/Penguin, 1969.

MacDonald, Michael. *Mystical Bedlam: Madness, Anxiety and Healing in Seventeenth-Century England.* Cambridge: Cambridge University Press, 1981.

MacDonald, Michael, and Terence R. Murphy. *Sleepless Souls: Suicide in Early Modern England.* Oxford: Clarendon Press, 1990.

MacKenzie, Charlotte. *Psychiatry for the Rich: A History of Ticehurst Private Asylum.* London: Routledge, 1992.

Mason, Alfred Bishop, ed. *Horace Walpole's England as His Letters Picture It.* Boston and New York: Houghton Mifflin, 1930.

McKendrick, Neil, John Brewer, and J. H. Plumb. *The Birth of a Consumer Society: The Commercialization of Eighteenth-Century England.* Bloomington: Indiana University Press, 1982.

Mitchison, Rosalind. *Sexuality and Social Control: Scotland 1660–1780.* Oxford: Basil Blackwell, 1989.

Morris, Arthur David. *The Hoxton Madhouses.* March, Cambridge: Goodwin Bros., 1958.

Mowl, Tim. *Horace Walpole: The Great Outsider.* London: John Murray, 1996.

Mullan, John. *Sentiment and Sociability: The Language of Feeling in the Eighteenth Century.* Oxford: Clarendon Press, 1988.

Nicholson, Colin. *Writing and the Rise of Finance: Capital Satires of the Early Eighteenth Century.* Cambridge Studies in Eighteenth-Century English Literature and Thought. Cambridge and New York: Cambridge University Press, 1994.

Oliver, Edith. *Alexander the Corrector: The Eccentric Life of Alexander Cruden.* London: Faber and Faber and New York: Viking, 1934.

Parry-Jones, William Ll. *The Trade in Lunacy: A Study of Private Madhouses in England in the Eighteenth and Nineteenth Centuries.* London: Routledge and Kegan Paul, 1972.

Peterson, Dale Alfred. *A Mad Peoples' History of Madness.* Pittsburgh: University of Pittsburgh Press, 1982.

Phillips, H. Temple. "The History of the Old Private Lunatic Asylum at Fishponds, Bristol, 1740–1859." M.Sc. thesis, Bristol University, 1973.

Porter, Roy. *English Society in the Eighteenth Century*. London: Penguin, 1982.

———, ed. *The Faber Book of Madness*. London: Faber and Faber, 1991.

———. *Health for Sale: Quackery in England 1660–1850*. Manchester and New York: Manchester University Press, 1989.

———. *Mind-Forg'd Manacles: A History of Madness in England from the Restoration to the Regency*. London: Athlone, 1987.

———, ed. *Patients and Practitioners: Lay Perceptions of Medicine in Preindustrial Society*. Cambridge: Cambridge University Press, 1985.

———, ed. *The Popularization of Medicine 1650–1850*. London: Routledge, 1992.

———. *A Social History of Madness: Stories of the Insane*. London: Weidenfeld and Nicolson, 1987.

Porter, Roy, and Dorothy Porter. *In Sickness and in Health: The English Experience 1650–1850*. London: Fourth Estate, 1988.

———. *Patient's Progress: Doctors and Doctoring in Eighteenth-Century England*. Oxford: Polity, 1989.

Rivers, Isabel. *Reason, Grace, and Sentiment: A Study of the Language of Religion and Ethics in England, 1660–1780*. Cambridge: Cambridge University Press, 1991.

Robinson, Daniel. *Wild Beasts and Idle Humours: The Insanity Defense from Antiquity to the Present*. Cambridge, Mass.: Harvard University Press, 1996.

Rousseau, George S., and Roy Porter, eds. *Sexual Underworlds of the Enlightenment*. 1987. Manchester: Manchester University Press, 1992.

Scull, Andrew, ed. *Madhouses, Mad-Doctors and Madmen: The Social History of Psychiatry in the Victorian Era*. Philadelphia: University of Pennsylvania Press, 1981.

———. *The Most Solitary of Afflictions: Madness and Society in Britain, 1700–1900*. London and New Haven: Yale University Press, 1993.

Scull, Andrew, Charlotte MacKenzie, and Nicholas Hervey. *Masters of Bedlam: The Transformation of the Mad-Doctoring Trade*. Princeton: Princeton University Press, 1996.

Shapin, Steven. *A Social History of Truth: Civility and Science in Seventeenth-Century England*. Chicago: University of Chicago Press, 1994.

Sharpe, James. *Instruments of Darkness: Witchcraft in England 1550–1750*. London: Hamish Hamilton, 1996.

Showalter, Elaine. *The Female Malady: Women, Madness and English Culture 1830–1980*. New York: Pantheon Books, 1985. London: Virago Press, 1987.

Skultans, Veida. *English Madness: Ideas on Insanity 1580–1890*. London, Boston, and Henley: Routledge and Kegan Paul, 1979.

Smith, Roger. *Trial by Medicine: Insanity and Responsibility in Victorian Trials*. Edinburgh: Edinburgh University Press, 1981.

Spellman, W. M. *The Latitudinarians and the Church of England, 1660–1700*. Athens and London: University of Georgia Press, 1993.

Stone, Lawrence. *Road to Divorce: England 1530–1987*. Oxford: Oxford University Press, 1990.

Suzuki, Akihito. "Mind and Its Disease in Enlightenment British Medicine." Unpublished Ph.D. diss., University of London, 1992.

Tucker, Susie I. *Enthusiasm: A Study in Semantic Change.* Cambridge: Cambridge University Press 1972.

Walker, Nigel. *Crime and Insanity in England.* Vol. 1. Edinburgh: Edinburgh University Press, 1968.

Ward, Karen. "'Moon Madness': A Study to Investigate the Relationship between Human Behaviour and the Phases of the Moon." Unpublished Ph.D. diss., University of Nottingham, 1997.

ARTICLES, PAPERS, AND BOOK CHAPTERS

Allderidge, Patricia. "Sketches in Bedlam." *Proceedings of the First European Congress on the History of Psychiatry and Mental Health Care, 's-Hertogenbosch, The Netherlands, 24–26 October 1990.* Ed. Leonie de Goei and Joost Vijselaar. Rotterdam: Erasmus Publishing, 1993. 76–82.

Andrews, Jonathan. "Case Notes, Case Histories, and the Patient's Experience of Insanity at Gartnavel Royal Asylum, Glasgow, in the Nineteenth Century." *Social History of Medicine* 11 (1998): 255–81.

———. "'Hardly a Hospital but a Charity for Pauper Lunatics'? Therapeutics at Bethlem in the Seventeenth and Eighteenth Centuries." *Medicine and Charity before the Welfare State.* Ed. Jonathan Barry and Colin Jones. Studies in the Social History of Medicine. London: Routledge, 1991. 63–81.

———. "Identifying and Providing for the Mentally Disabled in Early Modern London." *From Idiocy to Mental Deficiency.* Ed. David Wright and Anne Digby. London and New York: Routledge, 1996. 65–92.

———. "'In her vapours [or] indeed in her Madness'? Mrs Clerke's Case: An Early Eighteenth-century Psychiatric Controversy." *History of Psychiatry* 1 (1990): 125–43.

———. "The Lot of the 'Incurably' Insane in Enlightenment England." *Eighteenth Century Life* 12.3 (February 1988): 1–18.

———. "The Politics of Committal to Early-Modern Bethlem." *Medicine in the Enlightenment.* Ed. Roy Porter. Amsterdam: Rodopi, 1995. 6–63.

———. "A Respectable Mad-Doctor: Richard Hale, F.R.S. (1670–1728)." *Notes and Records of the Royal Society of London* 44 (1990): 169–203.

Beckett, J. V. "An Eighteenth-Century Case History: Carlisle Spedding 1738." *Medical History* 26 (1982): 303–06.

Brown, Theodore M. "The Changing Self-Concept of the Eighteenth-Century London Physician." *Eighteenth-Century Life* 7.2 (January 1982): 31–40.

Charon, Rita. "To Build a Case: Medical Histories as Traditions in Conflict." *Literature and Medicine* 11 (1992): 115–32.

Croxson, Bronwyn. "The Public and Private Faces of Eighteenth-Century London Dispensary Charity." *Medical History* 41 (1997): 127–49.

Cunningham, Andrew. "Pathology and the Case-History in Giambattista Morgagni's 'On the Seats and Causes of Diseases Investigated Through Anatomy' (1761)." *Medizin, Gesellschaft und Geschichte—Jahrbuch des Instituts fuer Geschichte der Medizin der Robert Bosch Stiftung. Bd. 14.* Ed. Robert Jütte. Stuttgart: F. Steiner, 1991. 37–61.

Davies, Owen. "Methodism, the Clergy, and the Popular Belief in Witchcraft and Magic." *History* 82 (1997): 252–65.

Fessler, A. "The Management of Lunacy in Seventeenth-Century England, An Investigation of Quarter-Sessions Records." *Proceedings of the Royal Society of Medicine* 49 (1956): 901–07.

Fissell, Mary E. "The Disappearance of the Patient's Narrative and the Invention of Hospital Medicine." *British Medicine in an Age of Reform*. Ed. Roger French and Andrew Wear. London and New York: Routledge, 1991. 91–109.

———. "Readers, Texts, and Contexts: Vernacular Medical Works in Early Modern England." *The Popularisation of Medicine, 1650–1850*. Ed. Roy Porter. London and New York: Routledge, 1992. 72–96.

———. "The 'Sick and Drooping Poor' in Eighteenth-Century Bristol and its Region." *Social History of Medicine* 2 (1989): 35–58.

Foyster, Elizabeth. "Wrongful Confinement in Eighteenth-Century England: A Question of Gender?" Social and Medical Representations of the Links between Insanity and Sexuality. University of Wales, Bangor, July 1999.

Hay, Douglas. "Property, Authority and the Criminal Law." *Albion's Fatal Tree: Crime and Society in Eighteenth Century England*. Ed. D. Hay, P. Linebaugh, J. Rule, E. P. Thompson, and C. Winslow. New York: Pantheon, 1975. 17–63.

Heyd, Michael. "Medical Discourse in Religious Controversy: The Case of the Critique of 'Enthusiasm' on the Eve of the Enlightenment." *Medicine as a Cultural System*. Ed. Michael Heyd and Hans-Joerg Rheinberger. Spec. issue of *Science in Context* 8.1 (Spring 1995): 133–57.

———. "Robert Burton's Sources on Enthusiasm and Melancholy: From a Medical Tradition to Religious Controversy." *History of European Ideas* 5 (1984): 17–44.

Hunter, Richard, and Ida Macalpine. Introduction to the facsimile edition of William Battie, *A Treatise on Madness,* and John Monro, *Remarks on Dr Battie's Treatise on Madness*. London: Dawson's, 1962.

———. "William Battie, M.D., F.R.S., Pioneer Psychiatrist." *The Practitioner* 174 (1955): 208–15.

Jackson, Stanley W. "Robert Burton and Psychological Healing." *Journal of the History of Medicine and Allied Sciences* 44 (1989): 160–78.

Jefferiss, F. J. G. "Extracts from a Biography of Dr Thomas Monro." *Dr Thomas Monro (1759–1833) and the Monro Academy*. London: Victoria and Albert Museum, 1976.

Jewson, Nicholas D. "The Disappearance of the Sick Man from Medical Cosmology." *Sociology* 12 (1976): 225–44.

———. "Medical Knowledge and the Patronage System in Eighteenth-Century England." *Sociology* 10 (1974): 369–85.

Kass, Amalie M. "'Called to her at three o'clock am': Obstetrical Practice in Physician Case Notes." *Journal of the History of Medicine and Allied Sciences* 50 (1995): 194–229.

Lane, Joan. "'The doctor scolds me': The Diaries and Correspondence of Patients in Eighteenth-Century England." *Patients and Practitioners: Lay Per-*

ceptions of Medicine in Pre-industrial Society. Ed. Roy Porter. Cambridge: Cambridge University Press, 1985. 205–48.

Langbein, J. H. "Albion's Fatal Flaw." *Past and Present* 99 (1983): 96–120.

Larsen, Oeivind. "Case Histories in Nineteenth-Century Hospitals—What Do They Tell the Historian? Some Methodological Considerations with Special Reference to McKeown's Criticism of Medicine." *Medizin, Gesellschaft und Geschichte—Jahrbuch des Instituts für Geschichte der Medizin der Robert Bosch Stiftung. Bd. 14.* Ed. Robert Jütte. Stuttgart: F. Steiner, 1991. 127–48.

Lawrence, Christopher. "Incommunicable Knowledge: Science, Technology, and the Clinical Art in Britain, 1850–1914." *Journal of Contemporary History* 20 (1985): 502–20.

Longfield-Jones, G. M. "The Case History of 'Sir H. M.'" *Medical History* 32 (1988): 449–60.

Loudon, Irvine S. L. "The Origins and Growth of the Dispensary Movement in England." *Bulletin of the History of Medicine* 55 (1981): 322–42.

Macalpine, Ida, and Richard Hunter. "Smollett's Reading in Psychiatry." *Modern Languages Review* 51 (July 1956): 409–11.

———. "Tobias Smollett, M.D. and William Battie, M.D." *Journal of the History of Medicine and Allied Sciences* 11 (1956): 102–03.

MacDonald, Michael. "Insanity and the Realities of History in Early Modern England." *Lectures on the History of Psychiatry.* Ed. R. M. Murray and T. H. Turner. The Squibb Series. London: Gaskell/The Royal College of Psychiatrists, 1990. 60–77.

———. "The Medicalization of Suicide in England: Laymen, Physicians, and Cultural Change, 1500–1870." *Framing Disease: Studies in Cultural History.* Ed. Charles E. Rosenberg and Janet Golden. New Brunswick, N.J.: Rutgers University Press, 1992. 85–103.

———. "Popular Beliefs about Mental Disorder in Early Modern England." *Münstersche Beiträge zur Geschichte und Theorie der Medizin.* Ed. Wolfgang Eckhart and Johanna Geyer-Kordesch. Münster: Burgverlag, 1982. 148–73.

———. "Religion, Social Change and Psychological Healing in England, 1600–1800." *The Church and Healing.* Ed. W. Shiels. Oxford: Basil Blackwell, 1982. 101–25.

———. "The Secularization of Suicide in England 1660–1800." *Past & Present* 111 (May 1986): 50–100.

MacDonald, Michael, and Donna T. Andrew. "The Secularization of Suicide in England 1660–1800." *Past & Present* 119 (May 1988): 158–70.

McCandless, Peter. "Liberty and Lunacy: The Victorians and Wrongful Confinement." *Madhouses, Mad-Doctors and Madmen: The Social History of Psychiatry in the Victorian Era.* Ed. Andrew Scull. Philadelphia: University of Pennsylvania Press, 1981. 339–61.

Micale, Mark S. "Paradigm and Ideology in Psychiatric History Writing: The Case of Psychoanalysis." *Journal of Nervous and Mental Disease* 184 (1996): 146–52.

Mullett, Charles F. "The Lay Outlook on Medicine in England circa 1800–1850." *Bulletin of the History of Medicine* 25 (1951): 169–77.

Nicolson, Malcolm. "The Art of Diagnosis: Medicine and the Five Senses."

Companion Encyclopedia of the History of Medicine. Ed. William F. Bynum and Roy Porter. Vol. 2. London and New York: Routledge, 1993. 801–25.

Noll, Steven. "Patient Records as Historical Stories: The Case of Caswell Training School." *Bulletin of the History of Medicine* 68 (1994): 411–28.

Nowell-Smith, Harriet. "Nineteenth-Century Narrative Case Histories: An Inquiry into Stylistics and History." *Canadian Bulletin of Medical History* 12 (1995): 47–67.

Porter, Roy. "Foucault's Great Confinement." *History of the Human Sciences* 3.1 (1990): 47–54.

———. " 'The Hunger of Imagination': Approaching Samuel Johnson's Melancholy." *The Anatomy of Madness.* Ed. William F. Bynum, Roy Porter, and Michael Shepherd. Vol. 1. London: Tavistock, 1985. 63–88.

———. "Lay Medical Knowledge in the Eighteenth Century: The Evidence of the 'Gentleman's Magazine.' " *Medical History* 29 (1985): 138–68.

———. "The Patient in England, c. 1660–c. 1800." *Medicine in Society: Historical Essays.* Ed. Andrew Wear. Cambridge and New York: Cambridge University Press, 1992. 91–118.

———. "The Patient's View: Doing Medical History from Below." *Theory and Society* 14 (1985): 175–98.

———. "The Prophetic Body: Lady Eleanor Davies and the Meaning of Madness." *Women's Writing: The Elizabethan to Victorian Period* 1.1 (1994): 51–63.

———. "The Rage of Party: A Glorious Revolution in English Psychiatry?" *Medical History* 29 (1983): 35–50.

———. "Reforming the Patient in the Age of Reform: Thomas Beddoes and Medical Practice." *British Medicine in an Age of Reform.* Ed. Roger French and Andrew Wear. London and New York: Routledge, 1991. 9–44.

Rack, Henry D. "Doctors, Demons and Early Methodist Healing." *The Church and Healing.* Ed. W. J. Sheils. Oxford: Blackwell, 1982. 137–52.

Rippere, Vicky. "The Survival of Traditional Medicine in Lay Medical Views: An Empirical Approach to the History of Medicine." *Medical History* 25 (1981): 411–14.

Risse, Guenther B., and John Harley Warner. "Reconstructing Clinical Activities: Patient Records in Medical History." *Social History of Medicine* 5 (1992): 183–205.

Rosen, George. "Enthusiasm: 'a dark lanthorn of the spirit.' " *Bulletin of the History of Medicine* 42 (1968): 393–421.

Rushton, Peter. "Idiocy, the Family and the Community in Early Modern North-East England." *From Idiocy to Mental Deficiency.* Ed. David Wright and Anne Digby. London and New York: Routledge, 1996. 44–64.

———. "Lunatics and Idiots: Mental Disability, the Community, and the Poor Law in North-East England 1600–1800." *Medical History* 24 (1980): 34–50.

Rusnock, Andrea A. "The Weight of Evidence and the Burden of Authority: Case Histories, Medical Statistics and Smallpox Inoculation." *Medicine in the Enlightenment.* Ed. Roy Porter. Amsterdam and Atlanta: Rodopi, 1995. 289–315.

Sampson, Harold, Sheldon L. Messinger, and Robert D. Towne. "Family Process and Becoming a Mental Patient." *American Journal of Sociology* 68 (1962): 88–96.

Sawyer, Ronald C. "Friends or Foes? Doctors and Their Patients in Early Modern England." *History of the Doctor-Patient Relationship: Proceedings of the Fourteenth International Symposium on the Comparative History of Medicine—East and West.* Ed. Yosio Kawakita, Shizu Sakai, and Yasuo Otsuka. Tokyo: Ishiyaku EuroAmerica, 1995. 31–53.

Schiller, Francis. "Haslam of 'Bedlam,' Kitchiner of the 'Oracles': Two Doctors under Mad King George III, and Their Friendship." *Medical History* 28 (1984): 189–201.

Schupbach, William. "John Monro MD and Charles James Fox: Etching by Thomas Rowlandson." *Medical History* 27 (1983): 80–83.

Schwartz, Charlotte Green. "Perspectives on Deviance: Wives' Definitions of Their Husbands' Mental Illness." *Psychiatry* 20 (1957): 275–91.

Scull, Andrew. "Bethlem Demystified?" *Medical History* 43 (1999): 248–55.

———. "A Failure to Communicate? On the Reception of Foucault's *Histoire de la folie* by Anglo-American Historians." *Rewriting the History of Madness.* Ed. Arthur Still and Irving Velody. London: Routledge, 1992. 150–63.

———. "Psychiatry and Its Historians." *History of Psychiatry* 2 (1991): 239–50.

Sheridan, Richard B. "The Doctor and the Buccaneer: Sir Hans Sloane's Case History of Sir Henry Morgan, Jamaica, 1688." *Journal of the History of Medicine and Allied Sciences* 41 (1986): 76–87.

Smith, Leonard D. "Behind Closed Doors." *Social History of Medicine* 1 (1988): 301–27.

———. "Close Confinement in Mighty Prison: Thomas Bakewell and His Campaign against Public Asylums, 1810–1830." *History of Psychiatry* 5 (1994): 191–214.

———. "Eighteenth-Century Madhouse Practice: The Prouds of Bilston." *History of Psychiatry* 3 (1992): 45–52.

———. "To Cure Those Afflicted with the Disease of Insanity: Thomas Bakewell and Spring Vale Asylum." *History of Psychiatry* 4 (1993): 107–28.

Speak, Gill. "An Odd Kind of Melancholy: Reflections on the Glass Delusion in Europe (1440–1680)." *History of Psychiatry* 1 (1990): 191–206.

Steffan, Thomas. "The Social Argument against Enthusiasm (1650–1660)." *Studies in English* 21 (1941): 39–63.

Suzuki, Akihito. "Enclosing and Disclosing Lunatics in the Family Walls: Domestic Psychiatric Regime and the Public Sphere in Early Nineteenth-Century England." *Outside the Walls of the Asylum: The History of Care in the Community 1750–2000.* Ed. Peter Bartlett and David Wright. London: Athlone, 1999. 115–31.

———. "The Household and the Care of Lunatics in Eighteenth-Century London." *The Locus of Care.* Ed. Peregrine Horden and Richard Smith. London: Routledge, 1998. 153–75.

———. "Lunacy in Seventeenth and Eighteenth-Century England: Analysis of Quarter Sessions Records. Part I." *History of Psychiatry* 2 (1991): 437–56.

———. "Lunacy in Seventeenth and Eighteenth-Century England: Analysis of Quarter Sessions Records. Part II." *History of Psychiatry* 3 (1992): 29–44.

Thomas, E. G. "The Old Poor Law and Medicine." *Medical History* 24 (1980): 1–19.

Wear, Andrew. "The Meaning of Illness in Early Modern England." *History of the Doctor-Patient Relationship: Proceedings of the Fourteenth International Symposium on the Comparative History of Medicine—East and West.* Ed. Yosio Kawakita, Shizu Sakai, and Yasuo Otsuka. Tokyo: Ishiyaku EuroAmerica, 1995. 1–29.

Weindling, Paul. "Medical Practice in Imperial Berlin: The Casebook of Alfred Grotjahn." *Bulletin of the History of Medicine* 61 (1987): 391–410.

Whittaker, Christine B. "Chasing the Cure: Irving Fisher's Experience as a Tuberculosis Patient." *Bulletin of the History of Medicine* 48 (1974): 398–415.

Williamson, George. "The Restoration Revolt against Enthusiasm." *Studies in Philology* 2 (1933): 571–603.

Yarrow, Marian Radke, Charlotte Green Schwartz, Harriet S. Murphy, and Leila Calhoun Deasy. "The Psychological Meaning of Mental Illness in the Family." *Journal of Social Issues* 11 (1955): 12–24.

Zimerman, Everett. "Fragments of History and *The Man of Feeling* from Richard Bentley to Walter Scott." *Eighteenth-Century Studies* 23.3 (Spring 1990): 283–300.

Index

Text:	10/13 Sabon
Display:	Sabon
Compositor:	G & S Typesetters, Inc.
Printer and binder:	Data Reproductions Corporation

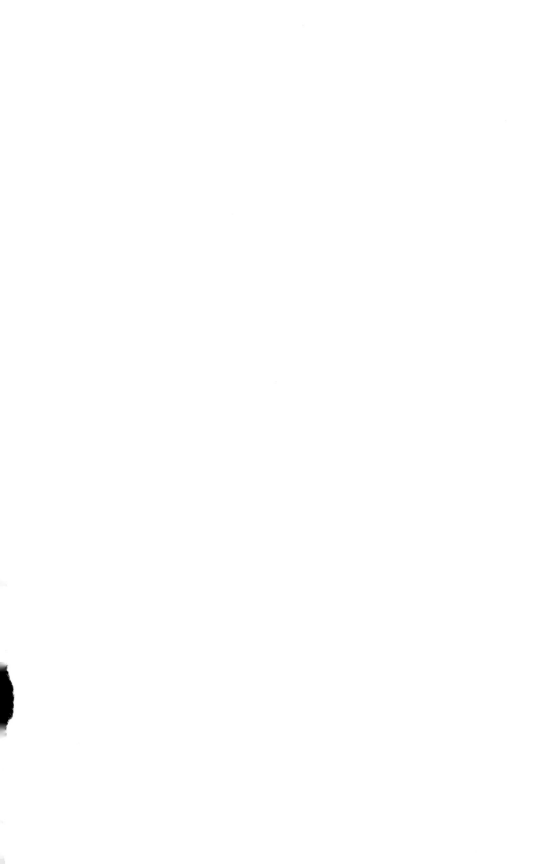